PERSPECTIVES ON
VASOPRESSIN

PERSPECTIVES ON
VASOPRESSIN

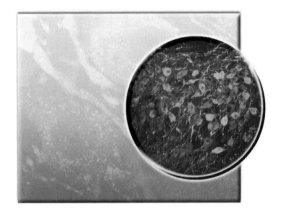

Editor

John Francis Laycock
Imperial College London, UK

Imperial College Press

Published by

Imperial College Press
57 Shelton Street
Covent Garden
London WC2H 9HE

Distributed by

World Scientific Publishing Co. Pte. Ltd.
5 Toh Tuck Link, Singapore 596224
USA office: 27 Warren Street, Suite 401-402, Hackensack, NJ 07601
UK office: 57 Shelton Street, Covent Garden, London WC2H 9HE

British Library Cataloguing-in-Publication Data
A catalogue record for this book is available from the British Library.

ISBN-13 978-1-84816-294-5
ISBN-10 1-84816-294-4

Printed in Singapore by Mainland Press Pte Ltd

Contents

Preface

Having spent much of my life studying the neurohypophysial hormone vasopressin, it is a great pleasure to have been involved in the production of a book giving various current perspectives on this hormone. It has been my good fortune to be able to invite a few long-standing friends and colleagues to contribute their knowledge and understanding of the hormone in particular areas of their expertise. I am very grateful to them all, particularly since they are all very busy people. There is some overlap between chapters on occasion but I think that this is generally appropriate since it allows each chapter to inform the reader independently without too much need for cross-reference between them. On the other hand, other relevant chapters are indicated when helpful to the reader. The end result is a text which covers most aspects of vasopressin research in a readily digestible format which I hope the reader will enjoy.

John F. Laycock

CHAPTER 1

INTRODUCTION TO VASOPRESSIN

John Laycock

Division of Neuroscience and Mental Health
Faculty of Medicine, Imperial College London
Charing Cross campus, London W6 8RF
Email: j.laycock@imperial.ac.uk

1. Brief Historical Perspective

We now know quite a lot about vasopressin. For instance, we have known for some time that it is a nonapeptide molecule associated chiefly with the hypothalamus and posterior lobe of the pituitary gland (the neurohypophysial system), and that it has a variety of physiological actions linked to specific receptors and intracellular second messenger systems. We know something about clinical conditions arising from an absence, or an excess, of its renal actions, and to a lesser extent its potential pathological role in other clinical conditions. We also know lots of other interesting facts about this molecule which may, or may not, be of physiological and clinical relevance. But how did we get here?

It is fascinating to see how the current perception of vasopressin is based on a number of different developing strands (e.g. hormone synthesis, structure, actions, receptors, clinical disease) which ultimately come together to give us the more complete canvas we see today. In particular, vasopressin research has played an important part in our present understanding of the process of neuromolecular synthesis and secretion, at least partly because the neurohypophysial neurones, the main physiological source of the hormone, are larger than the average nerve cell (magnocellular) and are therefore more readily manipulated.

Below, I have attempted to portray these various research strands from a chronological viewpoint as well as from the more logical, perhaps classical, progression of system components such as anatomical structure, synthesis, storage, release, etc. This brief and necessarily incomplete historical perspective covers the essential developments in vasopressin research up to the early 1980s, after which further details will be found in subsequent relevant chapters. While we think we know a lot about vasopressin today, the more we learn, the more we find we don't understand. This is particularly relevant with respect to the rapid advances being made following genetic and proteomic manipulations which will require yet more physiological studies to appreciate their significance.

As an endocrinologist, I shall refer generally to the hormone as vasopressin (VP) since this was the name originally given to the active principle derived from posterior pituitary extracts. However, the molecule is still sometimes given the name antidiuretic hormone (ADH), mainly by renal physiologists, in honour of its main recognised physiological, and clinically relevant, action.

2. General Development, Anatomy and Structure of the Neurohypophysial System

The pituitary gland, or hypophysis, is a small gland attached to the base of the brain. It was first described by Galen (129–216AD), who proposed that it drained phlegm from the brain to the nasopharynx. The embryological origin of the pituitary was described much later by Rathke in 1838, who described its development as a consequence of the fusion of an upward growth of the primitive buccal cavity (subsequently known as Rathke's pouch) with a downward growth from the brain, specifically from the hypothalamus. The internal structure of the gland conforms to its embryological origin: the anterior lobe (the adenohypophysis), which develops from Rathke's pouch, is comprised of typical secretory cells, while the posterior lobe (the neurohypophysis) consists mainly of nerve fibres descending from the hypothalamus. In most vertebrates there is also an intermediate zone between the anterior and posterior lobes called the pars intermedia, which was first described by Peremeschko in 1867. In adult humans this lobe is almost non-existent, except in women during pregnancy.

The first anatomical studies demonstrating nerve fibres in the posterior, or neural, lobe of the pituitary gland were described by Ecker in 1853, and later by others such as Ramon y Cajal, who in 1894 identified a nucleus of nerve cell bodies situated behind the optic chiasma. This supraoptic nucleus, together with the paraventricular nucleus which lies around the third ventricle, provide the hypothalamic neurones whose axons traverse the basal part of the hypothalamic median eminence to enter the posterior lobe of the pituitary. These supraoptic and paraventricular neurones, as nerve bundles, are called the hypothalamo-neurohypophysial nerve tracts. They are initially myelinated but lose their myelin sheaves as soon as they enter the median eminence.

An interesting feature of the neurohypophysial axons is that they are larger than normal nerve axons and are thus referred to as magnocellular neurones. Another interesting feature is the presence of dilations, or swellings, along the nerve axons and at the nerve terminals, called Herring bodies. Herring was the first person to describe colloid droplets in the neural lobe in 1908. Other cell types are present within the neural lobe: glial cells, and cells called pituicytes (astrocytes) which are often seen closely associated with the nerve axons. Developmentally, magnocellular vasopressinergic neurones originate from cell precursors lining the third ventricle, which migrate first to the supraoptic region of the developing hypothalamus and then to the paraventricular, and other areas such as the suprachiasmatic nuclei.

Another vasopressinergic pathway which influences the pituitary gland consists of normal, smaller (parvocellular) neurones originating in the hypothalamic paraventricular nucleus and terminating in the median eminence region at the base of the hypothalamus. Vasopressin released

J. Laycock

by these neurones enters the primary capillary network in the median
eminence and is transported to its target cells in the anterior pituitary
(corticotroph cells) by the specialised portal system which links it to a
second capillary plexus distributed throughout the anterior pituitary.
Other vasopressinergic fibres originating mainly in the paraventricular,
but also from the suprachiasmatic, nuclei have axons terminating in
various other parts of the brain (Fig. 1).

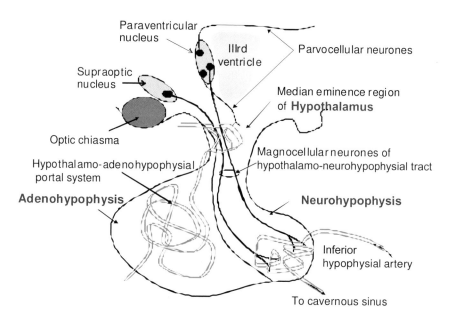

Figure 1. Cross-section of the hypothalamo-pituitary axis identifying the magnocellular
neurones of the neurohypophysis and the blood supply from the inferior hypophysial
artery. Also shown are the paraventricular parvocellular neurones which either terminate
on the walls of the primary capillary plexus in the median eminence or terminate on other
distant parts of the brain.

3. Synthesis, Storage and Release of Neurohypophysial Hormones

Vasopressin is detected as early as the tenth week of development in the human, following the extension of axons into the posterior lobe of the pituitary. Bargmann and Scharrer in 1951 were the first to hypothesise that the synthesis of the neurohypophysial hormones occurs in the neurone cell bodies located in the hypothalamic nuclei. The molecules then pass down the nerve axons to be stored and released from the terminals in the posterior pituitary. Evidence leading to the acceptance of this hypothesis was provided by the studies of Sachs and colleagues, who further proposed that vasopressin was initially synthesised in the neurones as an inactive precursor molecule and that the biologically active molecule appears during the formation and migration of granules within the cytoplasm (Sachs and Takabataki, 1964; Sachs *et al.*, 1969). The granules accumulate in the nerve terminals and in the Herring bodies. The structure of oxytocin was elucidated by du Vigneaud and colleagues (1953a) and independently by Tuppy (1953), who identified eight amino acids (nine when the cystine is replaced by two sulphide bond-linked cysteines after oxidation) made up into a ring of six amino acids and a short side branch of three amino acids. A remarkably similar structure was identified for vasopressin. This molecule is found in most mammals (including man), and consists of the same amino acids, except for the replacement of the leucine in the side branch of oxytocin by arginine, and isoleucine in the ring by phenylalanine (du Vigneaud *et al.*, 1953b; Acher and Chauvet, 1953). Du Vigneaud's team (du Vigneaud *et al.*, 1957) went on to identify the slightly modified vasopressin molecule in members of the Suina (e.g. pig) family, in which the arginine is replaced by lysine, hence reference to arginine vasopressin (AVP) or lysine vasopressin (LVP) (see Fig. 2).

We now know that the oxytocin and vasopressin molecules, like other polypeptide hormones, are post-translational products processed from larger prohormones which are enzymatically cleaved into the component

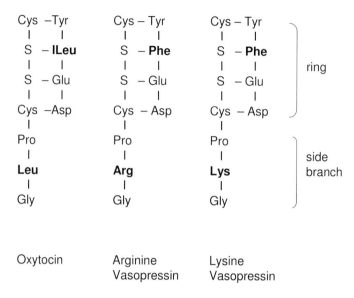

Figure 2. The amino acid sequences of oxytocin and the two mammalian forms of vasopressin.

hormones and their related proteins, the neurophysins (MW approximately 10,000) (Gainer *et al.*, 1977a, 1977b). Neurophysin I is the protein derived from the oxytocin precursor, while neurophysin II is a glycoprotein associated with vasopressin (Russell *et al.*, 1980). This processing occurs within the neurosecretory granules formed in the Golgi complex of the neurone cell bodies, with the relevant proteolytic enzymes identified within them (Gainer, 1983). An additional cleavage product from the provasopressin molecule is a glycopeptide of unclear function. All cleavage products are released into the general circulation (see Chapter 3).

In addition to the axonal transport of vasopressin and its associated molecules within granules, it is possible that some of these molecules are released from the granules and are transported directly down the axons. The neurohypophysial hormones are released from the storage granules to the exterior by the process of exocytosis, as originally proposed by Douglas and Poissner (1964). The process is the result of stimulus-secretion coupling, in which the stimulus activates the neurone and, as in other nerves, the action potential travels down the axon and depolarizes the terminal membrane, which leads to an influx of calcium ions. This is necessary for the subsequent fusion of the granule membrane with the neuronal cell membrane following Ca^{++}-calmodulin-dependent activation of a neuronal ATPase. Consequently, the granule contents are released into the blood vessels which lie in close proximity to the nerve terminals (Douglas, 1973).

More recently, it has become clear that vasopressin is also synthesized in other tissues, including the sympathetic ganglia (Hanley *et al.*, 1984), the adrenals (Nussey *et al.*, 1984; Guillon *et al.*, 1998), the ovaries (Fuller *et al.*, 1985; Stones *et al.*, 1996), the testis (Kasson *et al.*, 1985; Fillion *et al.*, 1993), the heart (Hupf *et al.*, 1999; Watanabe *et al.*, 2005) and even the thymus (Jessop *et al.*, 1995). Certainly there is plenty of evidence for the presence of vasopressin receptors (R) in all of these, and other, tissues, for example V1R in sympathetic ganglia (Kiraly *et al.*, 1986), V1aR and V1bR in adrenal medulla (Grazzini *et al.*, 1996; Guillon *et al.*, 1998), V1R in heart-derived myocytes (Reilly *et al.*, 1998; Brostrom *et al.*, 2000), V1aR, V1bR and V2R in the gastrointestinal tract (Monstein *et al.*, 2008) and V1R in the liver (Gopalakrishnan *et al.*, 1986). These findings certainly imply that vasopressin is a potential local autocrine regulator, if nothing else, in many tissue systems.

4. Vasopressin Assays

Fractionation and purification of posterior pituitary extracts was achieved initially using the extraction method described by Kamm *et al.* in 1928 which involved heating of the extract in 0.25% acetic acid. Identification of the two hormones oxytocin and vasopressin was made possible by the development of bioassays for oxytocic activity (e.g. rat uterine muscle contraction, milk ejection in the anaesthetized lactating rat) and vasoconstrictor or antidiuretic activities for vasopressin. The development of sensitive and specific assays has been an extremely important factor in the vast expansion of our knowledge of endocrinology over the last 50 years. Initially these assays were based on the biological responses of sensitive tissues or animal preparations, called bioassays.

It has long been appreciated that the measurement of vasopressin concentrations in biological fluids by means of dose-related vasoconstriction of arterial strips or increases in arterial blood pressure in an animal model is of limited practical value, as it is generally insensitive within the normal physiological range. One example is an assay using the proximal part of the guinea pig colon developed by Botting in 1965 which was reportedly quite sensitive (to as low as 1 microunit/ml), although published data indicate 100 microunits/ml as being the lowest effective concentration shown. In general, the more sensitive bioassays for vasopressin were developed using the antidiuretic action of the hormone as the dose-dependent measurable variable. This included the movement of water across amphibian skin or bladder, which is stimulated by vasopressin (Heller, 1941).

Since sodium transport across frog or toad skin is also stimulated by vasopressin, this too was measured using strips of skin (Morel et al., 1958), as determined by short-circuit current changes induced with different doses of hormone. However, the mainstay in vasopressin bioassays became the ethanol-anaesthetised water-loaded rat, with the hormone administered intravenously, as first described by Jeffers et al. in 1942. The use of ethanol as the anaesthetic was particularly advantageous because this drug also inhibits the endogenous release of vasopressin. The maintenance of the rat in a state of hydration also inhibited endogenous hormone release, making the preparation more sensitive for longer (Dicker, 1953). The first vasopressin radioimmunoassay was developed in the early 1970s (Robertson et al., 1970). Problems in getting specific sensitive antibodies for vasopressin delayed the widespread use of this technique for many years.

5. Physiological Actions

In 1895, Oliver and Schaffer administered a crude posterior pituitary extract to a dog which produced an increase in arterial blood pressure. They consequently named the active ingredient vasopressin. It took many years before the main physiological action, the antidiuretic effect, of vasopressin was described, following the important studies of Starling and Verney (1925), Pickford (1936) and other researchers. Vasopressin was then 'adopted' by renal physiologists for a while and it became commonly known as the Antidiuretic Hormone (ADH).

The micropuncture studies of Gottschalk and Mylle (1959) and others indicated that vasopressin must increase the permeability to water in the distal tubule of the renal nephron. Perfusion of rabbit collecting tubules with the hormone resulted in a threefold increase in water permeability (Grantham and Burg, 1966). Berliner and Bennett (1967) concluded that all the known effects of ADH at physiological concentrations could be explained by modifications of permeability to water that the hormone induces in the most distal parts of the nephron. While other renal sites and actions have now been identified (see Chapter 6), it is accepted that the collecting duct remains the principal region of the nephron where the antidiuretic effect of vasopressin is exerted.

But does vasopressin actually have any physiological effect on the cardiovascular system, and what about actions associated with the other vasopressinergic nerve pathways that have been described? Early work investigating the effect of vasopressin on isolated arterial strips indicated species, vessel and dose-specific effects (Dodd and Daniel, 1960). The intra-arterial infusion of vasopressin extracts (Pitressin) into the isolated hind limb of a dog produced quite pronounced vasoconstriction (Diana and Masden, 1965), while Rocha e Silva and Rosenberg (1969) showed that infusion of vasopressin in dogs at doses producing plasma concentrations comparable with those attained after haemorrhage are pressor, providing that the baroreceptor reflex is abolished. Altura (1973) compared the constrictor effects of various known vasoactive substances on the diameters of mesenteric arteriolar cross-sections and showed that vasopressin was more potent than any other known endogenous pressor agent, including angiotensin II. This, and later, work gradually re-established the neurohypophysial hormone as a pressor substance, and vasopressin is now its current generally accepted name (see Chapter 7). In the last 25 years, other actions of vasopressin have been described including its action as an adenohypophysial hormone (corticotrophin) releasing factor (see Chapter 9), the stimulation of factor VIII and von Willbrandt factor synthesis (see Chapter 7). In addition, there is now much interest in the central actions of this neuropeptide (see Chapter 10).

Interestingly, as indicated in Chapter 9, vasopressin can be considered a stress hormone, i.e. one that is released in response to various stressors. As such, and like most, if not all, other stress hormones, vasopressin promotes an increase in blood glucose concentration by stimulating hepatic glycogenolysis (Hems *et al.*, 1975; Hems *et al.*, 1978) predominantly in the perivenous zone (Schmeisch *et al.*, 2005). Vasopressin also stimulates tricarboxylic acid cycle activity (Patel, 1986).

Currently, it is increasingly appreciated that vasopressin has a number of disparate effects on the body, both peripheral and central, as indicated in Fig. 3.

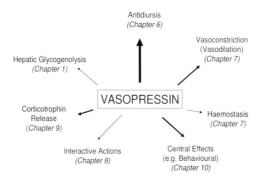

Figure 3. The principal known effects of vasopressin and the chapters which consider them in more detail.

6. Receptors and Mechanisms of Action

Three different receptors have now been identified for vasopressin and these are V1a, V1b and V2 receptors. The V1a receptor is found in many parts of the body, including the vasculature, heart, liver, kidneys, brain and platelets. The closely related V1b receptor is mainly specific to corticotroph cells in the anterior pituitary, while the V2 receptors are mainly located on the principal cells of the renal distal nephrons but also probably on endothelial cells. These receptor types are considered further in Chapters 4 and 5.

The ubiquitous second messenger system involving the action of the enzyme adenyl cyclase on adenosine triphostphate (ATP) with the resultant formation of cyclic adenosine monophosphate (cAMP) was first described for the catecholamine adrenaline by Sutherland and Rall in 1958. Later, Orloff and Handler (1964) proposed cAMP as the second messenger through which vasopressin exerted its antidiuretic effect. More details of the intracellular mechanisms stimulated by the arrival of vasopressin at the cell membrane have been provided over the last 30 years, following the rapid expansion of molecular and cellular biology. Of particular importance has been the determination of the vasopressin receptors and their relationships with the intracellular second messenger systems, of which the generation of cAMP is one and inositol triphosphate is another (see Chapter 4).

7. Circulation and Metabolism

In the blood, vasopressin is not believed to be associated with erythrocytes, as early reports indicated that it can be accounted for entirely in the plasma fraction, as determined by bioassay (Heller and Zaidi, 1957). However, data for its circulation as a protein-bound molecule were conflicting. Lauson (1967) concluded in a review that it was likely that most, if not all, of the vasopressin in blood circulates as the free unbound molecule. It is also accepted that since the necessary pH for vasopressin-neurophysin binding is far lower than the plasma pH, this co-released protein cannot play any part in the transportation of the hormone in the blood. Estimates of the half-life for vasopressin (8-arginine vasopressin) based on the loss of biological activity in blood range from 0.9 min in rat (Ginsburg, 1957) to 5.9 min in dog (Share, 1962) and 4.9 min in humans (Silver *et al.*, 1961).

More recently there have also been a number of reports indicating that the plasma vasopressin concentration actually represents only a small proportion of the total hormone content of the blood, with the major component located within the circulating platelets. One study showed that in rats, approximately 30% of circulating vasopressin was found in platelets (Lee-Kwon *et al.*, 1984), while other studies have suggested values ranging from approximately 50% in dogs (Share *et al.*, 1985) and in humans (Bichet *et al.*, 1987) to 90% in humans (Chesney *et al.*, 1985; Nussey *et al.*, 1986).

Clearance of vasopressin from the blood is associated mainly with renal and hepatic activities, as determined by studies in the whole animal or in isolated perfused organs. Interestingly, renal clearance estimates for vasopressin of between 50% (Ginsburg and Heller, 1953; Dicker, 1954) and 70% (Crawford and Pinkham, 1954) were determined from studies using nephrectomised rats. Some vasopressin appears unchanged in the urine, indicating that a considerable inactivation of the neurohypophysial hormone takes place in the kidneys. Values for the renal excretion of vasopressin vary (see Lauson, 1967). In one study, excreted vasopressin, expressed as a percentage of the dose of pitressin tannate in oil administered, varied from <1 to 5% (Laycock and Williams, 1973).

Clearance by the liver is also quite well established, following splanchnic vascular ligation studies (Ginsburg and Heller, 1953), and this accounts for most of the remaining removal of vasopressin from the blood. However, it is worth noting that some circulating vasopressin could be inactivated by a plasma vasopressinase, as suggested by Werle (1960), which might be an enzyme such as fibrinolysin. Furthermore, in pregnancy the increase in circulating oxytocinase correlates not only with the removal of oxytocin but also vasopressin from the blood (Croxatto, *et al.*, 1953). For more information, see Chapter 3.

8. Control of Release of Vasopressin

Studies by Verney (1947), O'Connor (1950) and other researchers were instrumental in identifying not only vasopressin's renal water reabsorption effect but also how this is linked to its release when the plasma osmolality increases, as first suggested by Chambers *et al.*, (1945). Initially the 'osmoreceptors' were located in the anterior hypothalamus (Jewell and Verney, 1957). Vasopressin is released by changes in plasma osmolality, but only by those solutes which remain in the extracellular fluid. Molecules which readily cross cell membranes such as urea have no effect. While it is now clear that the supraoptic (and presumably paraventricular) neuronal cell bodies are directly sensitive to changes in sodium ions in the extracellular medium (Leng *et al.*, 1981), it is generally accepted that the true osmoreceptors themselves lie outside the restrictive blood brain barrier. Indeed, various circumventricular organs such as the subfornical organ and the organum vasculosum of the lamina terminalis have been shown to mediate the changes in plasma osmolality with the release of neurohypophysial vasopressin (Thresher *et al.*, 1982).

Other influences on vasopressin secretion, particularly those associated with known neurotransmitters such as acetylcholine (Pickford, 1939) and catecholamines (O'Connor & Verney, 1945) have also been identified. These early studies were indicative of possible influences on the neurohypophysis, either via central nerve pathways or via the circulation. Central pathways were also implicated by studies of the effect of various stresses on water balance and vasopressin release (O'Conner and Verney, 1942). While conclusions drawn from early studies on the effect of blood loss on vasopressin release were variable, it became increasingly apparent that haemorrhage was a powerful stimulus (Ginsburg and Brown, 1956) and that the fall in blood pressure was the likely stimulus. Baroreceptor involvement was implicated in the release of vasopressin (and its consequent effect on arterial blood pressure) in various studies (Cowley *et al.*, 1974; Bisset and Chowdrey, 1984). See Chapter 11 for further information about mechanisms of control of neurohypophysial vasopressin secretion.

9. Clinical Aspects of Vasopressin

If vasopressin cannot exert its principal physiological action on the renal collecting ducts, then the final concentrating ability of the kidney is lost. The large volumes of dilute urine excreted in consequence gives rise to the condition of diabetes insipidus (the excretion of a large volume of tasteless, or insipid, urine). The absence or lack of circulating vasopressin because of a malfunctioning hypothalamo-neurohypophysial system results in the condition of central (hypothalamic), or cranial, diabetes insipidus. This form of the disease can nowadays be readily treated with a vasopressin agonist acting on V2 receptors. The other form of this disease, characterised by the presence of circulating vasopressin, but lacking collecting duct responsiveness to the hormone (target tissue insensitivity) is known as nephrogenic diabetes insipidus. This can only be partially treated at present. There is currently much interest in the use of vasopressin receptor antagonists in conditions such as hyponatraemia and congestive heart failure. The vasoconstrictor effect of vasopressin is also useful in the treatment of bleeding disorders such as oesophageal varices. Another clinical use of vasopressin is related to its effect on the synthesis of factor VIII and the von Willbrandt factor. These clinical aspects of vasopressin are discussed more fully elsewhere (Chapter 12).

10. Conclusion

We have known of the existence of the neurohypophysial peptide vasopressin for many years and we have appreciated the clinical consequences of its absence resulting from the loss of its principal physiological action in the renal collecting duct. However, we have learnt that this hormone has other peripheral effects, particularly its ability to vasoconstrict arteriolar smooth muscle, as a releasing hormone for the adenohypophysial hormone corticotrophin, and we are beginning to appreciate some of its central effects such as on different adaptive behaviours. Vasopressin and the neurohypophysial system have also been instrumental in our current understanding of neuropeptide secretion, storage and release. Future research will undoubtedly provide us with much more information about this interesting peptide and its involvement in physiological processes, and its likely clinical consequences.

Bibliography

Acher R., Chauvet J. (1953). La structure de la vasopressine du boeuf. *Biochem Biophys Acta* 12: 487–488

Altura B.M. (1973). Selective microvascular constrictor actions of some neurohypophysial peptides. *Eur J Pharmacol* 24: 49–60

Bargmann W., Scharrer E. (1951). The site of origin of the hormones of the posterior pituitary. *Am Sci* 39: 255–259

Berliner R.W., Bennett C.M. (1967). Concentration of urine in the mammalian kidney. *Am J Med* 42: 777–789

Bichet D.G., Arthus M-F., Barjon J.N., Lonergan M., Kortas C. (1987). Human platelet fraction arginine vasopressin. Potential physiological role. *J Clin Invest* 79: 881–887

Bisset G.W., Chowdrey H.S. (1984). A cholinergic link in the reflex release of vasopressin by hypotension in the rat. *J Physiol* 354: 523–545

Botting J.H. (1965). An isolated preparation with a selective sensitivity to vasopressin. *Br J Pharmacol Chemother* 24: 156–62

Brostrom M.A., Reilly B.A., Wilson F.J., Brostrom C.O. (2000). Vasopressin-induced hypertrophy in H9c2 heart-derived myocytes. *Int J Biochem Cell Biol* 32: 993–1006

Chambers G.H., Melville E.V., Hare R.S., Hare K. (1945). Regulation of the release of pituitrin by changes in the osmotic pressure of the plasma. *Am J Physiol* 144: 311–320

Chesney CM., Crofton J.T., Pifer D.D., Brooks D.P., Huch K.M., Share L. (1985). Subcellular localization of vasopressin-like material in platelets. *J Lab Clin Med* 106: 314–318

Cowley A.W., Monos E., Guyton A.C. (1974). Interasction of vasopressin and the baroreceptor reflex system in the regulation of arterial blood pressure in the dog. *Circ Res* 34: 505–514

Croxatto H., Vera C., Barnafi L. (1953). Inactivation of antidiuretic hormone by blood serum of the pregnant woman. *Proc Soc Exp Biol* 83: 784–786

Crawford J.D., Pinkham B. (1954). The removal of circulating antidiuretic hormone by the kidney. *Endocrinol* 55: 699–700

Diana J.N., Masden R.R. (1965). Effect of vasopressin infusion and sciatic nerve stimulation in isolated dog hindlimb. *Am J Physiol* 209: 390–396

Dicker S.E (1953). A method for the assay of very small amounts of antidiuretic activity with a note on the antidiuretic titre of rat's blood. *J Physiol* 122: 149–157

Dodd W.A., Daniel E.E. (1960). Electrolytes and arterial muscle contractility. *Circ Res* 8: 451–463

Douglas W.W. (1963). A possible method of neurosecretion. Release of vasopressin by depolarization and its dependence on calcium. *Nature* 197: 81–82

Douglas W.W. (1973). How do neurones secrete peptides? Exocytosis and its consequences including synaptic vesicle formation in the hypothalamo-neurohypophysial system. *Prog Brain Res* 39: 21–39

Douglas W.W., Poissner A.M. (1964). Stimulus-secretion coupling in a neurosecretory organ. The role of calcium in the release of vasopressin from the neurohypophysis. *J Physiol* 172: 1–18

Fillion C., Malassine A., Tahri-Joutei A., Allevard A.M., Bedin M., Gharib C., Hugues J.N., Pointis G. (1993). Immunoreactive arginine vasopressin in the testis: immunocytochemical localization and testicular content in normal and experimental cryptorchid mouse. *Biol Reprod* 48: 786–792

Fuller P.J., Clements J.A., Tregear G.W., Nicolaidis I., Whitfield P.L., Funder J.W. (1985). Vasopressin-neurophysin II gene expression in the ovary: studies in Sprague-Dawley, Long-Evans and Brattleboro rats. *J Endocrinol* 105: 317–321

Gainer H. (1983). Precursors of vasopressin and oxytocin. In The Neurohypophysis: structure, function and control. *Pro In Brain Res* 60: 205–215

Gainer H., Sarne Y., Brownstein J.J. (1977a). Neurophysin in biosynthesis: conversion of a putative precursor during axonal transport. *Science* 195: 1354–1356

Gainer H., Sarne Y., Brownstein J.J. (1977b). Biosynthesis and axonal transport of rat neurohypophysial proteins and peptides. *J Cell Biol* 73: 366–381

Ginsburg M. (1957). The clearance of vasopressin from the splanchnic vascular area and the kidneys. *J Endocrinol* 16: 217–226

Ginsburg M., Brown L..M (1956). Effect of anaesthetics and haemorrhage on the release of neurohypophysial antidiuretic hormone. *Br J Pharmacol* 14: 327–333

Ginsburg M. & Heller, H. (1953). The clearance of injected vasopressin from the circulation and its fate in the body. *J Endocrinol* 9: 283–291

Gopalakrishnan V., Triggle C.R., Sulakhe P.V., McNeill J.R (1986). Characterization of a specific high affinity [3H] arginine 8 vasopressin-binding site on liver microsomes from different strains of rat and the role of magnesium. *Endocrinol* 118: 990–997

Gottschalk C.W., Mylle M. (1959). Micropuncture study of the mammalian urinary concentrating mechanism: evidence for the countercurrent hypothesis. *Am J Physiol* 194: 927–936

Grantham J.J, Burg M.B. (1966). Effect of vasopressin and cyclic AMP on permeability of isolated collecting tubules. *Am J Physiol* 211: 255–259

Grazzini E., Boccara G., Joubert D., Trueba M., Durroux T., Guillon G., Gallo-Payet N., Chouinard L., Payet M.D., Serradeil-LeGal C. (1998). Vasopressin regulates adrenal functions by acting through different vasopressin receptor subtypes. *Adv Exp Med Biol* 449: 325–334

Grazzini E., Lodboerer A.M., Perez-Martin A., Joubert D., Guillon G. (1996). Molecular and functional characterization of V1b vasopressin receptor in rat adrenal medulla. *Endocrinol* 137: 3906–3914

Guillon G., Grazzini E., Andrez M., Breton C., Trueba M., Serradeil-LeGal C., Boccara G., Derick S., Chouinard L., Gallo-Payet N. (1998). Vasopressin: a potent autocrine/paracrine regulator of mammal adrenal functions. *Endocr Res* 24: 703–710

Hanley M.R., Benton H.P., Lightman S.L., Todd K., Bone E.A., Fretten P., Palmer S., Kirk C.J. & Michell R.H. (1984). A vasopressin-like peptide in the mammalian sympathetic nervous system. *Nature* 309: 358–261

Heller H. (1941). Differentiation of an (amphibian) water balance principle from the antidiuretic principle of the pituitary gland. *J Physiol* 100: 125–141

Heller H., Zaidi S.M. (1957). The metabolism of exogenous and endogenous antidiuretic hormone in the kidney and liver *in vivo*. *Br J Pharmacol Chemother* 12: 284–292

Hemms D.A., Whitton P.D., Ma G.Y. (1975). Metabolic actions of vasopressin, glucagon and adrenalin in the intact rat. *Biochim Biophys Acta* 411: 155–164

Hemms D.A., Rodrigues L.M., Whitton P.D. (1978). Rapid stimulation by vasopressin, oxytocin and angiotensin II of glycogen degradation in hepatocyte suspensions. *Biochem J* 172: 311–317

Herring P.T. (1908). A contribution to the comparative physiology of the pituitary body. *Quart J Exp Biol* 1: 261–280

Hupf H., Grimm D., Riegger G.A.J., Schunkert H. (1999). Evidence for a vasopressin system in the rat heart. *Circ Res* 84: 365–370

Jeffers W.A., Livezy M.M., Austin J.H. (1942). Method for demonstrating the antidiuretic action of minute amounts of pitressin: statistical analysis of results. *Proc Soc Exp Biol* 50: 184–188

Jessop D.S., Murphy D., Larsen P.J (1995). Thymic vasopressin (AVP) transgene expression in rats: a model for the study of thymic AVP hyper-expression in T cell differentiation. *J Neuroimmunol* 62: 85–90

Jewell P.A., Verney E.B. (1957). An experimental attempt to determine the site of the neurohypophysial osmoreceptors in the dog. *Phil Trans B* 240: 197–324

Kamm O. (1928). The dialysis of pituitary extracts. *Science* 67: 199–200

Kasson B.G., Meidan R., Hsueh A.J. (1985). Identification and characterization of arginine vasopressin-like substances in the rat testis. *J Biol Chem* 260: 5302–5307

Kiraly M., Audigier S, Tribollet E., Barbaris C., Dolivo M., Dreifuss J.J. (1986). Biochemical and electrophysiological evidence of functional vasopressin receptors in the rat superior cervical ganglion. *Proc Natl Acad Sci* 83: 5335–5339

Lauson H.D. (1967). Metabolism of antidiuretic hormones. *Am J Med* 42: 713–744

Laycock J.F., Williams P.G. (1973). The effect of vasopressin (Pitressin) administration on sodium, potassium and urea excretion in rats with and without diabetes insipidus (DI) with a note on the excretion of vasopressin in the DI rat. *J Endocrinol* 56: 111–120

Lee-Kwon W.J., Share L., Crofton J.T., Brooks D.P. (1984). Effect of angiotensin II on vasopressin in plasma and platelets in SH and WKY rats. *Clin Exp Hypertens A* 6: 1653–1672

Leng G., Mason W.T., Dyer R.G. (1981). The supraoptic nucleus as an osmoreceptor. *Neuroendocrinol* 34: 7–82

Monstein H.J., Truesdsson M., Ryberg A., Ohlsson B. (2008). Vasopressin receptor mRNA expression in the human gastrointestinal tract. *Eur Surg Res* 40: 34–40

Morel F., Maetz J., Lucerain C. (1958). The action of two neurohypophysial peptides on the active transport of sodium and the net flux of water across the skin of various species of anuran frogs and toads. *Biochim Biophys Acta* 28: 619–626

Nussey S.S., Ang V.T., Bevan D.H., Jenkins J.S. (1986). Human platelet arginine vasopressin. *Clin Endocrinol* 24: 427–433

Nussey S.S., Ang V.T., Jenkins J.S., Chowdrey H.S., Bisset G.W. (1984). Brattleboro rat adrenal contains vasopressin. *Nature* 310: 64–66

O'Conner W.J. (1950). The role of the neurohypophysis of the dog in determining urinary changes and the antidiuretic activity of urine following administration of sodium chloride. *Quart J exp Physiol* 36: 21–48

O'Conner W.J. Verney E.B (1942). The effect of removal of the posterior lobe of the pituitary on the inhibition of water diuresis by emotional stress. *Quart J Exp Physiol* 31: 393–408

O'Conner W.J., Verney E.B. (1945). The effect of increased activity of the sympathetic system in the inhibition of water diuresis by emotional stress. *Quart J Exp Physiol* 33: 77–90

Oliver G., Schafer E.A. (1895). On the physiological action of extracts of pituitary body and certain other glandular organs: preliminary communication. *J Physiol* 18: 277–279

Orloff J., Handler J.S. (1964). The cellular action of antidiuretic hormone. *Am J Physiol* 36: 686–697

Patel T.B. (1986). Hormonal regulation of the tricarboxylic acid cycle in the isolated perfused rat liver. *Eur J Biochem* 159: 15–22

Pickford M. (1936). Inhibition of water diuresis by pituitary (post lobe) extract and its relation to the water load of the body. *J Physiol* 87: 291–297

Pickford M. (1939). The inhibitory effect of acetylcholine on diuresis in the dog and its pituitary transmission. *J Physiol* 95: 226–238

Ramon y Cajal J. (1894). Alcunas contribuciones al conoscimeito del os ganglios del cerebro. III Hipofisis. *Ann Soc Exp Hist Nat* 2

Reilly B.A., Brostrom M.A. Brostrom C.O. (1998). Regulation of protein synthesis in ventricular myocytes by vasopressin. The role of sarcoplamic/endoplasmic reticulum Ca2+ stores. *J Biol Chem* 273: 3747–3755

Robertson G.L., Klein L.A., Roth J., Gorden P. (1970). Immunoassay of plasma vasopressin in man. *Proc Nat Acad Sci* 66: 12988–1305

Rocha e Silva M. Jr., Rosenberg M. (1969). The release of vasopressin in response to haemorrhage and its role in the mechanism of blood pressure regulation. *J Physiol* 202: 535–557

Russell J.T., Brownstein M.J., Gainer H. (1980). Biosynthesis of vasopressin, oxytocin and neurophysins: isolation and characterization of two common precursors (prepressophysin and preoxyphysin). *Endocrinol* 107: 1880–1891

Sachs H., Fawcett P., Takabatake Y., Portanova R. (1969). Biosynthesis and release of vasopressin and neurophysin. *Recent Prog Horm Res* 25: 447–491

Sachs H., Takabatake Y. (1964). Evidence for a precursor in vasopressin biosynthesis. *Endocrinology* 75: 943–948

Share L. (1962). Vascular volume and blood level of antidiuretic hormone. *Am J Physiol* 202: 791–794

Share L., Crofton J.T., Brooks D.P., Chesney C.M. (1985). Platelet and plasma vasopressin in dogs during hydration and vasopressin infusion. *Am J Physiol* 249: R313–R316

Silver L., Schwartz I.E., Fong C.T.O., Debons A.F., Dahl L.K. (1961). Disappearance of plasma radioactivity after injection of H3 or I131 labelled arginine vasopressin. *J Appl Physiol* 16: 1097–1099

Schmeisch A.P., de Olivera D.S., Ide I.T., Suzuki-Kemmelmeier F., Bracht A. (2005). Zonation of the metabolic action of vasopressin in the bivascularly perfused rat liver. *Regul Pept* 129: 233–243

Starling E.H., Verney E.B. (1925). The secretion of urine as studied on the isolated kidney. *Proc Roy Soc Med B* 97: 321–363

Stones R.W., Vials A., Milner P., Beard R.W., Burnstock G. (1996). Release of vasoactive agents from the isolated perfused human ovary. *Eur J Obstet Gynecol Reprod Biol* 67: 191–196

Sutherland E.W., Rall T.W. (1958) Fractionation and characterization of a cyclic adenine ribonucleotide formed by tissue particles. *J Biol Chem* 232: 1077–1091

Thrasher T.N., Keil L.C., Ramsey D.J. (1982). Lesions of the organum vasculosum of the lamina terminalis (OVLT) attenuate osmotically induced drinking and vasopressin secretion in the dog. *Endocrinol* 110: 1837–1839

Tuppy H. (1953). The amino acid sequence in oxytocin. *Biochim Biophys Acta* 11: 449–450

Verney E.B. (1947) The antidiuretic hormone and the factors which determine its release. *Proc Roy Soc Med B* 135: 25–106

du Vigneaud V., Ressler C., Tripett S. (1953a). The sequence of amino acids in oxytocin, with a proposal for the structure of oxytocin. *J Biol Chem* 205: 949–957

du Vigneaud V., Lawler H.C., Popenoe E.A. (1953b). Enzymic cleavage of glycinamide from vasopressin and a proposed structure for this pressor-antidiuretic hormone of the posterior pituitary. *J Am Chem Soc* 75: 4880–4881

du Vigneaud V., Bartlett M.F., Joell A. (1957). The synthesis of lysine vasopressin. *J Am Chem Soc* 79: 5572–5575

Watanabe I., Tani S., Nagao K., Anazawa T., Kawamata H., Ohguchi S., Kanmatsuse K., Kushiro T. (2005). Regulation of arginine vasopressin in the human heart. *Circ J* 69: 1401–1404

Werle E. (1960). Comment in discussion in: Polypeptides which affect smooth muscle and blood vessels. Ed. M.Schachter, 89–90

CHAPTER 2

COMPARATIVE AND EVOLUTIONARY ASPECTS
OF VASOPRESSIN

Jacques Hanoune

Institut Cochin, 22 Rue Méchain, 75014 Paris, France
Email: jacques.hanoune@inserm.fr

1. Introduction

The evolution of the vertebrates is uniquely correlated with their adaptation to the surrounding environment. The early proto-vertebrates lived in a salt water environment similar to their own extracellular fluid, so they could ingest salty water without endangering the composition of their own *milieu intérieur*. When the early vertebrates migrated into fresh water, they required a system which would permit filtration of the excess fluid from the blood and also to preserve their sodium content. The successive development of a primitive glomerulus, and later of proximal and distal tubules, allowed the kidney to emerge as a vital organ for the regulation of body fluid composition and volume (Schrier *et al.*, 2004).

Vasopressin, via its receptors, controls water distribution by modulating the function of a specific renal water channel, aquaporin 2 (see Chapter 6). We now have enough data for various animal species to enable us to try to understand how the various agents involved in this exquisitely precise regulatory pathway have evolved, or have been selected. In particular, the fact that multiple genes exist for each neuropeptide (including vasopressin), each receptor and each channel, leads one to ask whether all those various genes could have undergone a co-evolution in parallel with physiological functions. In particular, we are still lacking a coherent theory explaining the molecular basis of co-evolution, and specifically of interacting neuropeptide-receptor pairs.

The sequences of the various subtypes of genes coding for neuropeptides, receptors or aquaporins exhibit a high degree of identity within the same subfamily. These genes have arisen by the duplication of one or more common ancestral genes, for example through the two or possibly three genome doublings that have occurred during the evolution of vertebrates (Darlison and Richter, 1999), in addition to other events such as gene silencing and mutation. The questions that are currently being debated deal with the possibility that the various regulatory pathway components might have influenced each other, and whether one component might have preceded another. More specifically, did the neuropeptide genes arise before those of their corresponding receptors, or is it the reverse? How has a water-retaining function emerged from peptides first involved in regulating sexual function in invertebrates? By what evolutionary manipulations has such a vital function as water balance been obtained? These are some of the various questions that we will examine in the present chapter.

2. Evolutionary Aspects of the Vasopressin Family

Vasopressin is part of a hormone superfamily that includes vasopressin, oxytocin and related peptides in vertebrates and invertebrates. The structures of oxytocin and vasopressin were first established by du Vigneaud and his colleagues (du Vigneaud *et al.*, 1953a; du Vigneaud *et al.*, 1953b). Since then, a series of related peptides has been characterized and sequenced in all animal species, especially by Acher's group (Acher *et al.*, 1994; Acher *et al.*, 1997; Acher, 2002). All of these hormones are nonapeptides that are similar in structure: a sequence of nine amino acids differing mainly in the nature of the amino-acid at position 8, this being a basic residue in vasopressin and vasopressin-related peptides, and a neutral one in oxytocin and oxytocin-related peptides. Residues in positions 1, 5, 6, 7 and 9 are shared by all members of the superfamily. All members are also characterized by an intra-chain S-S bond between the two cysteines in positions 1 and 6 which is indispensable for biological activity (Schally *et al.*, 1964) (Table 1).

Table 1. Structural characterization of the peptides of the oxytocin/vasopressin superfamily. Residues at positions 1, 5, 6, 7 and 9, indicated in bold face, are shared by all members of the superfamily.

Vasopressin-related peptides

Cys Phe Ile Arg **Asn Cys Pro** Lys **Gly-NH2**	Lys-conopressin	*Lymnaea stagnalis*
Cys Ile Ile Arg **Asn Cys Pro** Arg **Gly-NH2**	Arg-conopressin	*Conus striatus*
Cys Phe Val Arg **Asn Cys Pro** Thr **Gly-NH2**	Annetocin	*Eisenia foetida*
Cys Leu Ile Arg **Asn Cys Pro** Arg **Gly-NH2**	Inotocin	*Locusta migratoria*
Cys Tyr Ile Gln **Asn Cys Pro** Arg **Gly-NH2**	Vasotocin	Non-mammalian vertebrates
Cys Phe Phe Arg **Asn Cys Pro** Arg **Gly-NH2**	Phenypressin	Marsupials
Cy Tyr Phe Gln **Asn Cys Pro** Arg **Gly-NH2**	Arg-vasopressin	Mammals
Cys Tyr Phe Gln **Asn Cys Pro** Lys **Gly- NH2**	Lys-vasopressin	Suiformes

Oxytocin-related peptides

Cys Tyr Phe Arg **Asn Cys Pro** Ile **Gly-NH2**	Cephalotocin	*Octopus vulgaris*
Cys Tyr Ile Asn **Asn Cys Pro** Leu **Gly-NH2**	Aspargtocin	Sharks
Cys Tyr Ile Gln **Asn Cys Pro** Val **Gly-NH2**	Valitocin	Sharks
Cys Tyr Ile Ser **Asn Cys Pro** Gln **Gly-NH2**	Glumitocin	Rays
Cys Tyr Ile Arg **Asn Cys Pro** Val **Gly-NH2**	Asvatocin	Dogfish
Cys Tyr Ile Arg **Asn Cys Pro** Ile **Gly-NH2**	Phasvatocin	Dogfish
Cys Tyr Ile Ser **Asn Cys Pro** Ile **Gly-NH2**	Isotocin	Bony fishes
Cys Tyr Ile Gln **Asn Cys Pro** Ile **Gly-NH2**	Mesotocin	Amphibians, reptiles
Cys Tyr Ile Gln **Asn Cys Pro** Leu **Gly-NH2**	Oxytocin	Mammals

1   2   3   4   5   6   7   8   9

Acher's group clearly identified two molecular lineages: the isotocin-mesotocin-oxytocin line, which is associated with the regulation of reproductive function, and the vasotocin-vasopressin line associated with water balance. Vasopressin, oxytocin and their related peptides are coded by two related genes. They are initially synthesized as larger precursor (pre-prohormone) molecules in the hypothalamic nuclei of the neurohypophysial neurones. Following removal of the signal peptide, each remaining prohormone is cleaved to release the specific peptide and a highly conserved cysteine-rich neurophysin protein which is involved in the transport of the hormone along the axon. In the case of the vasopressin prohormone, a C-terminal glycoprotein called copeptin is also present. When cleaved from the parent molecule it may have a potential physiological role as a prolactin-releasing factor. This copeptin is absent from the oxytocin prohormone.

In invertebrates, members of the superfamily include the vasopressin-like diuretic hormone (or inotocin) from the locust *Locusta migratoria* and from the arthropod red flour beetle *Tribolium castaneum* (Stafflinger *et al.*, 2008), annetocin from the earthworm *Eisenia foetida*, conopressins from the gasteropod molluscs *Conus geographicus, Conus striatus* and *Lymnaea stagnalis* (von Kesteren *et al.*, 1992) and cephalotocin from the cephalopod *Octopus vulgaris*. Interestingly, inotocin is not present in other insects such as the fruit-fly, mosquito, silkworm and honeybee, but it is found in the parasitic wasp *Nasonia vitripennis*. In the adult *Tribolium*, the receptor for inotocin is localized in the brain and much less in the hindgut (Stafflinger *et al.*, 2008), but it might mediate a diuretic signalling pathway through an indirect regulation from the central nervous system (Aikins *et al.*, 2008). While inotocin exists in coleoptera, but not in diptera, lepidoptera and hymenoptera, the reverse is true for the neuropeptide corazonin and its receptor. Since the vasopressin and the corazonin receptors originated from a common ancestral receptor (Hauser *et al.*, 2008), it has been proposed that duplications developed during evolution, but the lack of evolutionary pressure made certain hormones superfluous. In fact, the vasopressin system was lost on two occasions during holometabolous insect evolution, and the archetypical *Drosophila* is not a good representative of all insects as it lacks vasopressin (Hauser *et al.*, 2008).

In Lys-conopressin, the hormone present in *Lymnaea stagnalis*, the basic lysine residue in position 8 is not important for activity since it can be artificially replaced by an aliphatic one (isoleucine) with no loss in potency. Furthermore, the deduced amino acid sequence for pre-proconopressin indicates that it is organized like the vasopressin precursor, with a signal sequence followed by conopressin, a conserved neurophysin and a divergent copeptin-homologous sequence at the C-terminus. Interestingly Lys-conopressin, although structurally related to vasopressin, actually controls reproductive function. Another conopressin sub-type has been recently discovered in the venom of *Conus tulipa* (Dutertre *et al.*, 2008). This novel peptide is characterized by the replacement of Pro7 by Leu and Gly9 by Val in its sequence. But more interestingly, it behaves as an antagonist to the V1a receptor. Thus it joins the short list of natural peptides which act as receptor inhibitors, the best example of which is the well-known agouti protein.

In vertebrates, phenypressin has been identified in marsupials, vasotocin in birds, mesotocin in amphibians, and isotocin, glumitocin, valitocin, aspargtocin, asvatocin and phasvatocin in various species of fish. Coelacanth and lungfish are the only two surviving lineages that arose between tetrapods and ray-finned fish. While lungfish contain vasotocin and (Phe2) mesotocin, coelacanth (*Latimeria menadoensis*) contains vasotocin and mesotocin. The genes coding for these peptides are linked in tandem in a tail-to-head orientation, while their homologues are in a tail-to-tail orientation in placental mammals and in a tail-to-head orientation of isotocin and vasotocin in pufferfish (*Fugu rubripes*). These results show that the gene locus for neurohypophysial hormones has undergone independent rearrangements in mammals and in fish (Gwee *et al.*, 2008).

Amphibians are intermediate between aquatic and terrestrial vertebrates. The tadpole has the osmoregulatory status of a freshwater fish, while the adult acquires a partially terrestrial system. With the skin becoming permeable to gas and water molecules, amphibians compensate for evaporative water loss by cutaneous water uptake, as well as by some reabsorption in the nephron and the urinary bladder, which appears for the first time in vertebrates. The amphibian nephron has not yet developed a loop of Henlé so the urine is hypotonic to plasma. The neurohypophysial hormones include vasotocin, mesotocin and, in a number of anuran amphibians, two different peptides, vasotocin-Gly (hydrin 2) and vasotocinyl-Gly-Lys-Arg (hydrin 1), which may be hormonally active. Both result from impairments in the processing of provasotocin, these being a decrease in a) intracellular carboxypeptidase activity for hydrin 1, and b) amidating activity for hydrin 2 (Acher *et al.*, 1997).

In mammals, two vasopressins have been identified, with either arginine or lysine as the basic residue at position 8. Arginine vasopressin is the hormone present in humans and in most mammals. In domestic pigs and certain other members of the Suina family, only Lys-vasopressin appears to be present, while both Lys- and Arg-vasopressin have been identified in wild boar and others. It has been suggested that the latter situation is due to a heterozygous form, while the former, through selective breeding, has been brought to a homozygous condition (Hoyle, 1998).

In invertebrates, as well as in the lowest vertebrates (jawless fish such as hagfish and lampreys), only one gene is present. Some time after the evolution of the Agnatha, a gene duplication led to the separation of the lineages for oxytocin and vasopressin analogues because all vertebrates, from Gnathostomata onwards possess the two peptides. Concerning the vasopressin lineage, vasotocin is present from Agnatha to birds, while vasopressin is present in mammals. It appears that, when the mammalian stock diverged from the reptilian stock 200 million years ago, a mutation replaced vasotocin with vasopressin (Hoyle, 1998).

The vasopressin system seems to have been lost in certain species of macropodid marsupials, such as the black-footed rock wallaby and the Lesueur's bettong, which have to rely on behavioural strategies such as exploiting the cool and humid refuge of caves and underground warrens in order to maintain fluid homeostasis in arid environments (King and Bradshaw, 2007).

3. Evolutionary Aspects of the Vasopressin Receptor Family

The membrane-bound vasopressin receptors have been characterized during the last 20 to 30 years, first pharmacologically through the use of ligands labelled with tritium at a high enough specific activity, and later structurally with the benefit of all the methodology of molecular biology. The V2 and V1a receptors were first cloned in 1992 (Birnbaumer *et al.*, 1992; Morel *et al.*, 1992, respectively), while the V1b (or V3) receptor was cloned in 1994 (Sugimoto *et al.*, 1994; de Keyzer *et al.*, 1994).

These receptors belong to an enormous family of G protein-coupled receptors (GPCR) involved in the recognition and transduction of messages as diverse as light and odorants, calcium ions, small molecules (amino acids, nucleotides, peptides), as well as proteins. In vertebrates, this family of receptors contains up to 2,000 members (more than 1% of the total genome). In *Caenorhabditis elegans,* the genome encodes more than 1,100 such receptors (5% of its genome) and GPCRs are known in plants, yeasts, slime moulds as well as in protozoa and the earliest metazoa (Bockaert and Pin, 1999). All of these receptors have a central core structure comprising seven transmembrane (TM) helices (TM 1 to 7) connected by three intracellular and three extracellular loops. A disulphide link between the first two external loops is highly conserved and is probably important for the stabilization of a restricted number of conformations of the seven TMs. A change in the conformation of the core domain is responsible for receptor activation.

The GPCRs can be classified into five families (Fig. 1) and the three main ones can be easily recognized from their amino acid sequences. Interestingly, receptors from different families share no sequence similarity, which supports the remarkable concept of molecular convergence (Bockaert and Pin, 1999). Family 1 contains most GPCRs,

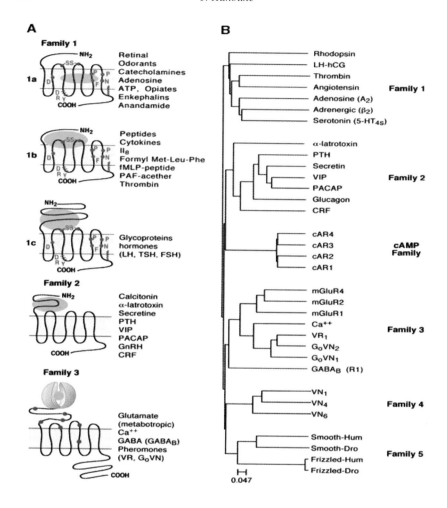

Figure 1. Classification and diversity of GPCRs (adapted from Bockaert and Pin, 1999). A. The three main families are easily recognized by comparing their amino-acid sequences, with receptors from different families not sharing any sequence similarity. All possess the same overall structure but differ by the presence or absence of an S-S bond between the external loops 1 and 2, and by the length of the external NH_2 tail. The ligand binding site is indicated by the orange zone. The vasopressin receptor belongs to family 2 together with the receptors for glucagon, secretin, PACAP and the black widow spider toxin α-latrotoxin. B. The dendrogram includes the other more distant families.

with Group 1a containing rhodopsin and β-adrenergic receptors, Group 1b, the receptors for various peptides including vasopressin and oxytocin, and Group 1c, the receptors for the glycoprotein hormones. Family 2, with the same structure but no sequence analogy, includes various receptors for glucagon, secretin and other polypeptides. Family 3 contains the calcium-sensing receptors, while Family 4 comprises the pheromone receptors. Family 5 includes receptors involved in development. The cAMP receptor family is separate, having been found only in *Dictyostelium. Discoideum.* This classification has been refined, but not fundamentally modified, by Fredriksson *et al.* (2003, 2005).

The phylogenic relationship of the various members of the vasopressin/oxytocin receptor family is depicted in Fig. 2. Of interest in this figure is the relative position of the two receptors cloned from the freshwater snail *Lymnaea stagnalis* (CPR1 and CPR2) which bind Lys-conopressin (van Kesteren *et al.*, 1996). Lys-conopressin is structurally related to vasopressin but is functionally similar to oxytocin: it does not depend on a basic residue being present at position 8 since Ile-conopressin is equally potent, and it controls reproductive functions. CPR1 and CPR2 have different distributions in the brain and in the peripheral issues. The CPR2 receptor is more closely related to the vertebrate vasopressin and oxytocin receptors than to CPR1. According to van Kesteren, the CPR2 receptor is a likely modern (vertebrate) representative of the ancestral receptor (van Kesteren *et al.*, 1998).

Phylogenic analysis shows that these two CPR receptors result from an ancient gene duplication that occurred before separate receptor types in vertebrates evolved. Also, according to van Kesteren (1998) "multiple receptors might have existed before the separation between the vasopressin and the oxytocin lineages evolved". However, as Darlison and Richter (1999) have pointed out, while an oxytocin-like peptide has not been found in *Lymnaea stagnalis,* such peptides have been found in other invertebrates (cephalotocin in octopus, annetocin in the earthworm). This is inconsistent with the hypothesis that the vasopressin and oxytocin genes arose by duplication after the radiation of the cyclostomes, and indicates that an oxytocin-like peptide might also exist in snails. The amino acid sequences of the receptor subtypes are generally more conserved than those of the related neuropeptides, and Darlison and Richter (1999) suggest that the receptors evolved as targets for peptides that were already present. In addition, as pointed out by Cho *et al.*, (2007), extensive sequencing of vertebrate neuropeptides and their receptor families reveals how they have achieved distinct ligand specificity during evolution while maintaining core ligand-receptor interaction sites. At least in the case of the vasopressin system, the question as to whether the ligand or the receptor came first is still open to debate.

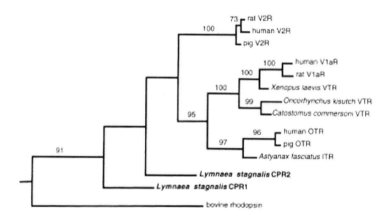

Figure 2. Phylogenic relationship of the members of the vasopressin/oxytocin family (adapted from van Kesteren *et al.* 1998). Numbers above the branches result from bootstrap analysis and are confidence limits for the positions of the branches. ITR, isotocin receptor; CPR, conopressin receptor; VTR, vasotocin receptor; OTR, oxytocin receptor.

A recent impetus in the study of evolutionary aspects of the vasopressin receptor has been provided by the current interest in the role that this receptor plays in mammalian social behaviour. This has been particularly well studied in the development of a mating system in the genus *Microtus*. It has been hypothesized that the differences in social behaviour were associated with extra- and inter-species variations in the distribution of the V1a receptor in the brain (Hammock *et al.*, 2005). In rodents, variation in a repetitive microsatellite element in the 5′ flanking region of the V1a receptor gene has been linked to those differences (Phelps and Young 2003; Hammock *et al.*, 2005). In humans, the same flanking region contains a tandem duplication of two microsatellite-containing elements, localized 3.5 kb upstream of the transcription start site. The second block contains a complex repetitive motif known as RS3 which is unrelated to the vole microsatellite (Donaldson *et al.*, 2008). It is highly polymorphic, yielding sixteen different alleles in the human population (Thibonnier *et al.*, 2000). It is possible that the RS3 region influences the expression of the receptor, which manifests as aspects of social behaviour in humans including altruism (Knafo *et al.*, 2008), partner bonding, marital problems and marital status (Walum *et al.*, 2008), essential hypertension (Hasan *et al.*, 2007) or autism (Insel, 2008). In addition, Fink *et al.* (2007) have stressed that high variability and non-neutral evolution of the coding sequence of the receptor, in particular the first exon, could also be associated with behavioural traits in voles and humans. An exonic polymorphism in the V1b receptor could be linked to panic disorder (Keck *et al.*, 2008).

4. Evolutionary Aspects of the Aquaporin Family

Living organisms are mainly composed of water, the consequence of which is that the organism somehow has to maintain its osmotic and electrochemical balance, and transport nutrients and metabolites across the cell membrane. Simple diffusion of water is too slow and too finite a phenomenon to account for the necessary movements of water in the presence of an osmotic gradient, and the concept of water channels was advanced some time ago (see short historical review by Calamita, 2005).

In 1987, a 28 kDa channel-like integral protein (CHIP28) in red blood cells was identified (Agre *et al.*, 1987). Later, this molecule was renamed aquaporin 1 (Agre *et al.*, 1993) after it had been shown to have the functional characteristic of a water channel in oocytes (Preston *et al.*, 1992). Since then, not only have at least eleven aquaporin-like molecules been identified in mammals, but aquaporins have been shown to be members of a much larger channel family comprising more than 450 identified isoforms. These channels, termed major intrinsic proteins (MIPs), are found in eubacteria, archaea, fungi, plants and animals (Zardoya, 2005; El Karkouri *et al.*, 2005). They are particularly abundant in plants and in vertebrates where they are restricted to fluid-conducting organs (kidney, lungs, secretory glands). It is clear that because of the vital role of these channels, they antedate the appearance of the vasopressin-signalling pathway which has endowed them with potential regulation via changes in their rate of synthesis, in activity or in subcellular localization.

The main characteristics of the 11 known aquaporins (AQP0 to AQP10) in mammals are depicted in Table 2. Four of them (AQP3, 7, 9 and 10) also transport glycerol or urea, and are classified as glycerol-uptake facilitators or aquaglyceroporins (GLP). A simple aquaporin family tree in humans is depicted in Fig. 3 (King *et al.*, 2004). According to phylogenic analysis, alternative main substrate-selective modes (AQPs and GLPs) were acquired very early in evolution by gene duplication and functional shift (Zardoya, 2005). Interestingly, in plants GLP orthologues are absent, while up to 35 different AQP genes have been identified in *Arabidopsis* and 31 in maize (Zardoya, 2005). Among the plant AQPs, one can distinguish four subfamilies: tonoplast intrinsic proteins (TIPs), plasma membrane intrinsic proteins (PIPs), small basic intrinsic proteins (SIPs) and NOD26-like intrinsic proteins (NIPs). The latter can also transport glycerol and belongs to a sister group of bacterial AQPs. They might have been acquired by horizontal gene transfer from bacteria at the evolutionary origin of plants (Zardoya, 2005).

Table 2. Permeability characteristics and distribution of the known mammalian aquaporin (AQP) analogues (adapted from King *et al.*, 2004).

Aquaporin	Permeability	Tissue distribution	Subcellular distribution*
AQP0	Water (low)	Lens	
AQP1	Water (high)	Red blood cell, kidney, lung, vascular endothelium, brain, eye	Plasma membrane
AQP2	Water (high)	Kidney, vas deferens	Apical membrane, intracellular vesicles
AQP3	Water (high), glycerol (high), urea (moderate)	Kidney, skin, lung, eye, colon	Basolateral membrane
AQP4	Water (high)	Brain, muscle, kidney, lung, stomach	Basolateral membrane
AQP5	Water (high)	Salivary, lacrimal and Sweat glands, lung, cornea	Apical membrane
AQP6	Water (low), intracellular anions ($NO_3^- > Cl^-$) vesicles	Kidney	
AQP7	Water (high), glycerol (high), urea (high), arsenite	Adipose tissue, kidney, testis	Plasma membrane
AQP8[#]	Water (high)	Testis, kidney, liver, pancreas, colon, small intestine	Plasma membrane, intracellular vesicles
AQP9	Water (low), glycerol (high), urea (high), arsenite	Liver, leukocytes, brain, testis	Plasma membrane
AQP10	Water (low), glycerol (high), urea (high)	Small intestine	Intracellular vesicles

*Homologues present in both apical and basolateral membranes are designated as having a plasma membrane distribution. #AQP8 might be permeated by water and urea.

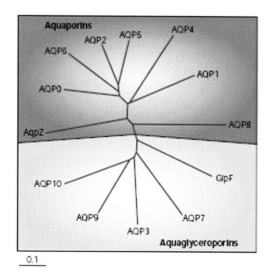

Figure 3. Aquaporin family tree (adapted from King *et al.*, 2004). This tree shows the relationship between the eleven human aquaporins (AQP) and the *Escherichia coli* analogues AqpZ and GlpF. The scale represents evolutionary distance: 0.1 equals 10 substitutions per 100 amino acid residues.

5. Conclusion

Control of water balance is certainly one of the most important regulatory mechanisms in all living organisms. The taxonomic range of aquaporins is extensive because they are found in all living forms, from bacteria and protozoa to mammals including humans. The additional regulation of those channels by neurohypophysial hormones occurred when evolution led animals to adapt to a fresh water environment, taking advantage of the fact that membrane-bound GCPR receptors were already available in a large variety of sequences and functions from the earlier appearance of protozoa and early metazoa. From this point of view, it is interesting to note that the mRNAs for AQP1 and arginne vasopressin receptor from the black porgy, *Acanthopagrus schlegeli*, are increased in parallel when the fish is transferred to an hypo-osmotic environment (An *et al.*, 2008).

Bibliography

Acher R., Chauvet J., Chauvet M.T., Rouillé Y. (1994). Unique evolution of neuphyseal hormones in cartilaginous fishes: possible implications for urea-based osmoregulation. *J Exp Zool* 284: 475–484

Acher R., Chauvet J., Rouillé Y. (1997). Adaptative evolution of water homeostasis regulation in amphibians: vasotocin and hydrins. *Biol Cell* 89: 283–291

Acher R. (2002). L'homéostase hydrique dans le vivant: organisation moléculaire, reflexes osmorégulateurs et evolution. *Ann Endocr* 63: 197–218

Agre P., Saboori A.M., Asimos A., Smith B.L. (1987). Purification and partial characerization of the Mr 30000 integral protein associated with the erythrocyte Rh (D) antigen. *J Biol Chem* 262: 17497–17503

Agre P., Sasaki S., Chrispeels M.J. (1993). Aquaporins: a family of water channel proteins. *Am J Physiol* 265: F461

Aikins M.J., Schooley D.A., Begum K., Detheux M., Beeman R.W., Park Y. (2008). Vasopressin-like petide and its receptor function in an indirect diuretic signalling pathway in the red flour beetle. *Insect Biochem Mol Biol* 38: 740–748

An K.W., Kim N.N., Choi C.Y. (2008). Cloning and expression of aquaporin 1 and arginine vasopressin receptor mRNA from the black porgy, *Acanthopagrus schlegeli:* effect of freshwater acclimation. *Fish Physiol Biochem* 34: 185–194

Birnbaumer M., Seibold A., Gilbert S., Ishido M., Barberis C., Antaramian A., Brabet P., Rosenthal W. (1992). Molecular cloning of the receptor for human antidiuretic hormone. *Nature* 357: 333–335

Bockaert J., Pin J.P. (1999). Molecular tinkering of G protein-coupled receptors: an evolutionary success. *EMBO J* 18: 1723–1729

Calamita G. (2005). Aquaporins: highways for cells to recycle water with the outside world. *Biol Cell* 97: 351–353.

Cho H.J., Acharjee S., Moon M.J., Oh D.Y., Vaudry H., Kwon H.B., Seong J.Y. (2007). Molecular evolution of neuropeptide receptors with regards to maintaining high affinity to their authentic ligands. *Gen Comp Endocrinol* 153: 98–107

Darlison M.G., Richter D. (1999). Multiple genes for neuropeptides and their receptors: co-evolution and physiology. *Trends Neurosci* 22, 81–88

Donaldson Z.R., Kondrashov F.A., Putnam A., Bai Y., Stoinski T.L., Hammock E.A.D., Young L.J. (2008). Evolution of a behavior-linked microsatellite-containing element in the 5′ flanking region of the primate AVPR1A gene. *BMC Evol Biol* 8: 180

Dutertre S., Croker D., Daly N.L., Andersson A., Muttenthaler M., Lumsden N.G., Craik D.J., Alewood P.F., Guillon G., Lewis R.J. (2008). Conopressin-T from *conus tulipa* reveals an antagonist switch in the vasopressin-like peptides. *J Biol Chem* 283: 7100–7108

El Karkouri K., Gueuné H., Delamarche C. (2005). MIP*DB*: a relational database dedicated to MIP family proteins. *Biol Cell* 97: 535–543

Fink S., Excoffier L., Heckle G. (2007). High variability and non-neutral evolution of the mammalian avpr1a gene. *BioMed Evol Biol*, 7: 176

Fredriksson R., Lagerström M.C., Lundin L.G., Schiöth H.B. (2003). The G-protein-coupled receptors in the human genome form fivemain families. Phylogenetic analysis, paralogon groups and fingerprints. *Mol Pharmacol*, 63: 1256–1272

Fredriksson R., Schiöth H.B. (2005). The repertoire of G-protein-coupled receptors in fully sequenced genomes. *Mol Pharmacol* 67: 1414–1425

Gwee P.C., Amemiya C.T., Brenner S., Venkatesh B. (2008). Sequence and organization of coelacanth neurophyseal hormone genes: evolutionary history of the vertebrate neurophyseal hormone gene locus. *BMC Evol Biol* 8: 93

Hammock E.A., Lim M.M., Nair H.P. Young L.J. (2005). Association of vasopressin 1a receptor levels with a regulatory microsatellite and behaviour. *Genes Brain Behav* 4: 289–301

Hammock E.A., Young L.J. (2005). Microsatellite instability generates diversity in brain and sociobehavioral traits. *Science* 308: 1630–1634

Hasan K.N., Shoji M., Sugimoto K., Tsutaya S., Matsuda E., Kudo R., Nakaji S., Suda T. Yasujima M. (2007). Association of novel promoter single nucleotide polymorphisms in vasopressin V1a receptor gene with essential hypertension in nonobese Japanese. *J Hum Hypertens* 21: 825–827

Hauser F., Cazzamali G., Williamson M., Park Y., Li B., Ranaka Y., Predel R., Neupert S., Schachtner J., Verleyen P., Grimmelikhuijzen C.J.P. (2008). A genome-wide inventory of neurohormone GPCRs in the red flour beetle *Tribolium castaneum*. *Front Neuroendocrinol* 29: 142–165

Hoyle C.H.V. (1998). Neuropeptide families: evolutionary perspectives. *Regul Pepides* 73: 1–33

Insel T.R. (2008). From species differences to individual differences. *Mol Psychiatry* 11: 424

Keck M.E., Kern N., Erhardt A., Unschuld P.G., Ising M., Salyakina D., Muller M.B., Knorr C.C., Lieb R., Hohoff C., Krakowitzky P., Maier W., Bandelow B., Fritze J., Deckert J., Holsboer F., Muller-Myhsok B., Binder E.B. (2008). Combined effects of exonic polymorphisms in CRHR1 and AVPR1B genes in a case/control study for panic disorder. *Am J Med Genet, B Neuropsychiatr Genet* 147: 1196–1204

van Kesteren R.E., Smit AB., Dirks RW., de With N.D., Geraerts W.PM., Joosse J. (1992). Evolution of the vasopressin/oxytocin superfamily: characterization of a cDNA encoding a vasopressin-related precursor, preproconopressin, from the mollusc *Lymnaea stagnalis*. *Proc Nat Acad Sci USA* 89: 4593–4597

van Kesteren R.E., Tensen C.P, Smit A.B., van Minnen J., Kolakowski L.F., Meyerhof W., Richter D., van Heerikhuizen H., Vreugdenhil E., Geraerts W.P. (1996). Co-evolution of ligand-receptor pair in the vasopressin/oxytocin superfamily of bioactive peptides. *J Biol Chem* 271: 3619–3626

van Kesteren R.E, Geraerts W.P. (1998). Molecular evolution of ligand-binding specificity in the vasopressin/oxytocin receptor family. *Ann New York Acad Sci* 839: 25–34

de Keyzer Y., Auzan C., Lenne F., Beldjord C., Thibonnier M., Bertagna X., Clauser E. (1994). Cloning and characterization of the human V3 pituitary vasopressin receptor. *FEBS Letters* 356: 215–220

King L.S, Kozono D., Agre P. (2004). From structure to disease: the evolving tale of aquaporin biology. *Nature Rev Mol Cell Biol* 5: 687–698

King J.M., Bradshaw S.D. (2007). Comparative water metabolism of Barrow Island macropodid marsupials: hormonal versus behavioural-dependant mechanisms of body water conservation. *Gen Comp Endocrinol* 155: 378–385

Knafo A., Israel S., Darvasi A., Bachner-Melman R., Uzefovsky F., Cohen L., Feldman E., Lerer E., Laiba E., Raz Y., Nemanov L., Gritsanko I., Dina C., Agam G., Dean B., Bornstein G., Ebstein R.P. (2008). Individual differences in the allocation of funds in the dictator game associated with length of the arginine vasopressin 1a receptor RS3 promoter region and correlation between RS3 length and hippocampal mRNA. *Genes Brain Behav* 7: 266–275

Morel A., O'Carroll A.M., Brownstein M.J., Lolait S.J. (1992). Molecular cloning and expression of a V1a arginine vasopressin receptor. *Nature* 356: 523–526

Phelps S.M, Young L.J. (2003). Extraordinary diversity in vasopressin (V1a) receptor distributions among wild prairie voles (*Microtus ochrogaster*): patterns of variation and covariation. *J Comp Neurol* 466: 564–576

Preston G.M., Piazza-Carroll T., Guggino W.B., Agre P. (1992). Appearance of water channels in *Xenopus* oocytes expressing red cell CHIP28 protein. *Science* 256: 385–387

Schally A.V., Bowers C.Y., Kuroshima A. (1964). Effect of lysine vasopressin dimers on blood pressure and some endocrine functions. *Am J Physiol* 207: 378–384

Schrier R.W., Chen Y.C., Cadnapaphornchai M.A (2004). From finch to fish to man: role of aquaporins in body fluid and brain water regulation. *Neuroscience* 129: 897–904

Stafflinger E., Hansen K.K., Hauser F., Schneider M., Cazzamali G., Williamson M., Grimmelikhuijzen C.J.P. (2008). Cloning and identification of an oxytocin/vasopressin-like receptor and its ligand from insect. *Proc Nat Acad Sci USA* 105: 3262–3267

Sugimoto T., Saito M., Mochizuki S., Watanabe Y., Hashimoto S., Kawashima H. (1994). Molecular cloning and functional expression of a cDNA encoding the human V1b vasopressin receptor. *J Biol Chem* 269: 27088–27092

Thibonnier M., Graves M.K., Wagner M.S., Chatelain N., Soubrier F., Corvol P., Willard H.F., Jeunemaitre X. (2000). Study of V(1)-vascular vasopressin receptor microsatellite polymorphisms in human essential hypertension. *J Mol Cell Cardiol* 32: 557–564

du Vigneaud V., Bartlett M.F., Tripett S. (1953a). The sequence of amino acids in oxytocin with a proposal for the structure of oxytocin. *J Biol Chem* 205: 949–957

du Vigneaud V., Lawler H.C., Popenoe E.A. (1953b). Enzymatic cleavage of glycinamide from vaspressin and a proposed structure for this pressor-antiduiretic hormone of the posterior pituitary. *J Am Chem Soc* 75: 4880–4881

Walum H., Westberg L., Henningsson S., Neiderhiser J.M., Reiss D., Wigmar I., Ganiban J.M., Spotts E.L., Pedersen N.L., Eriksson J., Lichtenstein P. (2008). Genetic variation in the vasopressin receptor 1a gene (AVPR1A) associates with pair-bonding behavior in humans. *Proc Soc Nat Acad USA* 105: 14153–14156

Zardoya R. (2005). Phylogeny and evolution of the major intrinsic protein family. *Biol Cell* 97: 397–414

CHAPTER 3

THE NEUROHYPOPHYSIAL SYSTEM: SYNTHESIS AND METABOLISM OF VASOPRESSIN

Jacques Hanoune

Institut Cochin, 22 Rue Méchain, 75014 Paris, France
Email: jacques.hanoune@inserm.fr

1. Developmental Aspects of the Neuroendocrine Hypothalamus

Both vasopressin and oxytocin are synthesized in hypothalamic neurones, those producing vasopressin originating mainly from the supraoptic nucleus and those producing oxytocin mainly from the paraventricular nucleus, although each site is not exclusive regarding the neuropeptide produced. The supraoptic nucleus is wholly magnocellular, with large neurones (20–40 µm cell body diameter), while the paraventricular nucleus is divided into a lateral magnocellular part and a more medial parvocellular (9–15 µm cell body diameter) subdivision which has a different function from the magnocellular component (Burbach *et al.*, 2001).

The development of the neuroendocrine hypothalamus is characterised by a precise series of morphogenic milestones that culminate in the differentiation of the various neurosecretory cell lineages. As shown by Acampora *et al.* (1999), the homeobox-containing gene Orthopedia (Otp) is expressed in those neurones, giving rise to the paraventricular, supraoptic, anterior periventricular and arcuate nuclei throughout their development. Homozygous Otp −/− mice die soon after birth, displaying progressive impairment of crucial neuroendocrine events such as cell proliferation, cell migration and terminal differentiation of the parvo- and magno-cellular neurones of these nuclei (Acampora *et al.*, 1999). Moreover, Otp and Sim 1 genes, the latter being a bHLH-PAS transcription factor that directs terminal differentiation of the

39

paraventricular and supraoptic nuclei, act in parallel and are both required to maintain expression of Brn2, a member (together with Pit1) of the large family of POU domain transcription factors. Some of these bind to specific DNA sequences to cause temporal and spatial regulation of the expression of genes, many of which are involved in the regulation of neuronal development in the central nervous system of mammals. Expression of Brn2 is required for the cell lineages secreting oxytocin and vasopressin, as well as corticotrophin releasing factor. The complex hierarchy of genetic interactions among transcription factors selectively required for the development of specific cell lineages in the developing hypothalamus is depicted in Fig. 1.

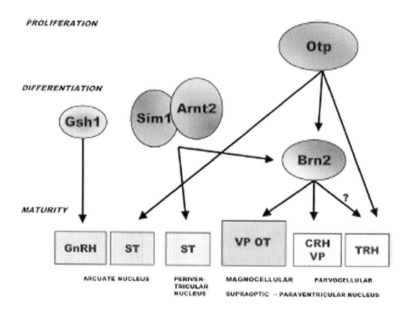

Figure 1. The hierarchy of transcription factors controlling the developing cell lineages in the hypothalamus. Otp and Sim are required from day E12 onward for neuroblast proliferation and lateral migration as well as for Brn2 expression. Brn2 is required for the terminal development of the oxytocin and vasopressin cell lineages (adapted from Burbach *et al.*, 2001).

During development, the vasopressin neurones in the supraoptic nucleus positively auto-control their electrical activity via dentritic release of the hormone. The effect of this auto control is maximal during the second post-natal week when the dendritic tree transiently increases and glutamatergic postsynaptic potentials appear (Chevaleyre *et al.*, 2000; 2002). Likely effects of the dendritic release of neurohypophysial hormones in the adult are currently the subject of much interest (see Chapter 11).

2. Biosynthesis

a) *Gene structure*

The genes that direct the synthesis of both vasopressin and oxytocin are located on the same chromosome (chromosome 20p13 in man; Ivell and Richter, 1984) in tandem arrangement and in reverse order (Fig. 2). The intergenic distance between the two genes ranges from 3 to 12 kb in mouse, man and rat (Gimp and Fahrenholz, 2001). This type of arrangement probably results from the duplication of an ancestral gene, as described in Chapter 2, followed by an inversion of one of them. The vasopressin locus in the rat contains long interspersed repeated DNA elements (LINEs) whose potential role on the expression of the hormone is unknown (Schmitz *et al.*, 1991; Burbach *et al.*, 2001).

The intergenic region (IGR) is probably the site of critical enhancer elements necessary for the hypothalamus-specific expression of vasopressin. This 'IGR hypothesis' has been confirmed by various transgenic experiments (Fields *et al.*, 2003). Reducing the 5′ flanking region in the mouse vasopressin gene from 3.5 kbp to 288 bp did not alter its expression in hypothalamic slices. The use of various constructs with the vasopressin or oxytocin promoters driving a green fluorescent protein reporter gene expression showed that the IGR was necessary for vasopressin and oxytocin gene expression in hypothalamic slices (Fig. 2). The sequence in the IGR responsible for both vasopressin and oxytocin gene expression is located in a 178 bp domain immediately downstream of exon 3 of the vasopressin gene. A variety of Fos/Jun family member proteins stimulate transcription of the vasopressin gene through an activation protein-1 (AP1) site (−134/−128) in the 5′ promoter region (Yoshida *et al.*, 2006). Additionally, another domain 430 bp downstream of exon 3 of the oxytocin gene contains a positive regulatory element for oxytocin gene expression (Fields *et al.*, 2003).

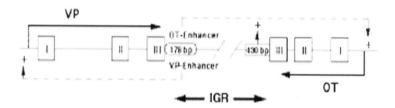

Figure 2. Relationship between the vasopressin and oxytocin genes. The two genes lie in tandem arrangement and in reverse order on the same chromosome. The solid arrows refer to the direction of trancription under the influence of each promoter. The dotted arrows refer to the hypothalamic specific enhancing influences. The intergenic region contains the putative enhancer domain for the vasopressin and oxytocin genes in a 178 bp segment immediately downstream of the exon 3 of the vasopressin gene. An additional oxytocin enhancer domain is located in the 430 bp downstream of the exon 3 of the oxytocin gene (adapted from Fields *et al.*, 2003).

Due to the complexity of the mammalian genome and in particular the large amount of 'junk' DNA that is interspersed in the intergenic and intronic sequences, it is of interest to compare it with that of a simpler genome, for example that of the pufferfish Fugu, which contains only 390 Mbp with very few repetitive elements (less than 10% of the genome). The magnocellular neurones of the preoptic nucleus of the fish express, in separate cells, isotocin and vasotocin, the teleost equivalents of oxytocin and vasopressin, respectively. Transgenic rats have been produced expressing the isotocin/vasotocin genes. The isotocin gene was expressed only in the rat oxytocin neurones and was upregulated in response to withdrawal of dietary water in parallel with the endogenous oxytocin gene (Venkatesh *et al.*, 1997). These results demonstrate the conservation of regulatory mechanisms between species such as rat and

Fugu, which inhabit widely different environments (Murphy *et al.*, 1998).

The mammalian vasopressin gene consists of three exons separated by two introns, and comprises about 2 kb (Fig. 3). Exon A codes for a signal peptide, vasopressin, a three amino acid spacer (Gly-Lys-Arg) and the first nine N-terminal amino acids of neurophysin II; exon B codes for the central, highly conserved (amino acids 10–76) region of neurophysin II, exon C codes for the C-terminal part of neurophysin, a monobasic cleavage site (Arg) and a glycoprotein (39 amino acids) of unknown function, called copeptin. In contrast to vasopressin, exon C of the oxytocin gene only codes for the C-terminal amino acids of neurophysin I. The neurophysin domain, especially the domain coded by exon B, is well conserved and exists in all vertebrate and invertebrate species. Furthermore, the two segments in the neurophysin sequence show a 66% analogy at the nucleotide level. This indicates that the primordial neurophysin gene itself arose from a partial gene duplication of an initially smaller structure (Capra *et al.*, 1972). The secondary structure of neurophysin also indicates a two-domain organization of the molecule (Burman *et al.*, 1989). Neurophysin contains 14 cysteine residues which are conserved with almost equal interdistances. The strong conservation of the neurophysin domain of the various vasopressin-related prohormones confirms that the mammalian oxytocin/vasopressin family evolved from a common ancestral molecule by gene duplication.

i) *The vasopressin promoter*
While the physiological regulation of the mammalian vasopressin gene expression is well known, studies concerning the vasopressin promoter have been limited by the difficulty in studying gene expression in a small population of neurones without any corresponding cell lines. Most studies have relied on transgenic animals or heterologous cell lines (Burbach *et al.*, 2001) and have dealt with regulation by cyclic AMP or glucocorticoids.

GENE

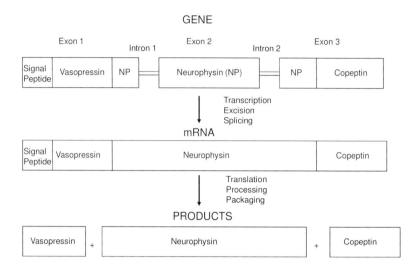

Figure 3. Synthesis steps of vasopressin. Neurophysin and the terminal glycopeptide copeptin are co-released with vasopressin.

The vasopressin promoter responds positively to cyclic AMP after transfection in cultured cells. A cyclic AMP analogue stimulates by twofold the luciferase activity of P19 cells transfected with the −174+44 sequence of the 5′-flanking region of the gene (Verbeeck *et al.*, 1990). In another study using a transfected JEG-3 cell line, an analysis with deletion mutants of the promoter showed that two cyclic AMP response element (CRE)-like sequences (−227 to −220 bp and −123 to −116 bp) contribute to this regulation (Iwasaki *et al.*, 1997). A similar CRE site has also been identified in the bovine vasopressin promoter, located at −120 to −112 and which is involved in the gene response to changes in water balance (Pardy *et al.*, 1992).

Glucocorticoids have been shown to suppress the increase in vasopressin promoter activity mediated by cyclic AMP analogues (Iwasaki *et al.*, 1997). This effect depended on the presence of the glucocorticoid receptor without its binding to DNA. However, a bovine vasopressin transgene in transgenic mice is negatively regulated by glucocorticoids, probably through a direct binding of the receptor to sequences between 150 and 300 bp upstream of the start site (Burke *et al.*, 1997). Interestingly, chronic hypoosmolarity induces glucocorticoid receptor expression in the vasopressin magnocellular neurones (Berghorn *et al.*, 1995), a phenomenon concomitant with the onset of the negative feedback on vasopressin transcription. This supports the hypothesis that the vasopressin gene could be directly inhibited by glucocorticoids. The opposing actions of glucocorticoids and cyclic AMP have also been reported in parvocellular neurones of the paraventricular nucleus in rat hypothalamic cultures (Kawahara *et al.*, 2003).

Finally, vasopressin promoter activity has been shown to be reduced by inhibitory forms of the cyclic AMP-responsive element modulator (CREM) family (Burbach *et al.*, 2001) and through ligand activation of the androgen or oestrogen receptors (Adan and Burbach, 1992).

A number of single nucleotide polymorphisms (SNPs) have been detected in the vasopressin locus in the rat, and two of them are embedded in cis-regulatory elements. In particular, one specific SNP/A (−1276)G/ confers reduced binding of the transcriptional repressor CArG binding factor A (CBF-A), which corresponds to an overexpression of vasopressin *in vitro* and *in vivo*, and could be responsible for high anxiety-related behaviour (Murgatroyd *et al.*, 2004). No such data are available for humans.

In the rat, the vasopressin poly (A) tail is unusually long and increases in length from 200 to 400 residues during stimulation of vasopressin gene expression *in vivo*, for example by 3 days of dehydratation (Carrazana *et al.*, 1988; Murphy and Carter, 1990; Carter and Murphy, 1991). In the mouse, an equivalent osmotic stimulus does not alter the poly (A) length of either vasopressin or oxytocin (Murphy and Carter, 1990). Bovine vasopressin RNA transfected into rat brain undergoes a dramatic lengthening of the poly (A) tail after dehydration. Transgene expression is also seen in rat adrenal cortex where it is also increased during dehydration, but without any change in the poly (A) tail (Si-Hoe *et al.*,

2001). The effect of dehydration on the poly (A) tail is therefore species and tissue specific. Although there is no information on the physiological role of the vasopressin poly (A) length shift, it might influence translational efficiency and/or message stability.

b) *Processing of the mature peptide*

Synthesis of the vasopressin precursor occurs in the cell bodies of specific magnocellular and parvocellular neurones of the supraoptic and paraventricular nuclei of the hypothalamus. The exact biochemical steps during the post-translational processing of vasopressin are not well elucidated but are very probably similar to what is known for the processing of other peptides (Walter and Blobel, 1981; Rose and Doms, 1988).

The large primary protein precursor is processed into the three polypeptides that are produced in equal amounts. Preprovasopressin is first cleaved into a signal peptide and provasopressin. After translation, the prohormone is inserted into the endoplasmic reticulum and eight disulphide bridges are formed within its rather short protein sequence. Then the carboxy terminal domain of the precursor is glycosylated and the product packaged into vesicles, which then pass down the axons. During this migration, basic endopeptidases cleave the provasopressin into the copeptin glycopeptide of 39 amino acids, the disulphide-rich neurophysin II protein of 93 amino acids and the active hormone (Russel *et al.*, 1980). Neurophysin II is essential for the proper targeting, packaging and storage of vasopressin before release into the bloodstream (Ginsburg and Ireland, 1966). Neurophysin II has a very strong binding affinity for vasopressin at acidic pH such as in the neurosecretory granules (pH 5.5). Dissociation of the complex is facilitated when it is released from the neurosecretory vesicules and enters plasma where the pH is 7.4. This strong affinity has been used to purify vasopressin through columns of neurophysin-sepharose.

Transport of the prohormone down the regulated neuronal secretory pathway involves a selective aggregation in the trans-Golgi network and the fact that neurophysin readily oligomerizes into dimers, tetramers and possibly higher order oligomers (Breslow, 1979; 1993), especially at acidic pH. According to the model proposed by De Bree (De Bree, 2000; De Bree *et al.*, 2000), the following events are involved in the trafficking of the vasopressin prohormone: a) it is first inserted into the endoplasmic reticulum in an unfolded form; b) there, both the hormone and the neurophysin domains are folded; c) the two domains then bind together, stabilizing the disulphide bridge; d) the prohormone dimerizes and is translocated to the Golgi apparatus; e) in the trans-Golgi network, it polymerizes and/or aggregates; f) the aggregate passes along the regulated secretory pathway; g) the prohormone is proteolyzed into the three polypeptide components during the initial stage of granule formation; h) the acidification of the granule leads to the condensation of the aggregate; i) the granule is transfered to the plasma membrane where a secretion-stimulus releases the three mature polypeptides into the bloodstream.

i) *The Brattleboro rat*
Brattleboro rats are characterized by the absence of vasopressin in the circulation and a large urinary output with an excessive thirst (central diabetes insipidus; Valtin and Schroeder, 1964). Studies of the vasopressin gene revealed a deletion of a single base, guanine, in the neurophysin coding region (Schmale and Richter, 1984; Schmale *et al.*, 1984). The mutated gene was found to be transcribed and translated into a mutated provasopressin precursor. This mutation leads to an open reading-frame with the loss of the normal stop codon, resulting in an extended precursor with a mutated C terminus, including a poly-lysine sequence encoded by the poly-A tail (Ivell *et al.*, 1986). During fluid deprivation, the impaired regulation of vasopressin gene expression appears to be a secondary phenomenon rather than a primary one (Kim *et al.*, 1990). The precise processing and secretory mechanisms for vasopressin have not been fully delineated yet. Schmale *et al.* (1989) suggested that the mutated precursor does not reach the Golgi apparatus, maybe because the elongated C-terminus remains anchored in the membrane of the endoplamsic reticulum. Immunocytochemical studies in Brattleboro rats have also suggested a block in the secretory pathway (Guldenaar and Pickering, 1988; Krisch *et al.*, 1986).

An extensive assessement of the consequences of various mutations of wild type and Brattleboro genes has led Kim *et al.* (1997) to the following interesting conclusions:

1) Vasopressin is processed and secreted more efficiently from the gene without the glycopeptide (GP) coding sequence than from the wild-type gene. This glycoprotein therefore plays a rather inhibitory role on the processing of vasopressin, and is actually lacking in the gene region coding for oxytocin.

2) The vasopressin coding region alone cannot be processed and secreted.

3) The Brattleboro construct with the same length as the wild-type vasopressin gene is not associated with vasopressin secretion.

4) The Brattleboro vasopressin gene with the same length as the combined vasopressin and neurophysin coding regions (still containing the guanyl deletion) is associated with vasopressin processing, but not to the level of the wild-type vasopressin gene.

5) The wild-type vasopressin gene with a stop codon at the same site as the guanyl deletion secretes less vasopressin than the wild-type gene.

These results suggest that an additional defect in the Brattleboro gene may relate directly to the guanyl deletion, in addition to the absence of the normal stop codon which results in an extended C terminus. A normal neurophysin coding region is necessary for optimal vasopressin processing, transport and secretion. In particular, the normal sequence of amino acids from the site of the guanyl deletion (site 64) is indispensable for the optimal processing of vasopressin. Because of the G deletion, amino acids 64 to 95 are mutated in the Brattleboro rat leading to the disappearance of any Gly (normally 3) or Cys (normally 7) in that region. As suggested from studies of the crystalline structure of bovine neurophysin (Chen *et al.*, 1991), correct folding of the polypeptide chain is necessary for the processing of the vasopressin precursor.

Interestingly in human central diabetes insipidus, genetic mutations have been found in the neurophysin coding region as well as in the signal peptide region (Repaske *et al.*, 1996), but no mutation has been found either in the vasopressin or the glycoprotein coding sequence. It is likely that the mutant precursors are retained in the endoplasmic reticulum (Ito *et al.*, 1997; Nijenhuis *et al.*, 1999; Si-Hoe *et al.*, 2000; Russell *et al.*, 2003; Christensen *et al.*, 2004), contributing to the cellular toxicity observed in these cases (Ito *et al.*, 1997; Russell *et al.*, 2003).

A further twist has been given to the biology of the Brattleboro rat by the discovery that a limited number of their magnocellular neurones exhibit a heterogenous phenotype, expressing immunoreactivity for a mutated precursor and also for an apparently normal vasopressin gene product. The number of those neurones increases with age, from 0.1% of the total number of vasopressin neurones at birth to 3% in 2-year-old Brattleboro rats (Evans *et al.*, 1994; Evans *et al.*, 2000). This is due to a +1 frameshift in the neurophysin domain that restores the reading frame, but leaves an altered 13–22 residue in the C-terminal of neurophysin. This frameshift, as well as another one due to a GA dinucleotide deletion, can also be found in some magnocellular neurones of wild-type rats (Evans *et al.*, 2000).

3. Control of Vasopressin Secretion

The secretion of vasopressin is mainly regulated by variations in plasma osmolality and blood volume. Additional factors are listed in Table 1.

a) *Control by extracellular osmolality and volaemia*
Because the principal physiological effect of vasopressin is the regulation of distal tubular water reabsorption, the most important control mechanisms for the release of this hormone are associated with changes in plasma osmolality and blood volume (and indirectly pressure). These aspects of control are also considered elsewhere (e.g. in Chapters 6 and 7).

Table 1. Factors regulating vasopressin secretion.

Stimulation	Inhibition
Major physiological changes	
Hyperosmolality	Hypoosmolality
Hypovolemia	Hypervolemia
Hypotension	
Additional factors	
Cerebrospinal fluid sodium increase	Hypothermia
Pain	α-adrenergic agonists
Nausea	GABA
Stress, lactation	Ethanol
Hypoglycaemia	Cortisol
Hyperthermia	Iodothyronines
Ageing	Atrial natriuretic peptide
Drugs	
Nicotine	Apelin
Opiates	Vasopressin
Barbiturates	
Sulfonylureas	
Antineoplastic agents	
Neurosteroids	

GABA, gamma aminobutyric acid.

b) *Additional factors*

i) *Neurotransmitters*

The fine control of the neurohypophysial secretion of vasopressin in the physiological situations described above involves mediation by various local neurotransmitters whose roles are essential. Some of them are listed in Table 2.

Acetylcholine, which is present in the supraoptic and paraventricular nuclei, is the major stimulator of vasopressin release in situations of hyperosmolality.

Hypovolemia and all other causes of stress (e.g. pain, hypoglycaemia) stimulate the release of noradrenaline within the hypothalamic nuclei which has a positive effect on vasopressin release. Hypovolemia also stimulates the generation of renin, and consequently angiotensin II, in the brain. This locally produced angiotensin II enhances the release of vasopressin in addition to stimulating thirst. Conversely, hypervolemia leads to a release of atrial natriuretic peptide (ANP) by the heart which, together with a homologous natriuretic peptide synthesised locally (brain natriuretic peptide, BNP), inhibits vasopressin release (Poole *et al.*, 1987).

Table 2. Effect of various centrally released chemicals on the secretion of vasopressin.

Neurotransmitter	Physiological context	Effect
Acetylcholine	Hyperosmolality	Stimulation
Noradrenaline	Hypovolaemia	Stimulation
Angiotensin II	Hypovolaemia	Stimulation
Noradrenaline	Stressors (e.g. pain, hypoglycaemia)	Stimulation
Dopamine	Nausea, vomiting	Stimulation
Atrial natriuretic peptide	Hypervolaemia	Inhibition
GABA	Local regulation	Inhibition
Vasopressin	Local regulation	Inhibition
Apelin	Local regulation	Inhibition
Chemokine	Local regulation	Inhibition

Dopamine, which is associated with nausea and vomiting, also stimulates vasopressin secretion. Gamma aminobutyric acid (GABA) inhibits the secretion of vasopressin (Saridaki *et al.*, 1989). Various other substances and drugs have also been reported to affect vasopressin release but their physiological significance is obscure (for a review see Carter and Lightman, 1985; Renaud and Bourquet, 1990). The same can be said for a possible effect by neurosteroids (Widmer *et al.*, 2003).

ii) *Vasopressin*

In addition to being released from the neurohypophysis into the bloodstream, vasopressin can also be released from the cell bodies and dendrites of the magnocellular neurones of the supraoptic nucleus (Ludwig, 1998) as discussed in Chapter 11. This central release occurs semi-independently of release from the axon terminals (Ludwig *et al.*, 2002) and is involved in pre- and post-synaptic regulation of electric activity and a negative autocontrol of vasopressin production (Kombian *et al.*, 1997). Vasopressin acts via specific V1a and V1b receptors (Hurbin *et al.*, 1998) to increase intracellular calcium ions (Dayathini *et al.*, 1996). Those paracrine and autocrine influences account for the rhythmic phasic pattern of vasopressin secretion (Brown and Bourque, 2006).

iii) *Apelin*

The possibility that local autoregulation of vasopressin secretion also occurs by locally released peptides has received novel confirmation following the discovery of apelin. Apelin is a peptide that has recently been isolated as the endogenous ligand of the human orphan APJ receptor, a G protein-coupled receptor that shares 31% amino-acid sequence identity with the angiotensin I receptor (O'Dowd *et al.*, 1993; Tatemoto *et al.*, 1998). Apelin naturally occurs in the brain and plasma as 13 and 17 amino acid fragments of a single propeptide precursor. Apelin and its receptor are widely distributed in the brain (Medhurst *et al.*, 2003) and are highly expressed in the supraoptic and paraventricular nuclei, colocalised with vasopressin neurones. Intracerebroventricular injection of apelin inhibits basal or dehydration-induced vasopressin release (Lee *et al.*, 2000; Reaux *et al.*, 2001). Both osmotic stimulation by salt-loading and water deprivation increased APJ receptor mRNA and vasopressin mRNA in magnocellular paraventricular and supraoptic nuclei. Furthermore, the peptide was colocalised with vasopressin in a small population of the vasopressin neurones (O'Carroll and Lolait, 2003). In the lactating rat, when hyperactivity of the vasopressinergic neurones occurs to protect fluid balance when optimal production of milk is required, the central administration of apelin decreases the secretion of vasopressin into the bloodstream and causes a diuresis (De Mota *et al.*,

2004). In addition, new roles have been established for apelin in lowering blood pressure, as a potent cardiac ionotrope, in modulating food and water uptake, in stress activation, and as a novel adipokine that is excreted from fat cells and regulates insulin (Lee *et al.*, 2006). Although vasopressin and apelin are located in the same neurones, a 24-hour dehydration in the rat leads to a hyperactivity of the vasopressinergic neurones, an increase in vasopressin and a decrease in apelin in the plasma (De Mota *et al.*, 2004), with an opposite pattern in the peptide content in the neurones (Reaux-Le Goazigo *et al.*, 2004). The intracellular accumulation of apelin is blocked by a selective V1 antagonist of the vasopressin receptor (Reaux-Le Goazigo *et al.*, 2004), which suggests a precise reciprocal cross-regulation of the two peptides, especially by osmotic stimuli (Azizi *at al.*, 2008; Llorens-Cortes and Moos, 2008; Llorens-Cortes and Kordon, 2008). Interestingly, apelin can also induce diuresis by a complex effect on the pre- and post-glomerular vasculature (Hus-Citharel *et al.*, 2008).

iv) *Chemokine*
Banisadr *et al.* (2003) have shown that the chemokine stromal cell-derived factor-1 (SDF-1+/CXCL12) and its receptor are selectively colocalized with vasopressin-expressing neurones and that SDF-1 could inhibit the vasopressin release by angiotensin or osmotic shock *in vivo* (Callewaere *et al.*, 2006). The level of the SDF-1 protein but not of its mRNA is markedly decreased in Brattleboro rats, in correlation with the amount of vasopressin expression (Callewaere *et al.*, 2008).

4. Extra-hypothalamic Expression of Vasopressin

Although expression of vasopressin is mainly in the hypothalamic neurones, a few extra-hypothalamic tissues do normally express the hormone, in particular the adrenal medulla, the testis, the heart and vasculature (see also Chapter 1). Many references can be found in a review by Murphy *et al.* (1993). Expression of vasopressin in some tumours is also well known and is a major example of the so-called paraneoplastic syndromes (this last aspect will be dealt with in more detail in Chapter 12, which is devoted to pathological aspects).

a) *Adrenal medulla*

Expression of vasopressin in the adrenal medulla was first demonstrated in both wild-type (Ang and Jenkins, 1984) and mutant Brattleboro (Nussey *et al.*, 1984) rats. This has been further confirmed by Perraudin *et al.* (1993) who demonstrated that vasopressin was produced in a discrete population of chromaffin cells of the adrenal medulla, as well as in a few cells within the cortex in humans. Since exogenous vasopressin stimulates the secretion of cortisol via the activation of a V1 receptor, it is suggested that vasopressin may be released together with catecholamines during stress and that it acts as a paracrine factor to locally modulate steroidogenesis, in addition to its well demonstrated action via the central release of adrenocorticotrophic hormone ACTH (see Chapter 8).

b) *Testis*

Vasopressin has been demontrated in the testis (Nicholson *et al.*, 1984; Kasson *et al.*, 1985). It has also been identified in the testis of the Brattleboro rat (Kasson and Hsueh, 1986), suggesting that the production of hypothalamic and peripheral vasopressin may involve different pathways. Immunoreactive vasopressin has been detected in the interstitial fluid of adult rat testis and its level decreases when spermatogenesis is disrupted (Porantz *et al.*, 1988). Northern blotting of the mRNA of rat testis with a specific vasopressin probe has detected a shorter message than that found in the hypothalamus, lacking in particular exon I, which encodes the vasopressin nonapeptide (Lefebvre and Zingg, 1991). No function could be found for this testicular vasopressin-like RNA (Foo *et al.*, 1991). Furthermore, a testis-specific promoter for the rat vasopressin gene has been described which allows for the transcription of a longer mRNA yet it is unable to function as a protein template (Foo *et al.*, 1994). Nevertheless, hypothalamic-like vasopressin mRNA has also been detected by a highly sensitive polymerase chain reaction (PCR) technique in the rat testis (Foo *et al.*, 1991), as well as in mouse Leydig cells (Tahri-Joutei and Pointis, 1989), where it is probably translated into normal vasopressin. Neither normal vasopressin nor the aberrant vasopressin gene products have been detected in the human or baboon testis (Ivell *et al.*, 1990). The function of the aberrant testicular vasopressin gene-derived transcripts is unknown (Gnessi *et al.*, 1997).

c) *Blood vessels and heart*

The presence of immunoreactive vasopressin has been reported in various blood vessels of several animal species (Lincoln *et al.*, 1990; Loesch *et al.*, 1991; Simon *et al.*, 1992) and this has been further confirmed by the identification of vasopressin mRNA in rat aorta (Simon and Kasson, 1995). There is also evidence for a vasopressin system in the rat heart (Hupf *et al.*, 1999). These authors have identified *de novo* synthesis of vasopressin in the heart as well as its release in the cardiac effluent. They have also shown that this synthesis is stimulated by stress such as cardiac overload, or nitric oxide (NO) synthesis, and occurs in concentrations sufficient to cause local as well as potentially systemic effects. Furthermore, the release of copeptin, the inactive fragment of the vasopressin presursor, has been shown to be an excellent predictor of outcome in advanced heart failure patients (Stoiser *et al.*, 2006). Interestingly, and conversely, vasopressin increases NO synthesis in cytokine-stimulated rat cardiac myocytes (Yamamoto *et al.*, 1997).

d) *Other organs*

Vasopressin is present in significant quantities in the ovaries of rats, cows and humans (Wathes *et al.*, 1982; Wathes *et al.*, 1983), in the ovary of the Brattleboro rat (Lim *et al.*, 1984), and is synthesized by isolated bovine ovarian cells (Swann *et al.*, 1984). Other organs where vasopressin can be found include the uterus (Ciarochi *et al.*, 1985), the thymus (Markwick *et al.*, 1986) and the pancreas (Amico *et al.*, 1988).

5. Peripheral Degradation and Metabolic Clearance

Vasopressin is present in the circulation at an average level of 1–2 pg/ml, a concentration that can increase more than 3- to 5-fold during water deprivation, and much more in response to stress such as hemorrhage, pain or nausea (Gines *et al.*, 1994). Vasopressin is not bound to plasma proteins but is present in platelets. Its concentration in platelet-rich plasma is 5-fold higher than in platelet-depleted plasma (Bichet *et al.*, 1987). Neurophysin II is also present in plasma and its level follows that of vasopressin. One can also find the C-terminal glycoprotein copeptin but these latter two polypeptides have no known functional role in peripheral tissues. However, copeptin is a reliable marker of vasopressin secretion (Szinnai *et al.*, 2007), correlating with the stress level (Katan *et al.*, 2008), and is elevated in critically ill patients (Jochberger *et al.*, 2006) including those with acute myocardial infarction (Khan *et al.*, 2007), hemorrhagic and septic shock (Morgenthaler *et al.*, 2007) or chronic heart failure (Neuhold *et al.*, 2008). It is a good surrogate marker for vasopressin (Morgenthaler *et al.*, 2008).

Vasopressin is degraded by several endothelial and circulating endo- and amino-peptidases and the plasma (chemical) half-life of vasopressin, like that of most peptide hormones, is quite short, being of the order of 5–15 minutes, the biological half-life being a little longer. The metabolic clearance of vasopressin is dependant on hepatic and renal blood fluxes. It increases with the plasma level and reaches 600 ml/min at a plasma concentration of 10 pg/ml in humans. The urinary clearance is about 5% of the total clearance, and the urinary excretion rate, at about 1 mg/day, is a good index of vasopressin secretion. Interestingly, vasopressin is a physiological substrate for the insulin-regulated aminopeptidase (IRAP) as its plasma level is increased two-fold in IRAP −/− mice (Wallis *et al.*, 2007).

Pregnancy is a specific physiological instance when the existence of a vasopressinase expressed at the maternal side of the placenta is responsible for very high circulating vasopressinase activity (Durr *et al.*, 1987). This vasopressinase activity increases as a function of the placental mass, and at the end of pregnancy may reveal a previously unknown, asymptomatic, pre-existing nephrogenic or central diabetes insipidus (Davidson *et al.*, 1993). In such cases, the vasopressin secretion cannot adapt to the increased metabolic clearance and a polyuricpolydypsic syndrome can appear at the end of pregnancy, especially in the case of multiple pregnancies. These polyuric states can be treated by the V2 receptor agonist desamino 8D-arginine vasopressin (DDAVP), which is resistant to the action of vasopressinase while vasopressin itself, which is rapidly degraded, is inactive (Davidson *et al.*, 1993).

Bibliography

Acampora D., Postiglione M.P., Avantaggiato V., Di Bonito M., Vaccarino F.M., Michaud J., Simeone A. (1999). Progressive impairment of developing neuroendocrine cell lineages in the hypothalamus of mice lacking the Orthopedia gene. *Genes Dev* 13: 2787–2800

Adan R.A., Burbach J.P (1992). Regulation of the vasopressin and oxytocin gene expression by estrogen and thyroid hormone. *Prog Brain Res* 92: 127–136

Amico J.A., Finn F.M., Haldar J. (1988). Oxytocin and vasopressin are present in human and rat pancreas. *Am J Med Sci* 296: 303–307

Ang V.T., Jenkins J.S. (1984). Neurohypophysial hormones in the adrenal medulla. *J Clin Endocrinol Metab* 58: 688–691

Azizi M., Iturrioz X., Blanchard A., Peyrard S., De Mota N., Chartrel N., Vaudry H., Corvol P., Llorens-Cortes C. (2008). *Am J Soc Nephrol* 19: 1015–1024

Banisadr G., Skrzydelski D., Kitabgi P., Rostene W., Parsadanaintz S.M. (2003). Highly regionalized distribution of stromal cell-derived factor-1/CXCL12 in adult rat brain: constitutive expression of cholinergic, dopaminergic and vasopressinergic neurons. *Eur J Neurosci* 18: 1593–1606

Berghorn K.A., Knapp L.T., Hoffman G.E., Sherman T.G. (1995). Induction of the glucocorticoid receptor in hypothalamic magnocellular neurons during chronic hypoosmolarity. *Endocrinology* 136: 804–807

Bichet D.G., Arthus M.F., Barjon J.N., Lonergan M., Kortas C. (1987). Human platelet fraction arginine-vasopressin. Potential physiological role. *J Clin Invest* 79: 881–887

Breslow E. (1979). Chemistry and biology of the neurophysins. *Ann Rev Biochem* 48: 251–274

Breslow E. (1993). Structure and folding properties of endophysin and its peptide complexes: biological implications. *Regul Peptides* 45: 15–19

Brown C.H., Bourque C.W. (2006). Mechanisms of rhythmogenesis: insights from hythalamic vasopressin neurons. *Trends Neurosci* 29: 108–115

Burbach J.P, Luckman S.M., Murphy D., Gainer H. (2001). Gene regulation in the magnocellular hypothalamo-neurohypophysial system. *Physiol Rev* 81: 1197–1267

Burke Z.D., Ho M.Y., Morgan H., Smith M., Murphy D., Carter D.A. (1997). Repression of vasopressin gene expression by glucocorticoids in transgenic mice: evidence of a direct mechanism mediated by proximal 5′ sequence. *Neuroscience* 78: 1177–1185

Burman S., Wellner D., Chait B., Chaudhary T., Breslow E. (1989). Complete assignment of neurophysin disulfides indicates pairing in two separates domains. *Proc Nat Acad Sci USA* 86: 439–433

Callewaere C., Banisadr G., Desarmenien M.G., Mechighel P., Kitabgi P., Rostene W.H., Melik Parsadaniantz S. (2006). The chemokine SDF-1/CXCL12 modulates the firing pattern of vasopressin neurons and counteracts induced vasopressin release through CXCR4. *Proc Nat Acad Sci USA* 103: 8221–8226

Callewaere C., Fernette B., Raison D., Mechighel P., Burlet A., Calas A., Kitabgi P., Melik Parsadaniantz S., Rostenbe W. (2008). Cellular and subcellular evidence for neuronal interaction between the chemokine stromal cell-derived factor-1/CXCL12 and vasopressin: regulation in the hypothalamo-neurohypophysial system of Brattleboro rats. *Endocrinology* 149: 310–319

Capra J.D., Kehoe J.M., Kotelchuck D., Walter R., Breslow E. (1972). Evolution of neurophysin proteins: the partial sequence of bovine neurophysin 1. *Proc Nat Acad Sci* 69: 431–434

Carrazana E.J., Pasieka K.B., Majzoub J.A. (1988). The vasopressin poly (A) tail is unusually long and increases during stimulation of vasopressin gene expression *in vivo. Mol Cell Biol* 8: 2267–2274

Carter D.A., Lightman S.L. (1985). Neuroendocrine control of AVP secretion. In Baylis P.H. and Padfield P.L. (eds): *The posterior pituitary: hormone secretion in health and disease*. pp. 53–118 Marcel Dekker, New York

Carter D.A., Murphy D. (1991). Rapid changes in poly(A) tail length of vasopressin and oxytocin mRNAs form a common early component of neurohypophysial peptide gene activation following physiological stimulation. *Neuroendocrinology* 53: 1–6

Chen L., Rose J.P., Breslow E., Yang D., Chang W.R., Fury W.F., Sax J.M., Wang B.C. (1991). Crystal structure of a bovine neurophysin II dipeptide complex at 2.8 A determined from the single-wavelength anomalous scattering signal of an incorporated iodine atom. *Proc Nat Acad Sci USA* 88: 4240–4244

Chevaleyre V., Dayanithi G., Moos F.C., Desarmenien M.G. (2000). Developmental regulation of local positive autocontrol of supraoptic neurons. *J Neurosci* 20: 5813–5819

Chevaleyre V., Moos F.C., Desarmenien M.G. (2002). Interplay between presynaptic and postsynaptic activities is required for dendritic plasticity and synaptogenesis in the supraoptic nucleus. *J Neurosci* 22: 265–273

Christensen J.H., Siggaard C., Corydon T.J., Robertson G.L., Niels G., Bolund L., Rittig S. (2004). Differential cellular handling of defective arginine vasopressin prohormones in cells expressing mutations of the AVP gene associated with autosomal dominant and recessive familial neurohypophyseal diabetes insipidus. *J Clin Endocrin Metab* 89: 4521–4531

Ciarochi F.F., Robinson A.G., Verbalis J.G., Seif S.M., Zimmermann E.A. (1985). Isolation and localization of neurophysin-like proteins in rat uterus. *Peptides* 6: 903–911

Davidson J.M., Sheills E.A., Philip P.R., Baron W.M., Lindheimer M.D. (1993). Metabolic clearance of vasopressin and an analog resistant to vasopressinase in human pregnancy. *Am J Physiol* 264: 121–129

Dayathini G., Widmer H., Richard P. (1996). Vasopressin–induced Ca^{2+} increase in isolated supraoptic cells. *J Physiol* 490: 713–727

De Bree F.M. (2000). Trafficking of the vasopressin and oxytocin prohormone through the regulated secretory pathways. *J Neuroendocrinol* 12: 589–594

De Bree F.M., Knight D., Howell L., Murphy D. (2000). Sorting of the vasopressin prohormone into the regulatory secretory pathway. *FEBS Lett* 475: 175–180

De Mota N., Reaux-Le Goazigo A., El Messari S., Chartrel N., Roesch D., Dujardin C., Kordon C., Vaudry H., Moos F., Llorens-Cortes C. (2004). Apelin, a potent diuretic neuropeptide counteracting vasopressin actions through inhibition of vasopressin neuron activity and vasopressin release. *Proc Nat Acad Sci* 101: 10464–10469

Durr J., Hoggard J., Hunt J., Schrier R. (1987). Diabetes insipidus in pregnancy associated with abnormally high circulating vaspressinase activity. *New Engl J Med* 316: 1070–1074

Evans D.A.P, van der Klej A.A.M., Sonnemans M.A., Burbach P.H., van Leewen F.W. (1994). Frameshift mutations at two hotspots in vasopressin transcripts in post-mitotic neurons. *Proc Nat Acad Sci* 91: 6059–6063

Evans D.A., De Bree F.M., Nijenhuis M., van der Klej A.A., Zalm R., Korteweg N., Van Leewen F.W., Burbach J.P. (2000). Processing of frameshifted vasopressin precursors. *J Neuroendocrinol* 121: 685–693

Fields R.L., House S.B., Gainer H. (2003). Regulatory domains in the intergenic region of the oxytocin and vasopressin genes that controls their hypothalmaus-specific expression. *J Neurosci* 23: 7801–7809

Foo N.C., Carter D., Murphy D., Ivell R. (1991). Vasopressin and oxytocin gene expression in rat testis. *Endocrinology* 128: 2110–2117

Foo N.C., Funkhouser J.M., Carter D.A., Murphy D. (1994). A testis-specific promoter in the rat vasopressin gene. *J Biol Chem* 269: 659–667

Gimpl G., Fahrenholz F. (2001). The oxytocin receptor system: structure, function and regulation. *Physiol Rev* 81: 629–683

Gines P., Abraham W., Schrier R. (1994). Vasopressin in pathological states. *Semin Nephrol* 4: 384–397

Ginsburg M., Ireland M. (1966). The role of neurophysin in the transport and release of neurophysial hormones. *J Endocrinol* 35: 289–298

Gnessi L., Fabbri A., Spera G. (1997). Gonadal peptides as mediators of development and functional control of the testis: an integrated system with hormones and local environment. *Endocrin Rev* 18 541–609

Guldenaar S.E.F., Pickering B.D. (1988). Mutant vasopressin precursor in the endoplasmic reticulum of the Brattleboro rat: ultrastructural evidence from individual vasopressin cells localized with the light microscope by use of a new gold/silver method for new immunostain enhancement. *Cell Tissue Es* 253: 671–677

Hupf H., Grimm D., Riegger G.A., Schunkert H. (1999). Evidence for a vasopressin system in the rat heart. *Circulation* 19: 365–370

Hurbin A., Boissin-Agasse L., Orcel H., Rabié A., Joux N., Desarmenien M.G., Richard P., Moos F.C. (1998). The V1a and V1b, but not V2, vasopressin receptor genes are expressed in the supraoptic nucleus of the rat hypothalamus, and the transcripts are essentially colocalized in the vasopressinergic magnocellular neurons. *Endocrinology* 139: 4701–4707

Hus-Citharel A., Bouby N., Frugiere A., Bodineau L., Gasc J.M., Llorens-Cortes C. (2008). Effect of apelin on glomerular hemodynamic function in the rat kidney. *Kidney Int* 74: 486–494

Ito M., Jameson J.L., Ito M. (1997). Molecular basis of autosomal dominant neurophyseal diabetes insipidus: cellular toxicity caused by the accumulation of mutant vasopressin precursors within the endoplasmic reticulum. *J Clin Invest* 99: 1897–1905

Ivell R., Reichter D. (1984). Structure and comparison of the oxytocin and vasopressin genes from rat. *Proc Nat Acad Sci USA* 81: 2006–2010

Ivell R., Schmale H., Krisch B., Nahke P., Richter D. (1986). Expression of a mutant vasopressin gene: differential polyadenylation and read-through of the mRNA 3′ end in a frame-shift mutant. *Eur Mol Biol Organ J* 5: 971–977

Ivell R., Furuya K., Brackmann B., Dawood Y., Khan-Dawood F. (1990). Expression of the oxytocin and vasopressin genes in human and baboon gonadal tissues. *Endocrinology* 127: 2990–2996

Iwasaki Y., Oiso Y., Saito H., Majzoub J.A. (1997). Positive and negative regulation of the rat vasopressin gene promoter. *Endocrinology* 138: 5266–5274

Jochberger S., Morgenthaler N.G., Mayr V.D., Luckner G., Wenzel V., Ulmer H., Schwarz S., Hasibeder W.R., Friesennecker B.E., Dünser M.W. (2006). Copeptin and arginine vasopressin concentrations in critically ill patients. *J Clin Endocrinol Metab* 91: 4381–4386

Lee D.K., Cheng R., Nguyen T., Fan T., Kariyawasan A.P., Liu Y., Osmons D.H., George S.R., O'Dowd B.F. (2000). Characterization of apelin, the ligand for the APJ receptor. *J Neurochem* 74: 34–41

Kahn S.Q, Dhillon O.S, O'Brien R.J., Struck J., Quinn, Morgenthaler N.G., Squire I.B., Davies J.E., Bergmann A., Ng L.L. (2007). C-terminal provasopressin (copeptin) as a novel and prognostic marker in acute myocardial infarction. Leicester Acute Mayocardial Infarction Peptide (LAMP) study. *Circulation* 115: 2103–2110

Kasson B.G, Meidan R., Hsueh A.J.W. (1985). Identification and characterization of arginine vasopressin like substances in the rat testis. *J Biol Chem* 260: 5303–5307

Kasson B.G., Hsueh A.J.W. (1986). Arginine vasopressin as an intragonadal hormone in Brattleboro rats: presence of a testicular vasopressin–like peptide and functional vasopressin receptors. *Endocrinology* 118: 23–31

Katan M., Morgenthaler N., Widmer I., Puder J.J., Konig C., Muller B., Christ-Crain M. (2008). Copeptin, a stable peptide derived from the vasopressin precursor, coorelmates with the individual stress level. *Neuro Endocrinol Lett* 29: 341–346

Kim J.K., Summer S.N., Wood W.M., Brown J.L., Schrier R.W. (1997). Arginine vasopressin secretion with mutants of wild-type and Brattleboro rats AVP gene. *J Am Soc Nephrol* 8: 1863–1869

Kim J.K., Soubrier F., Michel J.B., Bankir L., Corvol P., Schrier R.W. (1990). AVP gene regulation in the homozygous Brattleboro rat. *J Clin Invest* 86: 14–16

Kombian S.B., Mouginot D., Pittman Q.J. (1997). Dendritic released peptides act as retrograde modulators of afferent excitation in the supraoptic nucleus *in vitro*. *Neuron* 19: 903–912

Krisch B., Nahle P., Richter D(1986). Immunocytochemical staining of supraoptic neurons from homozygous Brattleboro rats by use of antibodies agoinst two domains of the mutated vasopressin precursor. *Cell Tissue Res* 244: 351–354

Kuwahara S., Arima H., Banno R., Sata I., Kondo N., Oiso Y. (2003). Regulation of vasopressin gene expression by cAMP and glucocorticoids in parvocellular neurons of the paraventricular nucleus in rat hypothalamic organotypic cultures. *J Neurosci* 23: 10231–10237

Lefebvre D.L., Zingg H.H. (1991). Novel vasopressin gene-related transcripts in rat testis. *Mol Endocrinol* 5: 645–652

Lee D.K., George S.R., O'Dowd B.F. (2006). Unravelling the roles of the apelin system: prospective therapeutic applications in heart failure and obesity. *Trends Pharmacol Sci* 27: 190–194

Lim A.T.W., Lolait S.J., Barlow J.W., Autelitano D.J., Toh B.H., Boublik J., Abraham J., Johnson C.I., Funder J.W. (1984). Immunoreactive arginine vasopressin in Brattleboro rat ovary. *Nature* 310: 61–64

Lincoln J., Loesch A., Burnstock G. (1990). Localization of vasopressin, serotonin and angiotensin II in endothelial cells of the renal and mesenteric arteries of the rat. *Cell. Tissue Res* 259: 341–344

Llorens-Cortes C., Moos F. (2008). Opposite effects of hypothalamic coexpressed neuropeptides, apelin and vasopressin in maintaining body-fluid homeostasis. *Prog Brain Res* 170: 559–570

Llorens-Cortes C., Kordon C. (2008). The neuroendocrine view of the angiotensin and apelin systems. *J Neuroendocrinol* 20: 279–289

Loesch A., Bodin P., Burnstock G. (1991). Colocalization of endothelin, vasopressin and serotonin in cultured endothelial cells of rabbit aorta. *Peptides* 12: 1095–1103

Ludwig M. (1998). Dendritic release of vasopressin and oxytocin. *Neuroendocrinology* 10: 881–889

Ludwig M., Sabatier N., Bull P.M., Landgraf R., Dayanithi G., Leng G. (2002). Intracellular calcium stores regulate activity-dependent neuropeptides release from dendrites. *Nature* 418: 85–89

Marwick A.J., Lolait S.J., Funder J.W. (1986). Immunoreactive arginine vasopressin in the rat thymus. *Endocrinology* 119: 1690–1696

Medhurst A.D., Jennings C.A., Robbins M.J., Davis R.P., Ellis C., Winborn K.Y., Lawrie K.W.M., Hervieu G., Riley G., Bolaky J.E., Herrity N.C., Murdock P., Darkers J.G. (2003). Pharmacological and immunohistochemical characterization of the APJ receptor and its endogenous ligand apelin. *J Neurochem* 84: 1162–1172

Morgenthaler N.G., Muller B., Struck J., Bergmann A., Redl H., Christ-Crain M. (2007). Copeptin, a stable peptide of the arginine vasopressin precursor, is elevated in hemorrhagic and septic shock. *Shock* 28: 219–226

Morgenthaler N.G., Struck J., Jochberber S., Dunser M.W. (2008). Copeptin: clinical use of a new biomarker. *Trends Endocrin Metab* 19: 43–49

Murgatroyd C., Wigger A., Frank E., Singlewald N., Bunck M., Holsboer F., Landgraf R., Spengler D. (2004). Impaired repression at a vasopressin promoter polymorphism underlies overexpression of vasopressin in a rat model of trait anxiety. *J Neurosci* 24: 7762–7770

Murphy D., Carter D.A. (1990). Vasopressin gene expression in the rodent hypothalamus: transcriptional and post-transcriptional responses to physiological stimulation. *Mol Endocrinol* 4: 1051–1059

Murphy D., Funkhouser J., Ang H.L., Foo N.C., Carter D. (1993). Extrahypothalamic expression of the vasopressin and oxytocin genes. *Ann NY Acad Sci* 689: 91–106

Murphy D., Si-Hoe S.L., Brenner S., Venkatesh B. (1998). Something fishy in the rat brain: molecular genetics of the hypothalamo-hypophysial system. *Bioessays* 20: 741–749

Nicholson H.D., Swann R.W., Burford G.D., Wathes D.C., Porter D.G., Pickering B. (1984). Identification of oxytocin and vasopressin in the testis, in adrenal tissue. Regul Peptides 8: 141–146

Nijenhuis M., Zahm R., Burbach J.P.H. (1999). Mutations in the vasopressin prohormone involved in diabetes insipidus impair endoplasmic reticulum export but not sorting. *J Biol Chem* 274: 21200–21208

Nussey S., Ang V.T.Y., Jenkins J.S., Chowdrey H.S., Bisset G.W. (1984). Brattleboro rat adrenal contains vasopressin. *Nature* 310: 64–66

O'Carroll A-M., Lolait S.J. (2003). Regulation of rat APJ receptor messenger ribonucleic acid expression in magnocellular neurones of the paraventricular and supraoptic nuclei by osmotic stimuli. *J Neuroendocrinol* 15: 661–666

O'Dowd B.F., Heiber M., Chan A., Heng H.H., Tsui L.C., Kennedy J.L., Shi X., Petronis A., George S.R., Nguyen T. (1993). A human gene that shows identity with the gene encoding the angiotensin receptor is located on chromosome 11. *Gene* 136: 355–360

Pardy K., Adan R.A., Carter D.A., Seah V., Burbach J.P., Murphy D. (1992). The identification of a cis-acting element involved in the cyclic AMP regulation of the bovine vasopressin gene expression. *J Biol Chem* 267: 21746–21752

Perraudin V., Delarue C., Lefebvre H., Contesse V., Kuhn J.M., Vaudry H. (1993). Vasopressin stimulates cortisol secretion from human adrenocortical tissue through activation of V1 receptors. *J Clin Endocrinol Metab* 76: 1522–1528

Pomerantz D.K., Jansz G.F., Wilson N. (1988). Disruption of spermatogenesis is associated with decreased concentration of immunoreactive arginine vasopressin in testicular fluid. *Biol Reprod* 39: 610–616

Poole C.J., Carter D.A., Vallejo M., Lightman S.L. (1987). Atrial natriuretic factor inhibits the stimulated *in vivo* and *in vitro* release of vasopressin and oxytocin in the rat. *J Endocrinol* 112: 97–102

Reaux A., De Mota N., Skultetyova I., Lenkei Z., El Messari S., Gallatz K., Corvol P. Palkovits M., Llorens-Cortes C. (2001). Physiological role of a novel neuropeptide, apelin, and its receptor in the rat brain. *J Neurochem* 77: 1085–1096

Reaux A., Le Goazigo A., Morinville A., Burlet A., Llorens-Cortes C., Beaudet A. (2004). Dehydratation-induced cross-regulation of apelin and vasopressin immunoreactivity levels in magnocellular hypothalamic neurons. *Endocrinology* 145: 4392–4400

Renaud L.P., Bourquet B.W. (1990). Neurophysiology and neuropharmacology of hypothalamic magnocellular neurons secreting vasopressin and oxytocin. *Prog Neurobiology* 36: 131–169

Repaske D.R., Summar M.L., Krishnamani M.R.S., Gültekin E.K., Arriazu M.C., Roubicek M.E., Blanco M., Isaac G.B., Phillips III J.A. (1996). Recurrent mutations in vasopressin-neuropohysin II gene cause autosomal dominant neurohypophyseal diabetes insipidus. *J Clin. Endocrin Metab* 81: 2328–2334

Rose J.K., Doms R.W. (1988). Regulation of protein export from the endoplasmic reticulum. *Ann Rev Cell Biol* 4: 257–288

Russell J.T., Brownstein M.J., Gainer H. (1980). Biosynthesis of vasopressin, oxytocin and neurophysins: isolation of two common precursors (propressophysin ands prooxyphysin). *Endocrinology* 107: 1880–1891

Russell T.A., Ito M., Yu R.N., Martison F.A., Weiss J., Jameson J.L. (2003). A murine model of autosomal dominant neurohypophyseal diabetes insipidus reveals progressive loss of vasopressin-producing neurons. *J Clin Invest* 112: 1697–1706

Saridaki E., Carter D.A., Lightman S.L. (1989). Ggamma Aminobutyric acid regulation of neurohypophysial hormone secretion in male and female rats. *J Endocrinol* 121: 343–349

Schmale H., Richter D. (1984). Single base deletion in the vasopressin gene is the cause of diabetes insipidus in Brattleboro rats. *Nature* 308: 705–709

Schmale H., Ivell R., Briendl M., Darner R., Richter D. (1984). The mutant vasopressin gene from diabetes insipidus (Brattleboro) rats is transcribed but the message is not efficiently translated. *EMBO J* 2: 3289–3293

Schmale H., Borowiak B, Holtgreve-Grez H., Richter D. (1989). Impact of altered protein structures on the intracellular traffic of a mutated vasopressin precursor from Brattleboro rats. *Eur J Biochem* 182: 621–627

Schmitz E., Mohr E., Richter D(1991). Rat vasopressin and oxytocin genes are linked by long interspersed repeated DNA elements (LINE): sequence and transcriptional analysis of LINE. *DNA Cell Biol* 10: 81–91

Si-Hoe S.L., de Bree F.M., Nijenhuis M., Davies J.E., Howell L.M.C., Tinley H., Waller S.J., Zeng Q., Zalm R., Sonnemans M., Van Leewen F.W., Burbach J.P.H., Murphy D. (2000). Endoplasmic reticulum derangement in hypothalamic neurons of rats expressing a familial neurohypophyseal diabetes insipidus mutant vasopressin transgene. *FASEB J* 14: 1680–1684

Si-Hoe S.L., Carter D., Murphy D. (2001). Species- and tissue-specific physiological regulation of vasopressin mRNA poly (A) tail length. *Physiol Genomics* 5: 1–9

Simon J.S., Brody M.J., Kasson B.G. (1992). Characterization of a vasopressin-like peptide in rat and bovine blood vessels. *Am J Physiol* 262: H799–H804

Simon J., Kasson B.G. (1995). Identification of vasopressin mRNA in rat aorta. *Hypertension* 25: 1030–1033

Stoiser B., Mortl D., Hulsmann M., Berger R., Struck J., Morgenthaler N.G., Bergmann A., Pacher R. (2006). Copeptin, a fragment of the vasopressin precursor, as a novel predictor of outcome in heart failure. *Eur J Clin Invest* 36: 771–778

Swann R.W., O'Shaughnessy P.J., Birkett S.D., Wathes D.C., Porter D.G., Pickering B.T. (1984). Biosynthesis of oxytocin in the corpus luteum. *FEBS Lett* 174: 262–268

Szinnai G., Morgenthaler N.G., Berneis K., Struck J., Muller B., Keller U., Christ-Crain M. (2007). Changes in the plasma copeptin, the C-terminal portion of arginine vasopressin during water deprivation and excess in healthy subjects. *J Clin Endocrinol Metab* 92: 3973–3978

Tahri-Joutei A., Pointis G. (1989). Developmental changes in vasopressin receptors and testosterone stimulation in Leydig cells. *Endocrinology* 125: 605–611

Tatemoto K., Hosoya M. , Habata Y., Fujii R., Kakegawa T., Zou M.X., Kawamata Y., Fukusumi S., Hinuma S., Kitada C., Kurokawa T., Onda H., Fijuno M. (1998). Isolation and characterization of a novel endogenous peptide ligand for the human APJ receptor. *Biochem Biophys Res Comm* 251: 471–476

Valtin H., Schroeder H.A. (1964). Familial hypothalamic diabetes insipidus in rats (Brattleboro strain). *Am J Physiol* 206: 425–430

Venkatesh B., Si-Hoe S.L., Murphy D., Brenner S. (1997). Transgenic rats reveal functional conservation of regulatory controls between Fugu isotocin and rat oxytocin genes. *Proc Nat Acad Sci* 94: 12462–12466

Verbeeck M.A., Adan R.A., Burbach J.P. (1990). Vasopressin gene expression is stimulated by cyclic AMP in homologous and heterologous expression systems. *FEBS Lett* 272: 89–93

Wallis M.G., Lankford M.F., Keller S.R. (2007). Vasopressin is a physiological substrate for the insulin-regulated aminopeptidase IRAP. *Am J Physiol* 293: 1092–1012

Walter P., Blobel G. (1981). Translocation of proteins across the endoplasmic reticulum. *J Cell Biol* 91: 545–550

Wathes D.C., Swann R.W., Pickering B.T., Porter D.G., Hull M.G.R., Drife J.O. (1982). Neurohypophyseal hormones in the human ovary. *Lancet* 2: 410–412

Wathes D.C., Swann R.W., Birkett S.D., Porter D.G., Pickering B.T. (1983). Characterization of oxytocin, vasopressin and neurophysin from bovine corpus luteum. *Endocrinology* 113: 693–698

Widmer H., Ludwig M., Bancel F., Leng G., Dayanithi G. (2003). Neurosteroid regulation of oxytocin and vasopressin release from the rat suproptic nucleus. *J Physiol* 548: 233–244

Yamamoto K., Ikeda U., Okada K., Kawahara Y., Okuda M., Yokoyama M., Shimada K. (1997). Arginine vasopressin increases nitric oxide synthesis in cytokine-stimulated rat cardiac myocytes. *Hypertension* 30: 1112–1120

Yoshida M., Iwasaki Y., Asai M., Takayasu S., Taguchi T., Itoi K., Hashimoto K., Oiso Y. 2006), Identification of a functional AP1 element in the rat vasopressin gene promoter. *Endocrinology* 147: 2850–2863

CHAPTER 4

VASOPRESSIN RECEPTORS, THE SIGNALLING CASCADE AND MECHANISMS OF ACTION

Jacques Hanoune

Institut Cochin, 22 Rue Méchain, 75014 Paris, France
Email: jacques.hanoune@inserm.fr

1. Introduction: A Short Historical Survey of Vasopressin Receptors

In 1895, the publication of a three-page article by Oliver and Schäfer on the pressor action of beef pituitary extract opened a century of research and discoveries, including that of its antidiuretic activity (von den Velden, 1913), which fundamentally changed our vision of renal physiology. One had to wait until much later to know the chemical structure of the hormones (Du Vigneaud *et al.*, 1953) and to start having access to labelled compounds that could identify and characterize their binding sites.

In 1959, Fong and colleagues obtained a randomly labelled hormone with a specific activity of 0.2–0.3 Ci/mM by exposing Lys-vasopressin to tritium gas under an electrical discharge (Fong *et al.*, 1959). They demonstrated that, following its administration to a rat, covalently bound radioactivity could be recovered from kidney particulate fractions. The following year, Schwartz *et al.* (1960) showed that tritiated Arg-vasopressin could bind to toad bladder and hypothesized that fixation of the hormone, and also its biological activity, depended on the formation of a hormone-plasma membrane covalent disulphide bridge, and that this site of physical interaction was also the site involved in its stimulation of transmembrane water transport. This elegant, but incorrect, hypothesis constituted an early attempt to define the interaction of a hormone and its receptor in a physiological context. However, it was subsequently discarded by the same authors (Schwartz and Rudinger, 1964) who demonstrated that a vasopressin analogue lacking a disulphide bridge, and therefore unable to establish a covalent binding with the cysteine residues of the membrane, was still able to increase toad bladder permeability to water.

In the early sixties, Orloff and Handler (1962) provided definite evidence for the implication of cyclic AMP as the second messenger in the action of vasopressin on the toad urinary bladder, thus fulfilling the criteria put forward by Earl Sutherland for such a mechanism (Sutherland and Robison, 1966). The presence of an adenyl cyclase sensitive to vasopressin in mammalian kidney was demonstrated the following year (Brown et al., 1963). It then took about ten years to demonstrate that most effects of vasopressin on organs other than the kidney were due to mechanisms independent of cyclic AMP (Hems and Whitton, 1973). In 1979, the hepatic effect of vasopressin was shown to be due to stimulation of phosphatidylinositol breakdown and the now established classification of the vasopressin receptors in two classes was proposed: V_1, acting through a rise of intracellular calcium and phosphatidylinositol breakdown, and V_2, acting through an increase of cyclic AMP (Mitchell et al., 1979).

At the same time, the production of labelled high specific activity vasopressin resulted in the definitive characterization of the vasopressin receptors. This was achieved in 1972 for ^{3}H Tyr^2-lysine-vasopressin (Pradelles et al., 1972) using a protocol whereby iodination of a tyrosyl residue was followed by the catalytic substitution of the iodine by tritium, the peptide being extensively purified by affinity chromatography on a sepharose-neurophysin column. This technique resulted in the achievement of obtaining a specific activity of the order of 10 Ci/mM. Tritiated Arg-vasopressin was obtained in 1977 (Flouret et al., 1977).

There are three different vasopressin receptor subtypes. In humans, the V1a (V1aR) receptor gene is located on chromosome 12q14-15, the V1bR gene on 1q32 and the V2R gene is located in the short arm of the X chromosome at Xq28 (Lolait et al., 1992; van den Ouweland et al.,

1992). In rats the three gene locations are 7q21, 13q13 and Xq37 respectively. The recent and very rapid progress in the field of molecular biology has allowed the complete elucidation of the structure of the vasopressin receptors: V1a in the rat (Morel *et al.*, 1992) and man (Thibonnier *et al.*, 1994); V1b (or V3) in the rat (Saito *et al.*, 1995) and in man (Sugimoto *et al.*, 1994; de Keyzer *et al.*, 1994); and V2 in rat (Morel *et al.*, 1993) and in man (Birnbaumer *et al.*, 1992). More recently, molecular modelling has been very useful for exploring the interaction sites of the vasopressin receptors with their ligands (Moulliac *et al.*, 1995). The most recent progress in the vasopressin field has been the development of various type-specific agonists and mainly antagonists for both V1 and V2 receptors (Serradeil-Le Gal *et al.*, 1993; Serradeil-Le Gal *et al.*, 1996). For a more detailed survey of the recent history of vasopressin receptor research, the reader is referred to the review by Jard (1998).

The bibliography dealing with vasopressin receptors probably amounts to several thousand publications. Obviously, we will not attempt to be exhaustive in that respect, and we will refer as much as possible to previous reviews when available or when the topic is now well known. Therefore, in the rest of the chapter we will cite mainly the most recent relevant findings.

2. Pharmacological Characterization of the Vasopressin Receptors

We will not detail all the various, now classical, binding experiments of the seventies using high specific activity tritiated ligands that resulted in the pharmacological characterisation of the receptors. The reader is referred to the original paper from Jard's group (Bockaert *et al.*, 1973) and to reviews by Jard (1983; 1998). We will simply recall that identification of "real" receptors is based on the universal criteria of saturability, reversibility and pharmacological specificity of ligand binding, and a tight correlation with a downstream physiological event such as enzyme activation or the production of a second messenger. The most important findings derived from these studies, which mainly dealt with the kidney and therefore with the V2 receptor, can be summarized as follows:

1. There is an important receptor reserve. The measured dissociation constant for vasopressin binding to its renal receptors is in the nanomolar range, far higher than the circulating vasopressin level (in the picomolar range), indicating the existence of a marked amplification between the primary signal and the antidiuretic response. This large receptor reserve allows for the rapid adjustment between renal water excretion and osmoregulatory conditions at low vasopressin secretion rates. This results in a rapid receptor occupancy, initiating further steps in vasopressin action in response to changes in circulating vasopressin levels. In fact, this would not be compatible with receptors which have a very high affinity. The changes in circulating vasopressin levels can be rapid and large, and therefore this implies the necessity of very efficient mechanisms for elimination and inactivation.

2. There is no strict correlation between the dissociation constants for the binding of various structural analogues of vasopressin and the corresponding antidiuretic effect measured *in vivo*. A large part of the signal amplification occurs at the adenylyl cyclase activation step. The K_{act} for enzyme activation is lower than the dissociation constant for hormone binding to the receptor K_D. In fact, the K_{act}/K_D ratio and maximal cyclase activation are dependent on the structure of the peptide tested. Differences in the efficacy of receptor/cyclase coupling are not always detectable in the *in vivo* antidiuretic assays, due to the fact that part of the amplification process occurs at a post-cyclic AMP step. Indeed, several vasopressin analogues which behave as partial agonists of very low intrinsic activity in the adenylyl cyclase assay do nevertheless elicit a full antidiuretic response *in vivo*.

3. There are marked differences in the respective ligand selectivities of renal receptors for different mammalian species.

3. Biochemical Characterization of the Vasopressin Receptors

Vasopressin receptors are plasma membrane proteins whose size varies from 371 to 424 amino acids and which comprise seven transmembrane helices linked by three extracellular and three intracellular loops. Within the same species, the three receptor types (V1a, V1b and V2) exhibit 45% sequence homology. Furthermore, these isoforms are highly conserved from one species to another, the homology being up to 90% for a given subtype. Vasopressin receptors belong to the 1b family of G protein-linked receptors as defined by Bockaert and Pin (1999). The members of this family are characterized by a disulfide bridge between the first and second extracellular loops and by a conserved arginine residue in the sequence Arg-Asp-Tyr located in the second intracellular loop. The binding site for the hormone involves the upper part of the transmembrane helices, the extracellular loops (including the disulfide bridge) and the N-terminal moiety (Fig. 1).

The biochemical analysis of the vasopressin receptors has shown an interesting difference between V1a and V2 receptors in terms of susceptibility to cellular proteases (Birnbaumer, 2000). The V1a receptor is highly sensitive to proteolysis and gives rise to a small 46 kDa fragment when studied after immunoprecipitation (Innamorati *et al.*, 1998a) while a molecular mass of 95 kDa is obtained after cross-linking with an iodinated ligand. In contrast, the V2 receptor is resistant to proteolysis and always has the same molecular size, whatever the technique used (Birnbaumer *et al.*, 1992; Sadeghi *et al.*, 1997; Innamorati *et al.*, 1998b). The main difference between the three isoforms is their coupling mechanism with the downstream intracellular signalling pathway: activation of adenylyl cyclase for the V2 type and activation of phospholipase C for the V1a and V1b types. The latter two receptors are also called V1 and V3 respectively, and we have to wait for a meeting of experts (to be held soon) to decide what nomenclature should be accepted. One should be aware that vasopressin is also capable of binding to the oxytocin receptor with a nanomolar affinity, while the reverse is not true (Guillon, 1989).

The essential characteristics of the three isoforms of the vasopressin receptors are depicted in Tables 1 and 2.

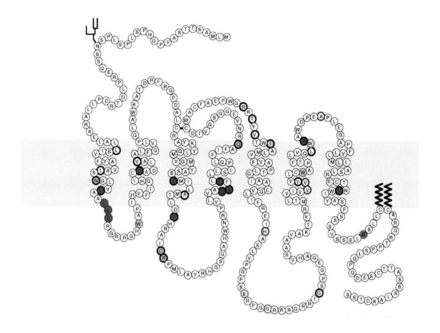

Figure 1. Schematic representation of the V2 receptor. The amino acid sequence of the receptor is depicted as its topographic localization through the plasma membrane. The receptor has a site for N-linked glycosylation at the extracellular N-terminus. The two cysteine residues present at the intracellular C-terminus are palmitoylated and are implicated in the membrane stability of the receptor. The mutations responsible for the retention of the receptor in the endoplasmic reticulum and responsible for nephrogenic diabetes insipidus are shown. The missence mutations are in black circles, the non-sense mutations in red circles and the deletions or insertions in blue circles. The colour-filled circles indicate those mutations that have been tested for the action of the pharmacological chaperones: green when surface expression and function were rescued and yellow when they were not (from Bernier et al., 2004).

To be thorough, it should also be noted that two other putative vasopressin receptors have been reported. They have no sequence similarity with the 'classical' ones and their physiological roles are undefined. They will be briefly dealt with at the end of this chapter.

Table 1. Main characteristics of the vasopressin receptors.

	V1a (V1)	V1b (V3)	V2
Chromosomal localization (man)	12(q14-15)	1(q32)	X(q28)
Size (aa) Man	418	424	371
Rat	424	425	371
Second messenger	IP3/Ca	IP3/Ca	Cyclic AMP
Tissue expression	Vascular smooth muscle	Adenohypophysis	Kidney
	Liver	Brain	Adrenals
	Adrenals	Pancreas	Endothelial cells
	Brain	Brain	
	Myometrium		
	Platelets		
	Kidney		
Main physiological response	Raised blood pressure	ACTH secretion	Antidiuresis
Selective agonist		dDAVP (human)	
Selective antagonist	SR 49059	SR 149415	SR 21463

4. Tissue Expression

a) *V1a receptor*

The V1a receptor is widely distributed in the organism as it can be found in liver, platelets, vascular smooth muscle cells, adrenal cortex and in the central nervous system (hippocampus, septum, amygdala). It has also been found in the mesangial cells in kidney as well as in several cell lines (3T3, A10, WRK-1, A7r5). By *in situ* hybridization, most of the V1a mRNA was found to be associated with vascular elements in the renal medulla (Ostrowki *et al.*, 1993). However, it is quite possible that the

V1a receptor is also expressed in the cortical collecting duct (Ammar *et al.*, 1992; Firsov *et al.*, 1994; Ecelbarger *et al.*, 1996). The main identified physiological effects are vasoconstriction with an increase in blood pressure, the regulation of renal medullary blood flow and a release of glucose from the liver by glycogenolysis. For reviews see Guillon, 1989; Thibonnier *et al.*, 1994; Young *et al.*, 1999; Knepper *et al.*, 2000).

Table 2. Main biological effects and sites of action of vasopressin.

Biological Effect	Site of Action	Receptor
Vasoconstriction	Vascular smooth muscle	V1a
Water reabsorption	Collecting duct	V2
ACTH secretion	Corticotroph cells	V1b
Steroidogenesis	Adrenal cortex	V1a
Catecholamine secretion	Adrenal medulla	V1b
Insulin secretion	Islet β cells	V1b
Inotropic effect	Cardiomyocyte	V1a
ANF secretion	Cardiomyocyte	V1a
Glycogenolysis	Hepatocyte	V1a
Aggregation	Platelet	V1a
Cell proliferation	Smooth muscle cells, mesangial cells, hepatocytes, etc.	V1a
Factor VII and von Willebrand factor		
Nitric oxide synthesis	Endothelial cells (?)	V2

ANF, atrial natriuretic factor.

b) *V1b (V3) receptor*

Unlike the V1a receptor, the V1b receptor is thought to be mainly localized in the adenohypophysis, where it is present on the surface of the corticotroph cells responsible for the secretion of ACTH (Jard *et al.*, 1986; Aguilera *et al.*, 1994; Aguilera and Rabadan-Diehl, 2000).

However, as noted by Birnbaumer (2000), it remains to be proven whether enhancing the secretion of ACTH is the only physiological role of the V1b receptor. In fact, at the peripheral level, it has been identified on a pharmacological basis in the adrenal medulla (Grazzini *et al.*, 1996) and in the pancreas (Lee *et al.*, 1995). Using *in situ* hybridization and immunochemistry, V1b receptors have also been found in heart, lung, thymus, uterus and mammary gland (Lolait *et al.*, 1995). In kidney, Saito *et al.* (2000) found an atypical receptor whose properties correspond to those of the V1b receptor. In the brain, the V1b receptor has been characterized by immunochemistry in hippocampus, putamen, cortex, thalamus and cerebellum (Hernando *et al.*, 2001). Finally, the presence of V1b receptors in hypophysial adenomas and in lung tumours has been identified (de Keyzer *et al,* 1996; 1997).

c) *V2 receptor*

The V2 receptors are essentially present in the kidney and have been extensively characterized by a variety of techniques, including cloning and sequencing (Butlen *et al.*, 1978; Guillon *et al.*, 1982; Birnbaumer *et al.*, 1992; Lolait *et al.*, 1992; Serradeil-Le Gal *et al.*, 2000). They have also been identified in human hypophysial tumours (de Keyzer *et al.*, 1995). The exact localization of the V2 receptor in the kidney is now well known. Aurbach and Chase (1968) first demonstrated that the vasopressin-sensitive adenyl cyclase was present in renal medullary homogenates. This was followed in 1975 by the elegant experiments performed in the laboratory of François Morel (Morel and Doucet, 1986). They clearly demonstrated the presence of vasopressin-sensitive adenyl cyclase in microdissected segments of the renal tubule (Imbert *et al.*, 1975a; 1975b). They showed that the activation by vasopressin occurred not only in collecting duct segments but also in the medullary and cortical thick ascending limbs of the loop of Henle and in the thin ascending limb in the inner medulla (Imbert-Teboul *et al.*, 1978). The distribution of hormone-sensitive adenyl cyclase activity along the human nephron demonstrates that the sensitivities to parathyroid hormone, calcitonin and vasopressin are uniquely, and differentially, localized (Chabardes *et al.*, 1980).

These results have been confirmed by a variety of different techniques: autoradiography (Stoeckel *et al.*, 1986; Marchingo *et al.*, 1988); reverse transcription polymerase chain reaction (Firsov *et al.*, 1994); *in situ* hybridization (Ostrowski *et al.*, 1992; 1993); and immunocytochemistry (Nonoguchi *et al.*, 1995). The latter study showed that the V2 receptor is localized not only in the basolateral membrane but also in the luminal (apical) membrane of the distal nephron. Vasopressin could act there by negative feedback following its action on the basolateral membrane of the inner medullary collecting duct (Nonoguchi *et al.*, 1995). In particular, this effect would be possible in the presence of tubular vasopressin which is excreted in the urine in a concentration-dependent manner (Laycock and Williams, 1973).

5. Vasopressin Receptors and G Proteins: An Overview

In this section, we shall focus on the overall functional interaction of the receptors with their G proteins because this knowledge is indispensable in order to understand the more structural aspects of the vasopressin receptors.

Membrane receptors such as the vasopressin receptors are members of the major G protein-coupled receptor (GPCR) family. They are involved in the recognition and transduction of messages as diverse as light, odorants, small molecules as well as proteins. They control the activity of enzymes, ion channels and transport of vesicles via the catalysis of the guanosine diphosphate to guanosine triphosphate exchange on the heteromeric G proteins (Fig. 2). Some of them can also form homo- or hetero-dimers, or interact with other membrane-bound proteins involved in their targeting, function or pharmacology. Some are unfaithful to G proteins and interact directly, via their C-terminal domain, with proteins containing PDZ and Enabled/VASP homology (EVH)-like domains (see Bockaert and Pin, 1999). However, no such promiscuous behaviour was known for the vasopressin receptors, at least until very recently (see below).

G proteins are essential in signal transduction as they transmit a positive or negative signal between the receptor and an intracellular effector,

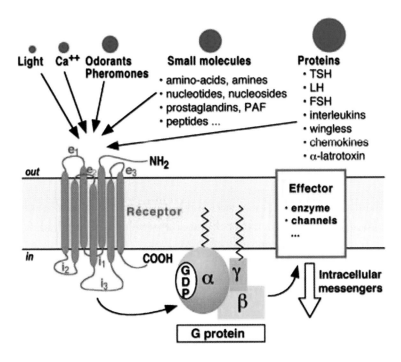

Figure 2. General scheme of the GPCRs which are able to interact with a large variety of external ligands and, through their interaction with the G proteins, modify the activity of various effectors to regulate the production of second messengers (Bockaert and Pin, 1999).

which may be an enzyme or a channel. Since the discovery of the role of GTP in cyclic AMP signalling (Rodbell *et al.*, 1971) the field has considerably expanded, with the elucidation of the trimeric structure of the GTP-binding proteins, their mechanism of action and their involvement with all seven-helix membrane receptors independent of the involvement of cyclic AMP (Fig. 2). Both Rodbell and Gilman, whose studies identified the molecular structure of these proteins demonstrating that they comprise three different subunits, were jointly rewarded with a joint Nobel prize in 1994 for their discoveries (see a short history of this accomplishment by Lefkowitz, 1994), constitute one of the most striking advances in the field of biology during the second half of the last century. The G proteins are considered in more detail in a later section (see below).

6. Structure of the Vasopressin Receptors

a) *General features*

The vasopressin and oxytocin receptors share the same general structure and display a marked degree of sequence identity, with up to 102 identical amino-acids out of the 370–420 that make up the human receptors. Furthermore, they display additional similar characteristics:

1. A disulphide bond between two highly conserved cysteine residues in the second and the third extracellular loops, which is required for the correct folding of the receptor.

2. Two well-conserved cysteine residues 124 and 205, probably implicated in the tertiary structure of the receptor since the alkylating agent N-ethylmaleimide can modify the binding of agonist ligands to the V1a and V2 receptors (Gopalakrishnan *et al.*, 1988; Pavo and Fahlrenholz, 1990; Thibonnier *et al.*, 1993).

3. Two cysteine residues which are well conserved have been shown to be palmitoylated in other G protein linked receptors. However, in the human V2 vasopressin receptor palmitoylation is not important for receptor binding and signalling (Sadeghi *et al.*, 1997) but may play a role in the binding of arrestin (Charest and Bouvier, 2003).

4. The asparagine residues present in the extracellular domains at position 14, 27 and 196 for the V1a receptor are glycosylated. Yet glycosylation plays a very small role, if any, in the overall function of the receptor including hormone binding, coupling to the G protein, desensitization and internalization (Jans *et al.*, 1992; Innamorati *et al.*, 1996).

b) *Modelling of vasopressin receptors*

Crystallography and nuclear magnetic resonance (NMR) are the best methods for identifying protein structure and function. However, they are of limited potential use when dealing with membrane-bound proteins such as the G protein linked receptors, and molecular modelling becomes the best method available. The first models used bacteriorhodopsin (Henderson *et al.*, 1990) as the template and were further improved when the crystallographic structure of a G protein linked receptor, bovine opsin (Schertler *et al.*, 1993; Palczewski *et al.*, 2000) confirmed the seven transmembrane helix bundle of these receptors. However, the hypotheses on which these theoretical models are based can be criticized (Hibert *et al.*, 1993) and need to be probed and strengthened by additional experimental tools (Hibert *et al.*, 1999; Barberis *et al.*, 1998). These other techniques include site-directed mutagenesis of the receptor, construction of chimeric receptors, labelling by photoaffinity and chemical modification of the ligands.

7. Structural Basis of the Receptor-Ligand Interaction

a) *Binding of agonists*

The electron density map of bovine opsin was used to build the optimized transmembrane domain of the vasopressin V1a receptor (Mouillac *et al.*, 1995). Surprisingly, the model suggested that vasopressin, in spite of its size, could be nearly completely buried within the central cleft of the receptor. Since then, this has been largely validated by site-directed mutagenesis experiments, which showed that the agonist binding site is located in a pocket delimited by several transmembrane domains (TM II–VII), about 15 Angström from the outside surface (Barberis *et al.*, 1998; Hibert *et al.*, 1999). Replacement of the conserved glutamine residues in TM II, III, IV and VI, and of the lysine residue in TM III, of the V1a vasopressin receptor decreased the affinity for the agonist considerably. Since these amino acids are conserved in all the vasopressin and oxytocin receptors, it has been proposed that the binding pocket is common to all receptor types in this family (Mouillac *et al.*, 1995). Indeed, this has also been demonstrated for the vasotocin receptor (Hausmann *et al.*, 1996).

In addition, residues located in the extracellular domain also interact with the hormone. This was already suggested by photoaffinity labelling of the first extracellular loop of the bovine vasopressin V2 receptor (Kojro *et al.*, 1993). The exocyclic, hydrophilic part of the hormone occupies the upper region of the cleft and the lateral chain of the arginine in position 8 interacts with the tyrosine residue in position 115 in the first extracellular loop of the V1a receptor (Chini *et al.*, 1995). Replacement of the tyrosine 115 with aspartic acid or phenylalanine, the amino acids naturally occurring in the human V2 or oxytocin receptors, results in a potent increase in V2 or oxytocin binding affinity (Chini *et al.*, 1995).

Similar results were obtained with the V2 bovine receptor (Ufer *et al.*, 1995). This also explains the low affinity of the porcine V2 receptor for desamino 8D-Arginine Vasopressin (DDAVP) which has a tyrosine residue at position 115 and not an asparagine. Along the same lines, Hawtin *et al.* (2002, 2005) demonstrated that the arginine located at position 46 within the N-terminus of the V1a vasopressin receptor was critical for binding vasopressin, but not for peptide or nonpeptide antagonists. Interestingly, the same group found that mutation of the glutamic acid in position 54 had an almost identical pharmacological effect as a mutation at arginine 46 (Hawkin *et al.*, 2005). In fact, the two residues function independently, providing two discrete epitopes for high-affinity binding and signalling and are highly conserved throughout the entire family of neurohypophysial peptide hormone receptors (Hawkin *et al.*, 2005).

A systematic analysis of the second extracellular loop of the V1a receptor (Conner *et al.*, 2007) revealed that four aromatic residues Phe189, Trp206, Phe209 and Tyr218 are important for agonist binding and receptor activation, and are highly conserved. Rodrigo *et al.* (2007) have recently taken advantage of the high resolution structure of bovine rhodopsin, the only GPCR crystallized to date, to develop analogue models for the V1a and V1b receptors. The results obtained are more precise, but essentially in line with those described above.

Chimeric constructs have also been made. Postina *et al.* (1996) proposed that all three extracellular loops are important in the discrimination between the binding of agonists and antagonists, on the basis of the exchange of extracellular domains between porcine V2 and oxytocin receptors. A similar approach has been used to relate part of the affinity of the vasotocin receptor for agonists to the second extracellular loop (Haussmann *et al.*, 1996). Small synthetic peptides mimicking the sequence of the supposed active region of the receptor have been used for the vasopressin V1a receptor. A twelve amino acid synthetic peptide from the sequence of the first extracellular loop of the V1a receptor inhibited both the binding of agonist and antagonist radioligands to the receptor and the activation of glycogen phosphorylase in isolated hepatocytes (Howl and Wheatley, 1996). Another synthetic peptide, 25 amino-acids long, analogous to the second extra-cellular loop of the V1a receptor, also inhibited ligand binding and production of second messenger (Mendre *et al.*, 1997). These results may indicate that the extracellular part of the receptor facilitates the initial capture of the ligand, whether agonist or antagonist (Barberis *et al.*, 1998).

Of course, mutations of the human V2 receptor found to be responsible for the appearance of nephrogenic diabetes insipidus also give interesting insights into vasopressin-receptor interaction. Mutation of Arg113 (located close to a cysteine involved in the disulphide bond) to Trp reduces receptor expression in transfected cells, as well receptor-ligand affinity and Gs coupling (Bichet *et al.*, 1993; Birnbaumer *et al.*, 1994). Another mutation, involving the deletion of the arginine in position 202 in the second extracellular loop of the human V2 receptor, gives rise to the same biological and clinical features (Ala *et al.*, 1998).

b) *Binding of antagonists*
The receptor domains involved in the binding of the various peptide or nonpeptide vasopressin antagonists are still relatively sketchy (Barberis *et al.*, 1998). In particular, from mutational studies it appears that the

sites involved in the binding of agonists are not those involved in the binding of antagonists (Mouillac et al., 1995; Postina et al., 1996). Combining the photolabelling data with predictions from molecular modelling studies, it was suggested that a peptide antagonist for the V1a receptor interacts with a hydrophobic cluster of aromatic residues situated in transmembrane domain VI (Phalipou et al., 1977) and also with the first extracellular loop (Phalipou et al., 1999). Cotte et al. (2000) took advantage of the existence of two peptides of similar chemical structure, vasopressin and $d(CH_2)_5(Tyr)Me)^2AVP$, agonist and antagonist, respectively. They demonstrated that the two analogues fit in the same cleft but interact with different residues. Tahtaoui et al. (2003) recently showed that an aromatic residue located in the transmembrane region V of the V1a receptor was responsible for the selective binding of the nonpeptide antagonist SR49059. Concerning the V1b receptor, Derick et al. (2004) reported that key amino-acids located in the transmembrane domains V and VII were responsible for the selective binding of the antagonist SSR149415.

We will describe in another chapter (Chapter 5) the marked differences between species regarding the binding of agonist and antagonist ligands. For example, Cotte et al. (1998) identified the residues in the second extracellular loop that are responsible for the selective binding of peptide agonists and antagonists in the V2 vasopressin receptor.

8. Domains Responsible for G Protein-Coupling Selectivity

Liu and Wess (1996) constructed chimeric receptors containing the intracellular loops of the V2 receptor in a V1a receptor background, and vice versa. The second intracellular loop of the V1a receptor is responsible for Gq/G11 coupling and the third intracellular loop of the V2 receptor is responsible for Gs coupling. Erlenbach and Wess (1998) demonstrated that two residues (glutamine and glutamic acid) located in the N-terminal part of the third intracellular loop contributed to the Gs coupling of the V2 receptor.

In one case of nephrogenic diabetes insipidus, the mutation responsible was found to be a replacement of the arginine in position 137 by a histidine in the V2 receptor (Rosenthal *et al.*, 1993). When tested *in vitro*, the receptor could not mediate the stimulation of adenylyl cyclise, although its ligand-binding activity remained unchanged. Since the Arg137 is located at the interface between the third transmembrane domain and the second intracellular loop of the V2 receptor, one may conclude that the second intracellular loop is also involved in the receptor/Gs coupling (Birnbaumer, 2000). The well conserved proline in position 322 in transmembrane domain VII of the human V2 vasopressin receptor is probably necessary to allow the relative movement within the helix bundle that is necessary for receptor activation (Barberis *et al.*, 1998). Mutation of this amino acid to serine leads to a mild phenotype with a mutant receptor still able to bind the hormone and to activate adenyl cyclase. Mutation with a histidine is responsible for a phenotype associated with the receptor being completely uncoupled from any signalling pathway (Tajima *et al.*, 1996). Conversely, replacement of the aspartic acid in position 136 of the V2 vasopressin receptor by alanine induces a constitutive activity of the receptor that permits the discrimination between antagonists with partial agonist and inverse agonist activities (Morin *et al.*, 1998).

9. Dimerization of Receptors

That GPCRs can oligomerize is now a well demonstrated phenomenon and a wide variety of studies have shown that they can form homo- and hetero-dimers (for reviews see Rashid *et al.*, 2004; Milligan, 2004; Prinster *et al.*, 2005). Using both co-immunoprecipitation and bioluminescence resonance energy transfer (BRET), Terrillon *et al.* (2003, 2004) and Devost and Zingg (2004) have established that both vasopressin V1a and V2 receptors, as well as the oxytocin receptors, exist as homo- and hetero-dimers in transfected human embryonic kidney 293T cells. The specificity of these interactions is highlighted by the fact that no heterodimerization has been detected between V1a and GABA receptors (Terrillon *et al.*, 2003).

The V1a/V2 interaction is functionally important, in that it has been shown to result in substantial co-internalization of the two receptors via a β-arrestin-dependent process. Dimerization is also potentially important for signal transduction. A cyclic peptide mimicking the third cytoplasmic loop of the vasopressin V2 receptor inhibited the adenylyl cyclase activity induced by vasopressin or GTP (Granier *et al.*, 2004). The peptide also converted the binding characteristics for vasopressin from a high to a low affinity without any effect on the maximal binding capacity. The peptide acts by directly decreasing the affinity of the receptor dimer for the agonist and also, through a direct interaction with the G protein by reducing its availability for GDP/GTP exchange, decreasing adenylyl cyclase activation. Nevertheless, as is the case for many of the studies dealing with receptor oligomerization, one should keep in mind that they often rely on *in vitro* cell transfection, and that physiological or clinical consequences are probably difficult to clearly demonstrate *in vivo*.

10. Signalling Pathways

a) *The heterotrimeric G protein*
GPCRs are called heterotrimeric because of their ability to recruit the intracellular G proteins and regulate their activity. The G proteins, capable of binding GTP, constitute fundamental elements of signal transduction which can transmit a stimulatory or inhibitory signal from the membrane-bound receptor to a downstream effector (enzyme or channel), thus initiating a cascade of intracellular events culminating in a physiological response. The role of the receptor is to shift the G protein from an inactive state to an active one, capable of positively or negatively modifying the activity of one or more intracellular effectors. The literature dealing with G proteins is immense and we will not try to fully describe the complex molecular physiology of the G proteins. Only a broad description is attempted here and the reader is referred to more detailed recent reviews (Gilman, 1987; Bourne *et al.*, 1991; Lefkowitz, 1994; Bourne, 1997; Bockaert and Pin, 1998; Cabrera-Vera *et al.*, 2003; Wettschureck and Offermanns, 2005).

The G proteins comprise three subunits: α, β and γ (see Table 3). The α sub-unit is the major one responsible for the specificity of signal transduction and exists in four large families: αs, αi, αq and α12. All of them possess a GTPase activity crucial for the activation cycle of the protein. When the receptor is not activated by its ligand, the G protein is in its trimeric form with the α subunit bound to GDP (state 1). The binding of the hormone modifies the conformation of the receptor, which can then associate with the G protein so that GDP is replaced by GTP (state 2). A correlate at the level of the receptor is the observed decrease in its affinity for the agonist in the presence of added GTP. Due to the attachment of GTP to the α subunit, the heterotrimeric complex is dissociated into an active αGTP subunit and a βγ complex. Both the α subunit and the βγ complex regulate their respective effectors. The GTPase activity of the α subunit hydrolyses GTP to GDP, thus allowing the cycle to go back to state 1.

The GTPase activity of isolated G proteins is much lower than that observed under physiological conditions and various effectors have been found to increase it. In particular, regulation is provided by another family of proteins, the regulators of G protein signalling (RGS), which enhance that activity and probably play a very important biological role (see Wieland and Mittmann, 2003). At least 30 RGS proteins, sharing a common domain of 120 amino acids and with various selectivities, are known. Their main action is to increase the GTPase activity of the α subunit, thus accelerating its return to basal state 1, and regulating the signalling mechanism by negative feedback.

Identification of the signalling pathway specifically linked to a definite receptor type is usually clear-cut: Gs for the V2 vasopressin receptor and the Gq/G11 family for the V1a and V1b receptors. However, one should keep in mind the possibility that spurious results can be obtained when unusually high levels of receptors are present in transfected cells. Thus when the level of V2 receptor is higher than 100,000 sites per cell, it can couple to phospholipase C, a non-physiological effect resulting from an inappropriate coupling event (Zhu *et al.*, 1994). In addition, a novel class of accessory proteins such as the activators of G protein signalling

(AGS) can activate the G proteins in the absence of a receptor and can influence GDP dissociation or nucleotide exchange, or form complexes with the subunits. Their role in physiology or in pathology is not yet known (see Sato *et al.*, 2006).

Among the signalling pathways that exist downstream of the G proteins, the most important are the cyclic AMP pathway controlled by Gαs, and the calcium/phosphatidyl inositol pathway controlled by Gαq. These two pathways are described in some detail below, but other pathways have also been shown to be influenced by the G proteins, at least *in vitro* or in simplified models. At present it is difficult to assess whether all of those additional pathways are actually important from a physiological point of

Table 3. Main effectors of the G protein subunits.

α subunits	
Gαs class	Increase AC (all types)
Gαi/o class	
Gαi (1, 2, 3)	Decrease AC (types 1, 3, 5, 6, 8, 9) and influence other effectors
Gαo	Decrease VDCC and increase GIRK
Gαz	Decrease AC (types 5, 6)
Gαgust	Increase PDE?
Gαq/11 class (q11, 14, 15/16)	Increase PLC,
Gα12/13 class	RhoGEF, etc.
β subunits β1 to β5 and	Decrease AC1, increase AC 2, 4, 7 and
γ subunits γ1 to γ14 complex	increase PLC, GIRK, GRK, PI3K and VDCC

AC, adenylyl cyclase; GIRK, G protein-regulated inward rectifier potassium channel; GRK, G protein-regulated kinase; PDE, phosphodiesterase; PLC, phospholipase C; PI3K, phosphatidylinositol 3 kinase; RhoGEF, Rho guanine nucleotide exchange factor; VDCC, voltage dependant Ca^{2+} channel.

view, or whether they result only from the conditions used in the experimental models. We will allude to some of these difficulties later for each vasopressin receptor isoform.

b) *The cyclic AMP pathway*

Cyclic AMP is made from ATP by a family of adenylyl cyclases (AC). At present at least nine closely related isoforms of the enzyme are known (see Hanoune and Defer, 2001). They share a large sequence homology. Each variant consists of two hydrophobic domains (with six transmembrane spans) and two cytoplamsic domains resulting in a pseudosymetrical protein. They are coded by nine independent genes and the different types are expressed as discrete patterns in only a limited number of tissues. Their regulatory properties are listed in Table 4.

Table 4. Regulatory properties of mammalian adenylyl cyclases.

AC isoform	Response to cAMP signalling pathway component					
	Gαs	Gαi	Gβγ	FSK	Calcium	Protein Kinases
AC1	↑	↓ (CaM- or FSK- stimulated activities)	↓	↑	↑ (CaM) ↓ (CaM kinase IV)	↑ PKC (weak) ↓ (CaM kinase IV)
AC2	↑	→	↑ (when stimulated by Gαs)			↑ (PKC)
AC3	↑	↓		↑	↑ (CaM) (*in vitro*) ↓ (CaM kinase II)	↑ (PKC) (weak) ↓ (CaM kinase II)
AC4	↑		↑	↑		↑ (PKC)
AC5	↑	↓	↓ (β1γ2)	↑	↓ (<1μM)	↓ (PKA) ↑ (PKCα/ζ)
AC6	↑	↓	↓ (β1γ2)	↑	↓ (<1μM)	↓ (PKA, PKC)
AC7	↑		↑	↑		↑ (PKC)
AC8	↑	↓ (Ca^{2+} rises)		↑	↑ (CaM)	→ (PKC)
AC9	↑	↓		↑(weak)	↓ (calcineurin)	
sAC	→	→		→		

↑ Positive regulatory response, ↓ negative regulatory response, → neutral regulatory response.

In addition to their ability to respond to Gαs and to forskolin, the different isoforms can receive signals from a variety of sources including other G protein subunits, protein kinases A (PKA), C (PKC) and calmodulin kinases, calcium and calcium/calmodulin.

Cyclic AMP is degraded via the activity of phosphodiesterases (PDEs). They are dimeric metallophosphohydrolases which catalyse the hydrolysis of cyclic nucleotides into their non-cyclic, inactive forms. This hydrolysis is the main mechanism for attenuating cyclic AMP signalling. At present, at least eleven isoforms have been identified, each having different specificities for cyclic AMP and/or cyclic GMP (see Table 5).

Table 5. Types of PDE as a function of their substrate.

Substrate	Type of PDE
Cyclic AMP	PDE4, PDE7, PDE8
Cyclic GMP	PDE 5, PDE6, PDE9
Cyclic AMP and GMP	PDE1, PDE2, PDE3, PDE10, PDE11

In most cases, the physiological effects of cyclic AMP are due to the phosphorylation of a protein catalyzed by a protein kinase. PKA comprises two regulatory subunits which inhibit the activity of two linked catalytic subunits. The binding of a molecule of cyclic AMP to each of the regulatory subunits leads to the release of the active catalytic subunits which are then able to phophorylate the tyrosine or threonine residues of proteins, whether enzymes or not, and then modify their activity. The so-called 'Carney Complex' is characterized by a mutation of the 1α isoform of the regulatory subunit, which leads to a compensatory increase in the other subunits and an enhanced response of the kinase to cyclic AMP. When the substrate of the phosphorylation event is cytoplasmic, effects can be readily observed in a matter of seconds. In other cases the effect can be protracted, for instance when the cyclic AMP regulates gene expression. Activated PKA is transferred to the nucleus and phosphorylates the regulatory protein cyclic AMP response element binding protein (CREB), which can then recruit the coactivator CBP, resulting in stimulation of the expression of genes and therefore the synthesis of new proteins (see Fig. 3).

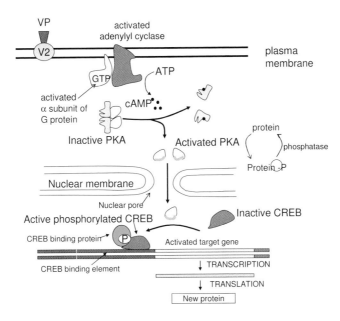

Figure 3. The cyclic AMP pathway associated with nuclear effects. The elements of the pathway are described in the text.

It should be emphasized that all effects of cyclic AMP are not simply due to the activation of PKA. The second messenger can also directly stimulate certain ion channels or bind to the exchange factors Epac 1 and 2, thus increasing the activity of the monomeric G protein Rap. In addition, the simple linear scheme of cyclic AMP-directed phosphorylation is now made more complex due to the existence of scaffolding proteins such as the A-kinase anchoring proteins (AKAPs). Approximately 50 such anchoring proteins have been identified. They can bind the regulatory subunits of PKA and are endowed with two properties: they can sequestrate PKA in a specific compartment of the cell (e.g. cell membrane, nucleus) and they can also bind to other signalling proteins. As an example, AKAP79 interacts at the same time with PKA, PKC and the PP2B calcium-dependent phosphatase in a site close to the plasma membrane while AKAP220 can bind PKA and phosphatase PP1. Recent advances in proteomics have demonstrated that no protein exists in isolation in the cytosol and that each one is part of a complex assembly of molecules. These networks or scaffoldings provide the ground for pre-existing or privileged connections between the various signalling pathways, thus counteracting the potentially unlimited, and often illegitimate, possibilities of cross-talks between different pathways.

c) *The calcium/phosphatidyl inositol pathway*
When the GPCR is linked to a Gαq protein, it activates the enzyme phospholipase PLCβ which catalyzes the hydrolysis of phosphatidylinositol-4,5-bisphosphate (PIP2), a phospholipid normally present in the plasma membrane, into two different second messengers, inositol triphosphate (IP3) and diacylglycerol (DAG). Inositol triphosphate can readily diffuse into the cytosol and, through its binding to calcium channels on the endoplasmic reticulum, allows the release of calcium from this intracellular storage site. Diacylglycerol, in the presence of calcium, directly activates PKC which then phosphorylates a series of protein substrates which may, or may not, differ from those of PKA. Diacylglycerol can also be cleaved into arachidonic acid, the precursor for prostaglandin synthesis (see Fig. 4).

The intracellular concentration of free calcium ions is normally very low (0.1 μm) and any increase in its concentration or in the frequency of its oscillations can have a marked signalling impact. In particular, calcium can bind to calmodulin and activate the calcium/calmodulin-dependent kinases which interestingly can also phosphorylate cyclic AMP response element binding protein (CREB). The calcium/IP3 pathway can be easily stopped through hydrolysis of IP3 or the reuptake of calcium. Hydrolysis of PIP2 can also occur either following activation of a plasma membrane tyrosine kinase receptor or activation of another phospholipase, PLCγ, to produce the same products, IP3 and DAG. Phosphatidylinositol-4,5-

bisphosphate can also initiate another signalling pathway, involving its IP3 kinase-induced phosphorylation into phosphatidylinositol-3,4,5-triphosphate (PIP3), another distinct second messenger. For example, PIP3 can activate the serine/threonine kinase Akt via a Plekstrin Homology (PH) domain. Other phospholipids can be hydrolyzed, such as phosphatidyl choline which can release DAG for several hours (while the release of DAG from IP3 is very rapid and transitory), or sphingomyelin, the precursor in ceramide synthesis.

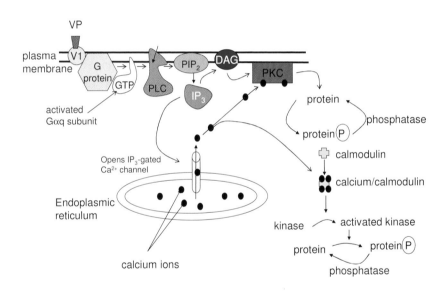

Figure 4. The V1 receptor-activated IP$_3$/DAG pathway. Only the pathway linked to the activation of PLC-β is described here. DAG, diacylglycerol; GTP, guanosyl triphosphate; PIP$_2$, phosphatidylinositol (4,5) bisphosphate; PKC, protein kinase C; PLC, phospholipase Cβ; V1, vasopressin V1 receptor. See the text for further details.

d) *The V2 receptor pathway*
The interaction of vasopressin with the renal V2 receptor leads to the activation of AC through the Gαs subunit, and results in the increased synthesis of cyclic AMP. Subsequent activation of PKA leads to the phosphorylation and translocation of aquaporin 2 to the luminal membrane, thus allowing water reabsorption to occur. This clear-cut and now classical pathway probably suffices to explain the bulk of the physiological action of vasopressin (see Chapter 6).

Among the various adenyl cyclase isoforms, Northern blot analysis and *in situ* hybridization demonstrated that AC6 was the predominant isoform in the adult rat kidney. AC4, AC5 and AC9 had a much lower expression (Shen *et al.*, 1997). AC4 was higher in the kidney cortex while AC5 and AC6 were higher in the medulla. Interestingly, AC activity was high in the fetus and declined in the adult (see Fig. 5). In the homozygote Brattleboro rat, the expression of all the cyclase isoforms was decreased. By the brilliant technique of microdissection, Morel and coworkers (Chabardes *et al.*, 1980) demonstrated that vasopressin stimulated adenyl cyclase activity in the terminal nephron segment, i.e. the late segment of the distal convoluted tubule, and the cortical and medullary collecting duct. In a further study using *in situ* hybridization (Helies-Toussaint *et al.*, 2000) the distribution of the AC5 and AC6 isoforms was studied in more detail in the rat outer medullary collecting duct. AC5 was expressed only in intercalated cells while AC6 was present in both intercalated and principal cells. In both cells the synthesis of cAMP was diminished by agents that increase the cellular entry of calcium, as should be expected for these calcium-inhibitable cyclase isoforms (Table 4).

The V2 vasopressin receptors are believed to be localized mainly in the basolateral membrane of the distal nephron. However, by an immunohistochemical study using a specific polyclonal antibody,

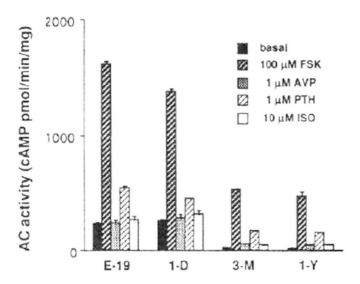

Figure 5. Distribution of AC6 mRNA in developing rat kidney examined by *in situ* hybridization. E-1, 19-day old fetus; 1-D, 1-day old neonate; 3-M, 3-month old; 1-Y, one-year old (from Shen *et al.*, 1997).

Nonoguchi *et al.* (1995) demonstrated the presence of the V2 receptor not only in the basolateral but also the luminal membrane (albeit at a lower density) of the distal nephron, especially in the terminal inner medullary collecting duct. The physiological meaning of such luminal receptors is still under discussion (Nonoguchi *et al.*, 1995).

In addition to the simple, and archetypal, scheme by which the V2 receptor activates adenyl cyclase, it appears now that the receptor can form a complex with β-arrestin-2 upon agonist stimulation (see below). This complex can then scaffold components of the extracellular signal-regulated kinase (ERK) cascade and sequester the activated ERK into cytoplasmic endocytic vesicles (Tohgo *et al.*, 2003). Formation of this complex is enhanced by the pamitoylation of the V2 receptor carboxy tail, and is dependent neither on the production of cyclic AMP (Charest and Bouvier, 2003) nor on the presence of G protein (Azzi *et al.*, 2003). Phosphorylation of the receptor by G protein-coupled receptor kinases

(GRKs) is a prerequisite for the formation of the receptor-β-arrestin complex. In the case of the V2 receptor, GRK 2 and 3 are responsible for most of the agonist-dependent receptor phosphorylation, desensitization and recruitment of β-arrestin, while GRK 5 and 6 appear exclusively to support β-arrestin-2-stimulated ERK activation (Ren *et al.*, 2005). Moreover, unlike the direct stimulation of ERK by G protein-dependent receptors, where the ERK pool is stimulated rapidly, is transient and translocates to the nucleus, the β-arrestin-dependent ERK activation is slower, sustained and apparently restricted to the cytoplasm (Ahn *et al.*, 2004).

The trafficking of aquaporin 2 is possibly the main site of regulation of vasopressin's physiological action, through the V2 receptor. In response to vasopressin, aquaporin 2 reaches the apical membrane where it facilitates water reabsorption. Cessation of the stimulus is followed by endocytosis of aquaporin through a clathrin-mediated process back to the initial intracellular storage sites, the vesicles. After the binding of vasopressin to its receptor, stimulation of PKA leads to the phosporylation of aquaporin at the site of at least two serine residues, Ser-256, the most studied, and also Ser-261, which was identified recently (Hoffert *et al.*, 2006). Binding of PKA to the PKA anchoring protein AKAP 18, or its variant AKAP18δ, appears to be required for the trafficking of aquaporin 2 (Henn *et al.*, 2004; 2005). Various studies have demonstrated that the administration of vasopressin induces a time- and dose-dependent increase in the phosphorylation of aquaporin 2 (Nishimoto *et al.*, 1999), and that at least three monomers of aquaporin should be phosphorylated for the aquaporin tetramer to be retained in the plasma membrane (Kamsteeg *et al.*, 2000).

Interestingly, the PKC-mediated endocytosis of aquaporin is independent of its phosphorylation state (van Balkom *et al.*, 2002). More surprising is the demonstration by Valenti *et al.* (2000) that aquaporin fusion to the plasma membrane could occur in the absence of phosphorylation by PKA, a result which needs to be clearly confirmed by other experimental approaches. This is all the more necessary as recent studies have indicated that phosphorylation of Ser-256 is important for its interaction with 70-kDa heat shock proteins and ultimately for the cytosolic aquaporin shuttle (Lu *et al.*, 2007). In addition, ubiquitination of the C-terminal tail of aquaporin at Lys-270 is important for internalization (Kamsteeg *et al.*, 2006). Finally, Fenton *et al.* (2008) have shown that aquaporin can also be phosphorylated at Ser-264, leading to a different aquaporin distribution in intracellular vesicles, but not in lysosomes.

Elevation of intracellular cyclic guanosine monophosphate (cGMP) in the kidney cells by either nitric oxide or atrial natriuretic peptide (Bouley *et al.*, 2000), or by inhibition of the cyclic GMP phosphodiesterase by sildenafil (Bouley *et al.*, 2005) leads to aquaporin insertion in the membrane, although one cannot eliminate the possibility that cyclic AMP is secondarily elevated under those conditions. The delivery of aquaporin to the membrane is dependent on elements of the cytoskeleton and in particular microtubules dynein and dynactin as well as actin. Inhibition of the small GTPase RhoA through PKA-dependent phosphorylation also appears to be a key element in aquaporin translocation (Tamma *et al.*, 2003). The docking and fusion of aquaporin 2 with the apical membrane requires a complex cascade of vesicle soluble N-ethylmaleimide-sensitive fusion protein attachment protein receptors (v-SNAREs) and target membrane SNAREs (t-SNAREs) such as VAMP-2, SNAP-23 or syntaxin-4.

The trafficking of aquaporins back and forth between cytoplasm and membrane is a very active field of research at present, all the more so since various mutations of the aquaporin 2 gene leading to missfolding of the protein, or its retention at internal sites during the trafficking process, have been reported. These mutations are described in chapter 12 dealing with nephrogenic diabetes insipidus. For further details on aquaporin trafficking, two recent reviews are available (Valenti *et al.*, 2005; Noda and Sasaki, 2005). See also Chapter 6.

e) *The V1a receptor pathway*
Most of the non-renal effects of vasopressin are due to its interaction with the V1a receptor. As early as 1974 Kirk and Hems demonstrated that the effect of vasopressin on liver was independent of the formation

of cyclic AMP. Later, Mitchell *et al.* (1979), Exton *et al.* (1981) and Kirk *et al.* (1981) demonstrated that vasopressin acted via activation of phosphatidyl-inositol metabolism and an increase in intracellular calcium. Bocckino *et al.* (1985) further demonstrated that vasopressin stimulated DAG accumulation in hepatocytes, while Wange *et al.* (1991) identified Gq as the G protein involved in the ligand-receptor coupling (Fig. 4).

In cultured cortical astrocytes, Zhao and Brinton (2002) showed that vasopressin induced an increase in the calcium content of both the cytoplasm and the nucleus. In parallel, stimulation of the V1a receptor can lead to the activation of phospholipase D which hydrolyzes phosphatidylcholine to phosphatidic acid and choline, and also of phospholipase A2, possibly via an αi subunit (Briley *et al.*, 1994). However, as noted by Birnbaumer (2000), the existence of this multiplicity of coupling reactions needs to be verified in cells that intrinsically express the V1a receptor, in order to rule out the possibility of inappropriate coupling promoted by the high levels of receptors that are present in transfected cells. This criticism should be kept in mind for all studies dealing with transfected cells. In fact, the main mechanism leading to the elevation of calcium via the Gq/G11 subunits is sufficient to explain the known physiological effects of vasopressin on glycogenolysis, vasoconstriction and hormonal secretion. The mitogenic responses that are observed in various systems (Mazzocchi *et al.*, 1993; Bhora *et al.*, 1994; Ghosh *et al.*, 2001) are readily linked to signalling pathways involving the MAP kinases and the PIP3 kinase.

f) *The V1b receptor pathway*
This pathway is rather similar to that of the V1a receptor. At first, though, it was thought that vasopressin could potentiate the production of cyclic AMP elicited by corticotrophin releasing hormone, CRH (Giguere and Labrie, 1982). However, this was subsequently invalidated by Holmes *et al.* (1984) and Guillon *et al.* (1987), who demonstrated that activation of the vasopressin receptor led to an increased production of IP3. As demonstrated by Thibonnier *et al.* (1997), vasopressin acts on the V1b receptor by stimulating PLCβ via activation of the protein Gq/G11.

The increased production of IP3 leads to an increase in intracellular calcium (Levy *et al.*, 1990; Won and Orth, 1994) and presumably to the usual downstream events. In their 1997 paper, Thibonnier *et al.* showed that, depending on its level of expression, the V1b receptor could couple to the Gq/G11 protein, either alone or in combination with Gi, or may also recruit Gs. Before accepting that the receptor could stimulate several signalling pathways via different G proteins (Thibonnier *et al.*, 2001), one should keep in mind the above mentioned caveat from Birnbaumer about the possibility of spurious data originating from studies using transfected cells. Interestingly, Rabadan-Diehl and Aguilera (1998) have shown that glucocorticoids could increase the efficiency of the coupling between the V1b receptor and PLC, in spite of a reduction in receptor numbers as confirmed by Young *et al.* (2003). This could be due to an increase in the amount of G11 protein (Cheung and Mitchell, 2002).

g) *The proteomic approach*

It is interesting to note that, at the present time of large-scale biology, the proteomic approach has also been used to identify, quantify and analyze a large number of proteins during vasopressin stimulation. While it is clear that this new technique is not a substitute for hypothesis-driven experimental designs, it has already led to some interesting but minor pieces of information (Leng, 2007; Hoorn *et al.*, 2008), which will have to be further validated in the future.

11. Pre- and Post-transcriptional Regulation of Vasopressin Receptor Expression

The number of receptors at the cell membrane is susceptible to regulation at the pre- or post-transcriptional level, and a few such effects are well known. An acute increase in circulating vasopressin in the rat leads to a marked and rapid reduction in the amount of mRNA for the V2 receptor in the kidney (Terashima *et al.*, 1998). Noteworthy is the fact that the expression of the aquaporin 2 mRNA was upregulated in spite of the downregulation of the V2 receptor. In a similar study Park *et al.*, (1998) reported that water restriction, which increases the circulating vasopressin concentration, leads to a regional time-dependent downregulation of V2 receptor mRNA and protein within the kidney. Izumi *et al.* (2008) have recently shown that the V2 receptor promoter activity could be downregulated via the V1a receptor pathway, at least in the LLC-PK1 cell line.

Concerning the V1a receptor, it has been reported to be regulated negatively by nitric oxide (Patel *et al.*, 2002) and glucose (Williams *et al.*, 1992) and positively by glucocorticoids via a stabilisation of its mRNA (Murasawa *et al.*, 1995) and/or by an action at the gene level (Watters *et al.*, 1996a and b).

Finally studies mainly done by Aguilera's group have tackled the regulation of V1b receptors as part of the adaptation of the hypothalamo-adenohypophysial (corticotroph) axis during stress (Aguilera *et al.*, 1994; 2000; Volpi *et al.*, 2004). A chronic stress (Rabadan-Diehl *et al.*, 1995) or the administration of glucocorticoids (Rabadan-Diehl and Aguilera, 1998) each lead to an increase in the amount of V1b receptor as well as a decrease in the amount of receptor protein in the plasma membrane. Two mechanisms by which the 5′-untranslated region of the V1b mRNA mediates either inhibition or activation of mRNA translation have been identified. An open reading frame in the 5′ region represses translation, while an internal ribosome entry site (IRES) activates it (Aguilera *et al.*, 2003, Rabadan-Diehl *et al.*, 2003). Stimulation of the IRES activity through a PKC mediated pathway results in an increased receptor protein level. At the gene level itself, the transcriptional regulation of the pituitary vasopressin V1b receptor involves a GAGA-binding protein which may provide a potential mechanism for a physiological regulation of V1b receptor transcription (Volpi *et al.*, 2002).

12. Downregulation of Vasopressin Receptors: Desensitization and Internalization

The number of seven-transmembrane receptors is maintained in a steady state within the membrane by the combination of new receptor synthesis, proteolytic degradation, constitutive internalisation and recycling back to the membrane. The binding of the hormone to its site leads to the desensitization of the receptor in response to a further hormonal challenge by a series of mechanisms that include a mere decrease of its affinity for the agonist, an internalisation with or without recycling to the membrane, an increased proteolytic degradation or ultimately a blockade of its synthesis at a pre- or post-transcriptional level.

These steps have been extensively studied with the β–adrenergic receptor as a model (Koenig and Edwardson, 1997; Böhm *et al.*, 1997; Lefkowitz and Shenoy, 2005) and it is expected, but not always well demonstrated, that the mechanisms involved are actually valid for the other GPCRs. Moreover, several experimental aspects have to be distinguished. *Stricto sensu*, desensitization refers to the loss of response following a hormonal stimulation which can be either short- or long-term. Internalization refers to the loss of membrane receptors and results from the combined effects of endocytosis and recycling. Down regulation is a more global phenomenon where the agonist-induced internalization is compounded with irreversible sequestration and intracellular proteolysis.

The mechanisms responsible for these events involve two main families of proteins, the GRKs and the arrestins (Lefkowitz and Shenoy, 2005). After binding the hormone, the receptor undergoes a conformational change and binds to a GRK (of which seven isoforms are known), which then phosphorylates the receptor on serine or threonine residues localized on the intracellular loops or on the C-terminal tail. This phosphorylation is able to diminish the receptor's affinity for the agonist and mainly leads to its subsequent binding to an arrestin (four isoforms are known). This physically prevents coupling of the receptor to its G protein and therefore to the transduction of the signal. Phosphorylation of the receptor can also be caused by kinases other than the GRKs, such as PKA or PKC, thus sustaining a desensitization process which is dubbed heterologous as opposed to the homologous one caused by the specific hormone via GRK.

In addition, arrestins can behave as adaptor proteins which facilitate the recruitment of receptors to the plasma membrane domains where the clathrin-coated pits develop prior to the endocytosis process. Arrestins play this role not by binding to clathrin itself but by interacting with other endocytic elements, including the adaptor protein AP2, the small guanosine triphosphatase ARF6 and its guanine nucleotide exchange factor ARNO, and the N-ethyl maleimide-sensitive fusion protein (NSF). Arrestins also bind to, and are ubiquitinated by, the E3 ubiquitin ligase Mdm2. The ubiquitination is required for arrestin-mediated endocytosis. In most cases, arrestin dissociates from the receptor after having targeted it to the clathrin-coated pit. In other cases, such as with the vasopressin V2 receptor, the tightly-bound arrestin dissociates from the receptor and accompanies it into the cell where the complex stays for extended periods of time within endosomal vesicles before being directed to lysosomes or being recycled. Arrestins can also recruit molecules such as Raf, Src, Erk, and JNK to eventually activate MAP kinases and cell division. Therefore arrestins would be involved at the same time in the termination of the hormonal signal and the stimulation of another signalling pathway. In this scheme (Lekowitz and Shenoy, 2005), the same receptor would first transmit a specific signal when binding to the hormone, and later, when desensitized, would have a more general action, for example on cell division.

Most of the recent references concerning the vasopressin receptors have dealt with the internalization process. Very early on, it was demonstrated by several techniques that the V2 receptor (Kirk, 1988; Hocher *et al.*, 1992) and the V1a receptor (Cantau *et al.*, 1988) were internalized. The overall desensitization process of the V2 receptor has been recently reproduced in an *in vitro* system of polarized renal collecting duct cells (Robben *et al.*, 2004). The molecular mechanisms involved in the desensitization process have been extensively studied in the case of the V2 receptor (V2R), and the phosphorylation of the receptor is well described in particular by the group of Birnbaumer (Innamorati *et al.*, 1997; 1998b; 1999; 2001; Wu *et al.*, 2008). The vasopressin-promoted internalization and phosphorylation of the V2 receptor has slower kinetics than the V1a receptor (Innamorati *et al*, 1998a) and the internalized receptor fails to return to the cell surface. The phosphorylation is catalyzed only by the GRKs, i.e. there is no heterologous desensitization (Birnbaumer *et al.*, 1992), and in contrast with the results for the V1a receptor, the phosphates remain associated with the protein for as long as 3 hours after removal of vasopressin from the medium (Innamorati *et al.*, 1999). Retention of the receptor inside the cell correlates with the permanence of phosphate groups attached to the Ser and Thr of the C-terminus because mutations that confer recycling to the V2 receptor accelerate the cleavage of phosphates from the protein (Innamorati *et al.*, 1998b; Le Gouill *et al.*, 2002). The role of the various GRKs, and in particular GRK5, has been studied (Bowen-Pigeon *et al.*, 2001, Innamorati *et al.*, 2001), as well as the role of the ADP ribosylation factor 6 (Madziva and Birnbaumer, 2006). As reported above, it appears that different GRKs are involved in the processing of the V2 receptor. GRK 2 and 3 are involved in the desensitization process *per se* (phosphorylation, recruitment of arrestin), while GRK5 is involved in ERK pathway stimulation (Ren *et al.*, 2005). Interestingly, while the vasopressin V2 receptor is internalized after vasopressin stimulation of renal epithelial cells, aquaporin 2 remains located in an 'endocytosis-resistant' membrane domain (Bouley *et al.*, 2006).

More recently, it has been shown (Yi *et al.*, 2007) that a 100 kDa protein called Alix (ALG-2-interacting protein X) interacts with the last 29 amino acids of the V2R C-terminus to increase the rate of its lysosomal degradation.

Internalization of the receptor is uniquely dependent on the binding of an agonist. However it has been shown to occur albeit at a slower rate in the presence of certain peptidic antagonists, but not in the presence of non-peptidic antagonists (Pfeiffer *et al.*, 1998). Also, as noted above, the V1a receptor recycles rapidly to the cell membrane (Innamorati *et al.*, 1998a; Bowen-Pidgeon *et al.*, 2001). A highly conserved "Asp-Arg-Tyr" triplet (the DRY triplet) in the distal region of the third transmembrane domain of the V1a vasopressin receptor appears important for the delivery of the receptor to the membrane as well as for its internalization (Hawtin, 2005).

13. Are There Other Vasopressin Receptors?

In 1995, Burnatowska-Hledin *et al.* isolated, by expression cloning, a cDNA clone coding for a protein of 780 amino acids. Expression of this protein in COS-1 cells revealed that it could bind vasopressin with a Kd of approximately 2 nM and activate a calcium second messenger pathway. This vasopressin-activated Ca^{2+} mobilizing (VACM-1) receptor has no amino acid sequence homology with the traditional vasopressin receptors and is expressed in numerous endothelial cells (Burnatowska-Hledin *et al.*, 1999), as well as in the renal medullary collected tubules. It is homologous with a newly discovered cullin family of proteins which are involved in the regulation of cellular signalling by calcium, cyclic AMP (Burnatowska-Hledin *et al.*, 2000) and the MAPK-dependant pathway (Sartor *et al.*, 2006). On the basis of molecular recognition theory, this predicts that binding domains of peptides and their corresponding receptor binding domains evolved from complementary strands of genes. Ruiz-Opazo *et al.* identified a novel, dual, angiotensin II/vasopressin receptor in 1995 and a vasopressin VI type receptor in 2001 (Herrera and Ruiz-Opazo, 2001). The dual AngII/AVP receptor (or AVR) responds with equivalent affinities to angiotensin II and vasopressin, is coupled to adenyl cyclase and cosegregates with salt-sensitive hypertension in the Dahl hypertensive rat model (Ruiz-Opazo *et al.*, 2002).

Two different teams have reported that both above mentioned receptors are expressed in the central nervous system of the rat where they might mediate some effects of vasopressin (Hurbin *et al.*, 2000, Ceremuga *et al.*, 2001). However, a clear characterization of these two receptors is still lacking and their physiological role remains to be fully assessed. This is all the more needed as Albrecht *et al.* (2003) have reported that

AVR is contained in a larger protein, PYPAF5 (or Nalp6), which is a member of a large family of proteins described only as cytosolic proteins, thus questioning the functional existence of AVR as a *bona fide* transmembrane receptor. However Herrera *et al.* (2008) very recently showed that the Nap6/PYPAF5 locus contains overlapping genes which are coding for two V2-type vasopressin isoreceptors, the angiotensin-vasopressin receptor AVR and another one which binds vasopressin but not angiotensin, called for that reason non-AVR or NAVR. Whether those newly identified receptors are responsible for the vasopressin effects which are thought not to be transduced by the classical V1a, V1b and V2 receptors (Sabatier *et al.*, 2004) is still an open question.

Bibliography

Abramow-Newerly M., Roy A.A., Nunn C., Chidiac P. (2006). RGS proteins have a signalling complex: interactions between RGS proteins and GPCRs, effectors and auxiliary proteins. *Cellular Signalling* 18: 579–591

Aguilera G., Pham Q., Rabadan-Diehl C. (1994). Regulation of pituitary vasopressin receptors during chronic stress: relationship to corticotroph responsiveness. *J. Neuroendocrinol.* 6: 299–304

Aguilera G., Rabadan-Diehl C. (2000). Vasopressinergic regulation of the hypothalamic-pituitary-adrenal axis: implications for stress adaptation. *Regul Pep* 96: 23–29

Aguilera G., Volpi S., Rabadan-Diehl C. (2003). Transcriptional and post-transcriptional mechanisms regulating the rat pituitary vasopressin V1b receptor gene. *J Mol Endocrinol* 30: 99–108

Ala Y., Morin D., Sabatier N., Vargas R., Cotte N., Déchaux M., Antignac C., Arthus M.F., Lonergan M., Turner M.S., Balestre M.N., Alonso G., Hibert M., Barberis C., Hendy G.N., Bichet D.G., Jard S. (1998). Functional studies of twelve mutant V2 vasopressin receptors related to diabetes insipidus: molecular basis of a mild clinical phenotype. *J Am Soc Nephrol* 9: 1861–1872

Ahn S., Shenoy S.K., Wei H., Lefkowitz R.J. (2004). Differential kinetic and spatial patterns of beta-arrestin and G protein-mediated ERK activation by the angiotensin II receptor. *J Biol Chem* 279: 35518–35525

Albrecht M., Domingues F.S., Schreiber S., Lengauer T. 2003, Identification of mammalian orthologs associates PYPF5 with distinct funtional roles, *FEBS Lett* 538: 173–177

Ammar A., Roseau S., Butlen D. (1992). Pharmacological characterization of V1a vasopressin receptors in the rat cortical collecting duct. *Am J Physiol* 262: 546–553

Aurbach G.D., Chase L.R. (1968). Renal adenylate cyclase anatomically separate sites for parathyroid hormone and vasopressin. *Science* 159: 545–547

Azzi M., Charest P.G., Angers S., Rousseau G., Kohout T., Bouvier M., Pineyro G. (2003). β-arrestin–mediated activation of MAPK by inverse agonists reveals distinct active conformation for G protein-coupled receptors. *Proc Nat Acad Sci USA* 100: 11406–11411

Van Balkom B.W., Savelkoul P.J., Markovitch D., Hofman E., Nielsen S., van der Sluijs P., Deen P.M. (2002). The role of putative phosphorylation sites in the targeting and shuttling of the aquaporin-2 water channel. *J Biol Chem* 277: 41473–41479

Barberis C., Mouillac B., Durroux T. (1998). Structural basis of vasopressin/oxytocin receptor function. *J Endocrinol* 156: 223–229

Bernier V., Bichet D.G., Bouvier M. (2004). Pharmacological chaperone action on G-protein-coupled receptors. *Curr Opin Pharmacol* 4: 528–533

Bhora F.Y., Kothary P.C., Imanishi H., Eckhouser F.E., Raper S.E. (1994). Vasopressin stimulates DNA synthesis in cultures rat hepatocytes. *J Surg Res* 57: 706–710

Bichet D., Arthus M., Lonergan M., Henry G., Paradis A., Fujiwara M., Morgan K., Gregory M., Rosenthal W., Didwania A., Antaramian A., Birnbaumer M. (1993). X-linked nephrogenic diabetes insipidus mutations in North America and the Hopewell hypothesis. *J Clin Invest* 92: 1262–1268

Birnbaumer M., Seibold A., Gilbert S., Ishido M., Barberis C., Antaramian A., Barbet P., Rosenthal W. (1992). Molecular cloning of the receptor for human antidiuretic hormone. *Nature* 357: 333–335

Birnbaumer M., Antaramian A., Themmen A.P., Gilbert S. (1992). Desensitization of the human V2 vasopressin receptor. Homologous effects in the absence of heterologous desensitization. *J Biol Chem* 267: 11783–11788

Birnbaumer M., Gilbert S., Rosenthal W. (1994). An extracellular congenital nephrogenic diabetes insipidus mutation of the vasopressin receptor reduces cell surface expression, affinity for ligand and coupling to Gs/adenylyl cyclase system. *Mol Endocrinol* 8: 886–894

Birnbaumer M. (2000). Vasopressin receptors. *Trends Endocrinol Metab* 11: 406–410

Bocckino S.B., Blackmore P.F., Exton J.H. (1985). Stimulation of 1,2diacylglycerol accumulation in hepatocytes by vasopressin, epinephrine and angiotensin II. *J Biol Chem* 260: 14201–14207

Bockaert J., Roy C., Rajerison R., Jard S. (1973). Specific binding of 3H lysine vasopressin to pig kidney plasma membranes: relationship of receptor occupancy to adenylate cyclase activation. *J Biol Chem* 248: 5922–5931

Bockaert J., Pin J.P. (1998). G pour communiquer: un success évolutif, *C. R. Acad Sci Paris* 321: 529–551

Bockaert J., Pin J.P. (1999). Molecular tinkering of G protein coupled receptors: an evolutionary success. *EMBO J* 18: 1723–1729

Böhm S.K., Grady E.F., Bunnett N.W. (1997). Regulatory mechanisms that modulate signalling by G-protein-coupled receptors. *Biochem. J* 322: 1–18

Bouley R., Breton S., Sun T., McLaughlin M., Nsumu N.N., Lin H.Y., Ausiello D.A., Brown D. (2000). Nitric oxide and atrial natriuretic factor stimulate cGMP-dependent membrane insertion of aquaporin 2 in renal epithelial cells. *J Clin Invest* 106: 1115–1126

Bouley R., Pastor-Soler N., Cohen O., McLaughlin M., Breton S., Brown D. (2005). Stimulation of AQP2 membrane insertion in renal epithelial cells *in vitro* and *in vivo* by the cGMP phosphodiesterase inhibitor sildenafil citrate (Viagra). *Am J Physiol Renal Physiol* 288: 1103–1112

Bouley R., Hawthorn G., Russo L.M., Lin H.Y., Ausiello A., Brown D. (2006). Aquaporin 2 (AQP2) and vasopressin type 2 receptor (VR2) endocytosis in kidney epithelial cells: AQP2 is located in 'endocytosis-resistant' membrane domains after vasopressin treatment. *Biol Cell* 98: 215–232

Bourne H., Sanders D.A., McCormick F. (1991). The GTPase super family: conserved structure and molecular mechanism. *Nature* 349: 117–127

Bourne H. (1997). How receptors talk to trimeric G proteins. *Curr Opin Cell Biol* 9: 134–142

Bowen-Pidgeon D., Innamorati G., Sadeghi H.M., Birnbaumer M. (2001). Arrestin effects on internalization of vasopressin receptors. *Mol Pharmacol* 59: 1395–1401

Briley E.N., Lolait S.J., Axelrod J., Felder C.C. (1994). The cloned vasopressin V1a receptor stimulates phospholipase A2, phospholipase C and phospholipase D through activation of receptor-operated calcium channels. *Neuropeptides* 27: 63–74

Brown E., Clarke D.L., Roux V., Sherman D.H. (1963). The stimulation of adenosine-3'5' monophosphate production by antidiuretic factors. *J Biol Chem* 238: 852–853

Burnatowska-Hledin M.A., Spielman W.S., Smith W.L., Shi P., Meyer J.M., Dewitt D.L. (1995). Expression cloning of an AVP-activated, calcium mobilizing receptor from kidney medulla. *Am J Physiol* 268: C1198–C1210

Burnatowska-Hledin M., Lazdins I.B., Listenberger L., Zhao P., Sharangpani A., Card B. (1999). VACM-1 receptor is specifically expressed in rabbit vascular endothelium and renal collecting tubules. *Am J Physiol* 276: C199–C209

Burnatowska-Hledin M., Zhao P., Capps B., Poel A., Parmelee K., Mungall C., Sharangpani A., Listenberger L. (2000). VACM-1, a cullin gene family member, regulates cellular signalling. *Am J Physiol* 279: C266–C273

Butlen D., Guillon G., Rajerison R.M., Jard S., Sawyer W.H., Manning M. (1978). Structural requirements for activation of vasopressin–sensitive adenylate cyclase, hormone binding, and antidiuretic actions: effects of highly potent analogues and competitive inhibitors. *Mol Pharmacol* 14: 1006–1017

Cabrera-Vera T.M., Vanhauwe J., Thomas T.O., Medkova M., Preininger A., Mazzoni M.R., Hamm H.E. (2003). Insights into G protein structure, function and regulation. *Endocrine Rev* 24: 765–781

Chabardes D., Gagnan-Brunette M., Imbert-Teboul M., Gontcharevskaia O., Montégut M., Clique A., Morel F. (1980). Adenylate cyclase responsiveness to hormones in various portions of the human nephron. *J Clin Invest* 65: 439–448

Cantau B., Guillon G., Alaoui M.F., Chicot D., Balestre M.N., Devilliers G. (1988). Evidence of two steps in the homologous desensitization of vasopressin-sensitive phospholipase C in WRK1 cells. Uncoupling and loss of vasopressin receptors. *J Biol Chem* 263: 10443–10450

Ceremuga T.E., Yao X.L., McCabe J.T. (2001). Vasopressin-activated calcium-mobilizing (VACM-1) receptor mRNA is expressed in peripheral organs and the central nervous system of the laboratory rat. *Endocrinol Res* 27: 433–445

Charest P.G., Bouvier M. (2003). Palmitoylation of the V2 vasopressin receptor carboxy tail enhances β-arrestin recruitment leading to efficient receptor endocytosis and ERK 1/2 activation. *J Biol Chem* 278: 41541–41551

Cheung R., Mitchell J. (2002). Mechanisms of regulation of G11α protein by dexamethasone in osteoblastic UMR 106-01 cells. *Am J Physiol Endocrinol Metab* 282: 24–30

Chini B., Mouillac B., Balestre M.N., Trumpp-Kallmeyer S., Hoflack J., Elands J., Hibert M., Manning M., Jard S., Barberis C. (1995). Tyr 115 is the key residue for determining agonist selectivity in the V1a vasopressin receptor. *Eur Mol Biol Org J* 14: 2176–2182

Conner M., Hawtin S.R., Simms J., Wootten D.L., Lawson Z., Conner A.C., Parslow R.A.,Wheatley M. 2007, Systematic analysis of the entire second extracellular loop of the V1a vasopressin receptor: key residues, conserved throughout a G-protein-coupled receptor family, identified. *J Biol Chem* 282: 17405–17412

Cotte N., Balestre M.N., Phalipou S., Hibert M., Manning M., Barberis C., Mouillac B. (1998). Identification of residues responsible for the selective binding of peptide antagonists and agonists in the V2 vasopressin receptor. *J Biol Chem* 273: 29462–29468

Cotte N., Balestre M.N., Aumelas A., Mahé E., Phalipou S., Morin D., Hibert M., Manning M., Durroux T., Barberis C. (2000). Conserved aromatic residues in the transmembrane region VI of the V1a vasopressin receptor differentiate agonist vs antagonist ligand binding. *Eur J Biochem* 267: 4253–4263

Defer N., Best-Belpmomme M., Hanoune J. (2000). Tissue specificity and physiological relevance of various isoforms of adenylyl cyclase. *Am J Physiol Renal Physiol* 279: 400–416

Derick S., Pena A., Durroux T., Wagnon J., Serradeil-Le Gal C., Hibert M., Rognan D., Guillon G. (2004). Key amino acids located within the transmembrane domains 5 and 7 account for the pharmacological specificity of the human V1b vasopressin receptor. *Mol Endocrinol* 18: 2777–2789

Devost D., Zingg H.H. (2004). Homo and heterodimeric complex formations of the human oxytocin receptor. *J Neuroendocrinol* 16: 372–377

Ecelbarger C.A., Chou C.L., Lolait S.J., Knepper M.A., Digiovanni S.R. (1996). Evidence for dual signaling pathways for V2 receptor in rat inner medullary collecting duct. *Am J Physiol Renal Physiol* 270: 623–633

Erlenbach I., Wess J. (1998). Molecular basis for the V2 vasopressin receptor/Gs coupling selectivity. *J Biol Chem* 273: 26549–26558

Exton J.H., Blackmore P.F., El-Refai M.F., Dehaye J.P., Strickland W.G., Cherrington A.D., Chan T.M., Assimacopoulos-Jeannet F.D., Chrisman T.D. (1981).

Mechanisms of hormonal regulation of liver metabolism. *Adv Cyclic Nucleotide Res* 14: 491–505

Fenton R.A., Moeller H.B., Hoffert J.D., Yu M.J., Nielsen S., Knepper M.A. (2008). Acute regulation of aquaprin-2phosphorylation at Ser-264 by vasopressin. *Proc Nat Acad Sci USA* 105: 3134–3139

Firsov D., Mandon B., Morel J., Merot S., Lemout S., Bellanger A.C., de Rouffignac C., Elalouf J.M., Buhler J.M. (1994). Molecular analysis of vasopressin receptors in the rat nephron. Evidence for alternative splicing of the V2 receptor. *Pflugers Arch* 429: 79–89

Flouret G., Terada S.H., Nakahara T., Hechter O. (1977). Iodinated neurohypophyseal hormones as potential ligands for receptor binding and intermediates in synthesis of tritiated hormones. *Biochemistry* 16: 2119–2123

Fong C.T.O., Schwartz I.L., Popenoe E.A., Silver L., Schloesser M.A. (1959). On the molecular binding of lysine vasopressin at its renal receptor sites. *J Am Soc Chem* 81: 2592–2593

Frederiksson R., Lagerstrom M.C., Lundin L.G., Schioth H.B. (2003). The G-protein-coupled receptors in the human genome form five main families. Phylogenetic analysis, paralogon groups and fingerprints. *Mol Pharm* 63: 1256–1272

Gilman A.G. (1987).G proteins: transducers of receptor-generated signals. *Ann Rev Biochem* 56: 615–649

Ghosh P.M., Mikhailova M., Bedolla R., Kreisberg J.I. (2001). Arginine vasopressin stimulates mesangial cell proliferation by activating the epidermal growth factor. *Am J Physiol Renal Physiol* 280: 972–979

Giguere V., Labrie F. (1982). Vasopressin potentiates cyclic AMP accumilation and ACTH release induced by corticotrophin-releasing factor (CRF) in rat anterior pituitary cells in culture. *Endocrinology* 111: 1752–1754

Gopolakrishnan V., McNeill J., Sulakhe P., Triggle C. (1988). Hepatic vasopressin receptor: differential effects of divent cations, guanine nucleotides and N-ethylmaleimide on agonist and antagonist interactions with the V1 subtype receptor. *Endocrinology* 1232: 922–931

Grazzini E., Breton C., Derick S., Andres M., Raufaste D., Rickwaert F., Boccara G., Colson P., Guerineau N.C., Serradeil-Le Gal C. (1999). Vasopressin receptors in human adrenal medulla and pheochromocytoma. *J Clin Endocrinol Metab* 84: 2195–2203

Grenier S., Terrillon S., Pascal R., Dénémé H., Bouvier M., Guillon G., Mendre C. (2004). A cyclic peptide mimicking the third intracellular loop of the V2 vasopressin receptor inhibits signalling through its interaction with receptor dimmer and G protein. *J Biol Chem* 279: 50904–50914

Guillon G., Butlen D., Cantau B., Barth T., Jard S. (1982). Kinetic and pharmacological characterization of vasopressin membrane receptors from human kidney medulla: relation to adenylate cyclase activation. *Eur J Pharmacol* 85: 291–304

Guillon G., Gaillard R.C., Kehrer P., Schoenenberg P., Muller A.F., Jard S. (1987). Vasopressin and angiotensin induce inositol lipid breakdown in rat adenohyphysial cells in primary culture. *Reg Pept* 18: 119–129

Guillon G. (1989). Récepteurs de la vasopressine, de l'ocytocine et de l'angiotensine II chez les mammifères. *Ann Endocrinol* 50: 425–433

Hanoune J., Defer N. (2001). Regulation and role of adenylyl cyclase isoforms. *Ann Rev Pharmacol Toxicol* 41: 145–174

Haussmann H., Richters A., Kreienkamp H., Meyerhof W., Mattei H., Lederis K., Zwiers H., Richter D. (1996). Mutational analysis and molecular modelling of the nonapeptide hormone binding domains of the Arg^8 vasotocin receptor. *Proc Nat Acad Sci USA* 93: 6907–6912

Hawtin S.R., Wesley V.J., Parslow R.A., Simms J., Miles A., McEvan K., Wheatley M. (2002). A single residue (arg46) located in the N-terminus of the V1a vasopressin receptor is critical for binding vasopressin but not peptide or nonpeptide antagonists. *Mol Endocrinol* 16: 600–609

Hawtin S.R., Wesley V.J., Simms J., Argent C.C.H., Latif K., Wheatley M. (2005). The N-terminal juxtamembrane segment of the V1a vasopressin receptor provides two independent epitopes required for high-affinity agonist binding and signalling. *Mol Endocrinol* 19: 2871–2881

Hawtin S.R. (2005). Charged residues of the conserved DRY triplet of vasopressin V1a receptor provide molecular determinants for cell surface delivery and internalization. *Mol Pharmacol* 68: 1172–1182

Hélies-Toussaint C., Aarab L., Gasc J.M.L., Verbavatz J.M., Chabardès D. (2000). Cellular localization of type 5 and type 6 ACs in collecting duct and regulation of cAMP synthesis. *Am J Physiol Renal Physiol* 79: 185–194

Hems D.A., Whitton P.D. (1973). Stimulation of glycogen breakdown and gluconeogenesis in the perfused rat liver. *Biochem J* 136: 705–709

Henderson R.J., Baldwin J., Ceska T.H., Zemlin F., Beckman L., Downing K. (1990). Model for the structure of bacteriorhodopsin based on high s-resolution cryomicroscopy. *J Mol Biol* 21: 899–929

Henn V., Edemir B., Stefan E., Wiesner B., Lorenz D., Theilig F., Schmlitt R., Vosselbein L., Tamma G., Beyermann M., Krause E., Herberg F.W., Valenti G., Bachmann, Rosenthal W., Krussmann E. (2004). Identification of a novel A-kinase anchoring protein 18 isoform and evidence for its role in the vasopressin-induce aquaporin shuttle in renal principal cells. *J Biol Chem* 279: 26654–26665

Henn V., Stefan E., Baillie G.S., Houslay M.D., Rosenthal W., Klussmann E. (2005). Compartmentalized camp signalling regulates vasopressin-mediated water reabsorption by controlling aquaporin 2. *Biochem Soc Trans* 33: 1316–1318

Hernando F., Schoots O., Lolait S.J., Burbach J.P. (2001). Immunohistochemical localization of the vasopressin V1b receptor in the rat brain and pituitary gland: anatomical support for its involvement in the central effect of vasopressin. *Endocrinology* 142: 1659–1668

Herrera V.L., Ruiz-Opazo N. (2001). Identification of a novel V1-type AVP receptor based on the molecular recognition theory. *Mol Med* 7: 499–506

Herrera V.L., Bagamasbad P., Didishvili T., Decano J.L., Ruiz-Opazo N. (2008). Ovrelapping genes in Nalp6/PAPF5 locus encodes two V2-type vasopressin isoreceptors: angiotensin-vasopressin receptor (AVR) and non-AVR. *Physiol Genomics* 34: 65–77

Hibert M., Trumpp-Kallmeyer S., Hoflack J. (1993). This is not a G protein-coupled receptor. *Trends Pharmacol Sci* 14: 7–12

Hibert M., Hoflack J., Strumpp-Kallmeyer S., Mouillac B., Chini B., Mahé E., Cotte N., Jard S., Manning M., Barberis C. (1999). Functional architecture of vasopressin/oxytocin receptors. *J Receptor Signal Trans Res* 19: 589–596

Hocher B., Merker H.J., Durr J.A., Schiller S., Gross P., Hensen J. (1992). Internalization of V2-vasopressin receptors in LLC-PKI cells: evidence for receptor-mediated endocytosis. *Biochem Biophys Res Comm* 186: 1376–1383

Hoffert J.D., Pisikin T., Wang G., Shen R.F., Knepper M. (2006). Quantitative phosphoproteomics of vasopressin-sensitive renal cells: regulation of aquaporin-2 phosphorylation at two sites. *Proc Nat Acad Sci USA* 103: 7159–7164

Holmes M.C., Antoni F., Szentendrei T. (1984). Pituitary receptors for corticotropin-releasing factor: no effect of vasopressin on binding or activation of adenylate cyclase. *Neuroendocrinology* 39: 162–169

Hoorn E.J., Pisitkun T., Yu M.J., Knepper M.A. (2008). Proteomics approaches for the study of cell signalling in the renal collecting duct. *Contrib Nephrol* 160: 172–185

Howl J., Wheatley M. (1996). Molecular recognition of peptide and non-peptide ligands by the extra-cellular domains of neurohyohysial hormones. *Biochemical J* 317: 577–582

Hurbin A., Orcal H., Ferraz C., Moos F.C., Rabie A. (2000). Expression of the genes encoding the vasopressin-activated calcium mobilizing receptor and the dual angiotensinII/vasopressin receptor in the rat central nervous system. *J Neuroendocrinol* 12: 677–684

Imbert M., Chabardes D., Montégut M., Clique A., Morel F. (1975a). Adenylate cyclase activity along the rabbit nephron as mesured in single isolated segments. *Pflugers Arch* 354: 213–228

Imbert M., Chabardes D., Montégut M., Clique A., Morel F. (1975b). Vasopressin dependent adenylate cyclase in single segments of rabbit kidney tubule. *Pflugers Arch* 357: 173–186

Imbert-Teboul M., Chabardes D., Montégut M., Clique A., Morel F. (1978). Vasopressin-dependent adenylate cyclase activities in the kidney medulla: evidence for two separate sites of action. *Endocrinology* 102: 1254–1261

Innamorati G., Sadeghi H., Birnbaumer M. (1996). Fully active nonglycosylated V2 vasopressin receptor. *Mol Pharmacol* 50: 467–473

Innamorati G., Sadeghi H., Eberle A.N, Birnbaumer M. (1997). Phosphorylation of the V2 vasopressin receptor. *J Biol Chem* 272: 2486–2492

Innamorati G., Sadeghi H., Birnbaumer M. (1998a). Transient phosphorylation of the V1a vasopressin receptor. *J. Biol Chem* 273: 7155–7161

Innamorati G., Sadeghi H.M., Tran N.T., Birnbaumer M. (1998b). A serine cluster prevents recycling of the V2 vasopressin receptor. *Proc Nat Acad Sci USA* 95: 2222–2226

Innamorati G., Sadegui H.,Birnbaumer M. (1999). Phosphorylation and recycling kinetics of G protein coupled receptors. *J Receptor Signal Transduct Res* 19: 315–326

Innamorati G., Le Gouill C., Balamotis M., Birnbaumer M. (2001). The long and the short Cycle. Alternative intracellular routes for trafficking of G-protein-coupled receptors. *J Biol Chem* 276: 13096–13103

Izumi Y., Nakayama Y., Mori T., Miyazaki H., Inoue H., Kohda Y., Inoue T., Nonoguchi H., Tomita K. (2008). Down-regulation of vasopressin V2 receptor promoter activity via V1a receptor pathway. *Am J Physiol* 292: 1418–1426

Jans D., Jans P., Luzius H., Fahrenholz F. (1992). N-glycosylation plays a role in biosynthesis and internalization of the adenylate cyclase stimulating vasopressin V2 receptor of LLC-PK1 renal epithelial cells: an effect of concanavalin A on binding and expression. *Arch Biochem Biophys* 294: 64–69

Jard S. (1983). Vasopressin isoreceptors in mammals: relation to cyclic AMP-dependent and cyclic AMP-independent transduction mechanisms. *Curr Topics in Membrane Transport* 18: 255–285

Jard S. (1998). Vasopressin receptors; a historical survey. *Adv Exp Med Biol* 449: 1–13

Jard S., Gaillard R.C., Guillon G., Marie J., Schoenenberg P., Muller A.F., Manning M., Sawyer W.H. (1986). Vasopressin antagonists allow demonstration of a novel type of vasopressin receptor in the rat adenohypophysis. *Mol Pharmacol* 30: 171–177

Kamsteeg E.J., Heijnen I., van Os C.H., Deen P.M. (2000). The subcellular localization of an aquaporin-2 tetramer depends on the stoichiometry of phosphorylated and non phosphorylated monomers. *J Cell Biol* 151: 919–930

Kamsteeg E.J., Hendriks G., Boone M., Konings I.B., Oorschot V, van der Sluijs P., Klumperman J., Deen P.M. (2006), Short-chain ubiquitination mediates the regulated endocytosis of the aquaporin-2 water channel. *Proc Nat Acad Sci USA* 103: 18344–18349

de Keyzer Y., Auzan C., Lenne F., Beldjord C., Thibonnier M., Bertagna X., Clauser E. (1994). Cloning and characterization of the human V3 pituitary vasopressin receptor. *FEBS Lett* 356: 215–220

de Keyzer Y., Auzan C., Beldjord C., Luton J.P., Clauser E., Bertagna X. (1995). Expression du récepteur vasopressinergique V2 dans les adénomes corticotropes humains: un rôle dans la sécrétion d'ACTH? *Ann Endocrinol* 56: 444–445

de Keyzer Y., Lenne F., Auzan C., Jegou S., René P., Vaudry H., Kuhn J.M., Luton J.P., Clauser E., Bertagna X. (1996). The pituitary V3 vasopressin receptor and the corticotroph phenotype in ectopic ACTH syndrome. *J Clin Invest* 97: 1311–1318 de Keyzer Y., René P., Lenne F., Auzan C., Clauser E., Bertagna X. (1997). V3 vasopressin receptor and corticotropic phenotype in pituitary and non pituitary tumors. *Horm Res* 47: 259–262

Kirk C.J., Hems D.A. (1974). Hepatic action of vasopressin: lack of a role for adenosine-3',5'-cyclic monophosphate. *FEBS Lett* 47: 128–131

Kirk C.J., Mitchell R.H., Hems D.A. (1981). Phosphatidylinositol metabolism stimulated by vasopressin. *Biochem J* 194: 155–165

Kirk K.L. (1988). Binding and internalization of a fluorescent vasopressin analogue by collecting duct cells. A. *J Physiol* 255: 622–632

Knepper M.A., Valtin H., Sands J.M. (2000). Renal action of vasopressin, In Handbook of Physiology. Section 7, Vol 3, Endocrine regulation of water and electrolyte balance, 496–529

Koenig J.A., Edwardson J.M. (1997). Endocytosis and recycling of G protein-coupled receptors. *Trends Pharmacol Sci* 18: 276–287

Kojro E., Eich P., Gimpl G., Fahrenholz F. (1993). Direct identification of an extracellular agonist binding site in the renal V2 vasopressin receptor family. *Biochemistry* 32: 13537–13544

Laycock J.F., Hanoune J. (1998). From vasopressin receptor to water channel: intracellular traffic, constraint and by-pass. *J Endocrinol* 159: 361–372

Laycock J.F., Williams P.G (1973). The effect of vasopressin (pitressin) administration on sodium, potassium and urea excretion in rats with and without diabetes insipidus (DI), with a note on the excretion of vasopressin in the DI rat. *J Endocrinol* 56: 111–120

Lee B., Yang C., Chen T.H., al-Azawi N., Hsu W.H. (1995). Effect of AVP and oxytocin on insulin release: involvement of V1b receptors. *Am J Physiol* 269: 1095–1100

Lefkowitz R.J. (1994). Rodbell and Gilman win 1994 Nobel prize for Physiology and Medicine. *Trends Pharmacol Sci* 15: 442–44

Lefkowitz R.J., Shenoy S.K. (2005). Transduction of receptor signals by β-arrestins. *Science* 308: 512–517

Le Gouill C., Innamorati G., Birnbaumer M. (2002). An expanded V2 receptor retention signal. *FEBS Lett* 532: 363–366

Leng G. (2007). Proteomics: inspiring new hypotheses in the vasopressin system. *Endocrinology* 148: 3039–3040

Levy A., Lightman S.L., Hoyland J., Mason W.T. (1990). Inositol phospholipids turnover and intra-cellular calcium responses to thyrotopin-releasing hormone, gonadotropin-releasing hormone and arginine vasopressin in pituitary corticotroph and somatotroph adenomas. *Clin Endocrinol* 33: 73–79

Liu J., Wess J. (1996). Different single receptors domains determine the distinct G protein coupling profiles of members of the vasopressin receptor family. *J Biol Chem* 271: 8772–8778

Lolait S.J., O'Carroll A.M., McBridge O.W., Konig M., Morel A., Brownstein M.J. (1992). Cloning and characterization of a vasopressin V2 receptor and possible link to nephrogenic diabetes insipidus. *Nature* 357: 336–339

Lolait S.J., O'Carrol A.M., Mahan L.C., Felder C.C., Button D.C., Young W.S., Mezey E., Brownstein M.J. (1995). Extra-pituitary expression of the rat V1b receptor gene. *Proc Nat Acad Sci USA* 92: 6783–6787

Lu H.A., Sun T.X., Matsuzaki T., Yi X.H., Eswara J., Bouley R., McKee M., Brown D. (2007). Heat shock protein 70 interacts with aquaporin-2 (AQP2) and regulates its trafficking. *J Biol Chem* 282: 28721–28732

Madziva M.T., Birnbaumer M. (2006). A role for ARF6 in the processing of G protein-coupled receptors. *J Biol Chem* 281: 12178–12186

Marchingo A.J., Abrahamls J.M., Woodcock E.A., Smith A.I., Mendelsohn F.A.O., Johnston C.I. (1988). Properties of ^{3}H-desamino-8-D-arginine vasopressin as a radioligand for vasopressin V_2-receptors in rat kidney. *Endocrinology* 122: 1328–1336

Mazzocchi G., Markowska A., Malendowicz L.K., Musajo F., Meneghelli V., Nussdorfer G.G. (1993). Evidence that endogenous arginine-vasopressin (AVP) is involved in the maintenance of the growth and steroidogenic capacity of rat adrenal zona glomerulosa. *J Steroid Biochem Mol Biol* 45: 251–256

Mendre C., Dufour M.N., Le Roux S., Seyer R., Guillou L., Callas B., Guillon G. (1997). Synthetic rat V1a vasopressin receptor fragments interfere with vasopressin binding via specific interaction with the receptor. *J Biol Chem* 272: 21027–21036

Milligan G. (2004). G protein-coupled receptor dimerization; function and ligand pharmacology. *Mol Pharmacol* 66: 1–7

Mitchell R.H, Kirk C.J., Billah M.M. (1979). Hormonal stimulation of phosphatidylinositol breakdown with particular reference to the hepatic effect of vasopressin. *Biochem Soc Trans* 7: 861–865

Morel F., Doucet A. (1986). Hormonal control of kidney functions at the cell level. *Physiol Rev* 66: 377–468

Morel A., O'Carroll A.M., Brownstein M.J. Lolait S.J. (1992). Molecular cloning and expression of a rat V1a arginine vasopressin receptor. *Nature* 356: 523–526

Morel A., Lolait S.J., Brownstein M.J. (1993). Molecular cloning and expression of rat V1a and V2 arginine vasopressin receptors. *Regul Peptides* 45: 53–59

Morin D., Cotte N., Balestre MN., Mouillac B., Manning M., Breton C., Barberis C. (1998). The D136A mutation of the V2 vasopressin receptor induces a constitutive activity which permits discrimination between antagonists with partial agonist and inverse agonist activities. *FEBS Lett* 441: 470–475

Moulliac B., Chini B., Balestre M.N, Elands J., Trumpp-Kallmeyer S., Hoflack J., Hilbert M., Jard S., Barberis C. (1995). The binding site of neuropeptide vasopressin V1a receptor. Evidence for a major localization within transmembrane regions. *J Biol Chem* 270: 25771–25777

Murasawa S., Matsubar H., Kizim K., Maruyam K., Mori Y., Inada M. (1995). Glucocorticoids regulate V1a vasopressin receptor expression by increasing mRNA stability in vascular smooth muscle cells. *Hypertension* 26: 665–669

Nishimoto G., Zelenina M., Aperia A., Nielsen S. (2000). Localization and regulation of PKA-phosphorylated AQP2 in response to V2 receptor agonist/antagonist treatment. *Am J Physiol Renal Physiol* 278: 29–42

Noda Y., Sasaki S. (2005). Trafficking mechanism of water channel aquaporin-2. *Biology Cell* 97: 885–892

Nonoguchi A., Owada A., Kobayashi N., Takayama M., Terada Y., Koike J., Ujiie K., Marumo F., Sakai T., Tomita K. (1995). Immunohistochemical localization of V2 vasopressin receptor along the nephron and functional role of luminal V2 receptor in terminal inner medullary collecting ducts. *J Clin Invest* 96: 1768–1778

Oliver G., Schäfer E.A. (1895). On the physiological action of extracts of pituitary body and certain other glandular organs. *J Physiol* 18: 277–279

Orloff J., Handler J.S. (1962). The similarity of effects of vasopressin, adenosine 3'5' phosphate (cyclic AMP) and theophylline on the toad bladder. *J Clin Invest* 41: 702–706

Ostrowski N.L., Lolait S.J., Bradley D.J., O'Carroll A.M., Brownstein M.J., Young W.S. (1992). Distribution of V1a and V2 vasopressin receptor messenger ribonucleic acids in rat liver, kidney, pituitary and brain. *Endocrinology* 131: 533–535

Ostrowski N.L., Young W.S., Knepper M.A., Lolait S.J. (1993). Expression of vasopressin V1a and V2 receptor messenger ribonucleic acid in liver and kidney of embryonic, developing and adult rats. *Endocrinology* 133: 1849–1859

Palczewski K., Kumasaka T., Hori T., Behnke C.A., Motoshima H., Fox B.A., Le Trong I., Teller D.C., Okada T., Stenkamp R.E. (2000). Crystal structure of rhodopsin, a G protein-coupled receptor. *Science* 289: 739–745

Park F., Koike G., Cowley A.W. (1998). Regional time-dependent changes in vasopressin V2 receptor expression in the rat kidney during water restriction. *Am J Physiol* 274: 906–913

Patel S., Gaspers L.D., Boucherie S., Memim E., Stellato K.A., Guillon G., Combettes L., Thomas A.P. (2002). Inducible nitric-oxide synthase attenuates vasopressin-dependent Ca signalling in rat hepatocytes. *J Biol Chem* 277: 33776–22782

Pavo I., Fahrenholz F. (1990). Differential inactivation of vasopressin receptor subtypes in isolated membranes and intact cells by N-ethylmaleimide. *FEBS Lett* 272: 205–208

Pfeiffer R., Kirsch J. Fahrenholz F. (1998). Agonist and antagonist-dependent internalization of the human vasopressin V2 receptor. *Exp Cell Res* 244: 327–339

Phalipou S., Cotte N., Carnazzi E., Seyer R., Mahe E., Jard S., Barberis C., Mouillac B.(1997). Mapping peptide-binding domains of the V1a vasopressin receptor with a photoactivatable linear peptide antagonist. *J Biol Chem* 272: 26536–26544

Phalipou S., Seyer R., Cotte N., Breton C., Barberis C., Hibert M., Mouillac B. (1999). Docking of linear peptide antagonist in the V1a vasopressin receptor.

Identification of binding domains by photoaffinity labelling. *J Biol Chem* 274: 23316–23327

Postina R., Kojro E., Fahrenholz F(1996). Separate agonist and peptide antagonist binding sites of the oxytocin receptor defined by their transfer into the V2 vasopressin receptor. *J Biol Chem* 271: 31593–31601

Pradelles P., Morgat J.L., Fromageot P., Camier M., Bonne D., Cohen, P., Bockaert J., Jard S. (1972). Tritium labelling of 8-lysine vasopressin and its purification by affinity chromatography on sepharose-bound neurophysins. *FEBS Lett* 26: 189–195

Prinster S.C., Hague C., Hall R.A. (2005). Heterodimerization of G protein-coupled receptors: specificity and functional significance. *Pharmacol Rev* 57: 289–298

Rabadan-Diehl C., Aguilera G. (1998). Glucocorticoids increase vasopressin V1b receptor coupling to phospholipase C. *Endocrinology* 139: 3220–3226

Rabadan-Diehl C., Lolait S.J., Aguilera G(1995). Regulation of pituitary vasopressin V1b receptor mRNA during stress in the rat. *J Neuroendocrinol* 7: 903–910

Rabadan-Diehl C., Volpi S., Nikodemova M., Aguilera G. (2003). Translational regulation of the vasopressin V1b receptor involves an internal ribosome entry site. *Mol Endocrinol* 17: 1959–1971

Rashid A.J., O'Dowd B.F., George S.R. (2004). Diversity and complexity of signalling through peptidergic G protein-coupled receptors. *Endocrinology* 145: 2645–2652

Ren X.R., Reiter E., Ahn S., Kim J., Chen W., Lefkowitz R.J. (2005). Different G protein-coupled receptor kinases govern G protein and β-arrestin mediated signalling of V2 vasopressin receptor. *Proc Nat Acad Sci USA* 102: 1448–1453

René P., de Keyser Y. (2002). The vasopressin receptor of corticotroph pituitary cells. *Prog Brain Res* 139: 345–357

Robben J.H., Knoers N.V.A.M., Deen P.M.T. (2004). Regulation of the vasopressin V2 receptor by vasopressin in polarized renal collecting duct cells. *Mol Biol Cell* 12: 5693–5699

Rodbell M., Birnbaumer L., Pohl S.L., Krans H.M. (1971). The glucagon-sensitive adenyl cyclase system in plasma membranes of rat liver. V. An obligatory role of guanyl nucleotides in glucagons action. *J Biol Chem* 246: 1877–1882

Rodrigo J., Pena A., Murat B., Trueba M., Duroux T., Guillon G., and Rognan D. (2007). Mapping the binding site of arginine vasopressin to V1a and V1b vasopressin receptors. *Mol Endocrinol* 21: 512–523

Rosenthal W., Antaramian A., Gilbert S., Birnbaumer M. (1993). Nephrogenic diabetes insipidus: a V2 vasopressin receptor unable to stimulate adenylyl cyclase. *J Biol Chem* 268: 13030–13033

Ruiz-Opazo N., Akimoto K., Herrera V.L.M. (1995). Identification of a novel dual angiotensinII/vasopressin receptor on the basis of molecular recognition theory. *Nature Med* 1: 1074–1081

Ruiz-Opazo N., Lpez L.V., Herrera V.L. (2002). The dual AngII/AVP receptor gene N119S/C163R variant exhibits sodium-induced dysfunction and cosegregates with salt-sensitive hypertension in the Dhal salt-sensitive hypertensive rat model. *Mol Med* 8: 24–32

Sabatier N., Shibuya I., Dayanithi G. (2004). Intracellular calcium increase and somatodendritic vasopressin release by vasopressin receptor agonists in the rat supraoptic nucleus: involvement of multiple transduction signals. *J Neuroendocrinol* 16: 221–236

Sadeghi H.M., Innamorati G., Dagarag M., Birnbaumer M. (1997). Palmitoylation of the V2 vasopressin receptor. *Mol Pharmacol* 52: 21–29

Saito M., Sugimoto T., Tahara A., Kawashima H. (1995). Molecular cloning and characterization of rat V1b vasopressin receptor: evidence for its expression in extra-pituitary tissues. *Biochem Biophys Res Comm* 212: 751–757

Saito M., Tahara A., Sugimoto T., Abe K., Furuichi K. (2000). Evidence that atypical vasopressin V(2) receptor in inner medulla of kidney is V(1b) receptor. *Eur J Pharmacol* 401: 289–296

Sarmiento J.M., Anazco C.C., Campos D.M., Prado G.N., Navarro J., Gonzalez C.B. (2004). Novel down-regulatory mechanism of the surface expression of the vasopressin V2 receptor by an alternative splice variant. *J Biol Chem* 279: 47017–47023

Sartor A., Kossoris J.B., Wilcox R., Shearer R., Zeneberg A.E., Zhao K., Lazdins I.B., Burnatowska-Hledin M.A. (2006). Truncated form of VACM-1/cul-5 with an extended 3′ untranslated region stimulates cell growth via a MAPK-dependent pathway. *Biochem Biophys Res Comm* 343: 1086–1093

Sato M., Blumer J.B., Simon V., Lanier S.M. (2006). Accessory proteins for G proteins: partners in signalling. *Ann Rev Pharmacol Toxicol* 46: 151–187

Schertler G., Villa C., Henderson R. (1993). Projection structure of rhodopsin. *Nature* 362: 770–772

Schwartz I.L., Schloesser M.A., Silver L., Fong C.T.O. (1960). Relation of the chemical attachment to physiological action of vasopressin. *Proc Nat Acad Sci USA* 46: 1288–1298.

Schwartz I.L., Rudinger J. (1964). Activity of neurohypophysial hormone analogues lacking a disulfide bridge. *Proc Nat Acad Sci USA* 52: 1044–1045

Serradeil-Le Gal C., Wagon J., Garcia C., Lacour C., Guiraudou P., Christophe B., Villanova G., Nisato D., Maffrand J.P., Le Fur G. (1993). Biochemical and pharmacological properties of SR 49059, a new, potent nonpeptide antagonist of rat and human vasopressin V1a receptors. *J Clin Invest* 92 : 224–231

Serradeil-Le Gal C., Lacour C., Valette G., Garcia G., Foulon L., Galindo G., Bankir L., Pouzet B., Guillon G., Barberis C. (1996). Characterization of SR 121463A, a highly potent and selective, orally active vasopressin V2 receptor antagonist. *J Clin Invest* 98: 2729–2738

Serradeil-Le Gal C., Raufaste D., Double-Cazenave E., Guillon G., Garcia C., Pascal M., Maffrand J.P. (2000). Binding properties of a selective tritiated V2 vasopressin receptor antagonist, H-SR 121463. *Kidney Int* 58: 1613–1622

Shen T.S., Suzuki Y., Poyard M., Miyamoto N., Defer N., Hanoune J. (1997). Expression of adenylyl cyclase mRNA in the adult, in the developing and in the Brattleboro rat kidney. *Am J Physiol* 273: 323–330

Stoeckel M.E., Freund-Mercier M.J., Palacios J.M., Richard P., Porte A. (1986). Autoradiographic localization of binding sites for oxytocin and vasopressin in the rat kidney. *J Endocrinol* 113: 179–182

Sugimoto T., Saito M., Mochizuki S., Watanabe Y., Hashimoto S., Kawashima H. (1994). Molecular cloning and functional expression of a cDNA encoding the V1b vasopressin receptor. *J Biol Chem* 269: 27088–27092

Surgand J.S., Rodrigo J., Kellenberger E., Rognan D. (2006). A chemogenomic analysis of the transmembrane binding cavity of human G-protein-coupled receptors. *Proteins* 62: 509–538

Sutherland E.W., Robison G.A. (1966). The role of cyclic-3',5'-AMP in responses to catecholamines other hormones. *Pharmacol Rev* 18:145–61

Tahtaoui C., Balestre M.N., Klotz P., Rognan D., Barberis C., Mouillac B., Hibert M. (2003). Identification of the binding sites of the SR49059 nonpeptide antagonist into the V1a vasopressin receptor using sulfydryl-reactive ligands and cysteine mutants as chemical sensor. *J Biol Chem* 278: 40010–40019

Tajima N., Nakae J., Takekoshi Y., Takahishi Y., Yuri K., Nagashima T., Fujieda K. (1996). Three novel A VPR2 mutations in three Japanese families with X-linked nephrogenic diabetes insipidus. *Pediatric Res* 39: 522–526

Tamma G., Klussmann E., Procino G., Svelto M., Rosenthal W., Valenti G. (2003). cAMP-induced AQP2 translocation is associated with RhoA inhibition through RhoA phosphorylation and interaction with RhoGDI. *J Cell Sci* 116: 1519–1525

Terashima Y., Kondo K., Mizuno Y., Iwasaki Y., Oiso Y. (1998). Influence of acute elevation of plasma AVP level on rat vasopressin V2 receptor and aquaporin 2 mRNA expression. *J Mol Endocrinol* 20: 281–285

Terrillon S., Durroux T., Mouillac B., Breit A., Ayoub M.A., Taulan M., Jockers R., Barberis C., Bouvier M. (2003). Oxytocin and Vasopressin V1a and V2 receptors form constitutive homo-and heterodimers during biosynthesis. *Mol Endocrinol* 17: 677–691

Terrillon S., Barberis C., Bouvier M. (2004). Heterodimerization of V1a and V2 vasopressin receptors determines the interaction with β-arrestin and their trafficking patterns. *Proc Nat Acad Sci USA* 101: 1548–1553

Thibonnier M., Goraya T., Berti-Mattera L. (1993). G protein coupling of human platelet V1 vascular vasopressin receptors. *Am J Physiol* 264: 1336–1344

Thibonnier M., Auzan C., Madhun Z., Wilkins P., Berti-Mattera L., Clauser E. (1994). Molecular cloning, sequencing and functional expression of a cDNA encoding the human V1a vasopressin receptor. *J Biol Chem* 269: 3304–3310

Thibonnier M., Preston J.A., Dulin N., Wilkins P.I., Berti-Matera L.N., Matera R. (1997). The human V3-pituitary receptor: ligand-binding profile and density-dependent signaling pathways. *Endocrinology* 138: 4109–4122

Thibonnier M., Coles P., Thibonnier A., Shoham M. (2001). The basic and clinical pharmacology of nonpeptide vasopressin receptor antagonists. *Ann Rev Pharmacol Toxicol* 41: 175–202

Tohgo A., Choy E.W., Gesty-Palmer D., Pierce K.L., Laporte S., Oakley R.H., Caron M.G., Lefkowitz R.J., Luttrell L.M. (2003). The stability of G protein-coupled receptor-arrestin interaction determines the mechanism and functional consequence of ERK activation. *J Biol Chem* 278: 6258–6267

Ufer E., Postina R., Gorbulev V., Fahrenholz F. (1995). An extracellular residue determines the agonist specificity of V2 vasopressin receptors. *FEBS Lett* 362: 19–23

Valenti G., Procino G., Carmosino M., Frigeri A., Mannucci R., Nicoletti I., Svelto M. (2000). The phosphatase inhibitor okadaic acid induces AQP2 translocation independently from AQP2 phosphorylation in renal collecting duct cells. *J Cell Sci* 113: 1985–1992

Valenti G., Procino G., Tamma G., Carmosino M., Svelto M. (2005). Aquaporin 2 trafficking. *Endocrinology* 146: 5063–5070

Van den Ouweland A.M., Knoop M.T., Knoers V.V., Markslag P.W., Rocchi M., Warren S.T., Ropers H.H., Fahrenholz F., Monnens L.A., van Oust B.A. (1992). Colocalization of the gene for nephrogenic diabetes insipidus (DIR) and the vasopressin type 2 receptor gene (AVPR2) in the Xq28 region. *Genomics* 13: 1350–1352

Von den Velden (1913). Die Nierenwirkung von Hypophysenextracten beim Menschen. *Berl Klin Wochenschr* 50: 2083

Du Vigneaud V., Lawler H.C., Popenoe E.A. (1953). Enzymatic cleavage of glycinamide from vasopressin and a proposed structure for the pressor-antidiuretic hormone of the posterior hypophysis. *J Amer Chem Soc* 75: 4880–4881

Volpi S., Rabadan-Diehl C., Cawley N., Aguilera G. (2002). Transcriptional regulation of the pituitary vasopressin V1b receptor involves a GAGA-binding protein. *J Biol Chem* 277: 27829–27938

Volpi S., Rabadan-Diehl C., Aguilera G. (2004). Vasopressinergic regulation of the hypothalamic pituitary adrenal axis and adaptation. *Stress* 7: 75–83

Wange R.L., Smercka A.V., Strenweiss P.C., Exton J.H. (1991). Photoaffinity labelling of two rat liver plasma membrane proteins with 32 gamma-azidoanilido GTP in response to vasopressin. Immunologic identification as alpha subunits of the Gq class of G proteins. *J Biol Chem* 266: 11409–11412

Watters J.J., Swank M.W., Wilkinson C.W., Dorsa D.M. (1996). Evidence for glucocorticoid regulation of rat vasopressin V1a receptor gene. *Peptides* 17: 67–73

Watters J.J., Wilkinson C.W., Dorsa D.M. (1996). Glucocorticoid regulation of vasopressin V1a receptors in rat forebrain. *Mol Brain Res* 38: 276–284

Wettschureck N., Offermanns S. (2005). Mammalian G proteins and their cell type specific functions. *Physiol Rev* 85: 1159–1204

Wieland T., Mittmann C. (2003). Regulators of G-protein signaling: multifunctional proteins with impact on signalling in the cardiovascular system. *Trends Ther* 97: 95–115

Williams B., Stai P., Schrier R.W. (1992). Glucose-induces downregulation of angiotensin II and arginine vasopressin receptors in cultures rat aortic vascular smooth muscle cells. Role of protein kinase C. *J Clin Invest* 90: 1992–1999

Won J.G., Orth D.N. (1994). Role of lipoxygenase metabolites of arachidonic acid in the regulation of adrenocorticotropin secretion by perifused rat anterior pituitary cells. *Endocrinology* 135: 1496–1503

Wu N., Macion-Dazard R., Nithianantham S., Xu Z., Hanson S.M., Vishnivetskiy S.A., Gurevitch V.V., Thibonnier M., Shoham M. (2006). Soluble mimics of the cytoplasmic face of the human V1-vascular vasopressin receptor bind arrestin2 and calmodulin. *Mol Pharmacol* 70: 249–258

Wu S., Birnbaumer M., Guan Z., 2008, Phosphorylation analysis of G protein-couples receptor by mass spectrometry: identification of a phosphorylation site in V2 vasopressin receptor. *Annal Chem* 80: 6034–6037

Yi X., Bouley R., Lin H.Y., Bechoua S., Sun T.X., Del Re E., Shioda T., Raychowdhury M.K., Lu H., Abou-Samra A.B., Brown D., Ausiello D.A. (2007). Alix (AIPI) is a vasopressin receptor VR2) interacting protein that increases lysosomal degradation of the V2R. *Am J Physiol* 292: 1303–1313

Young L.J., Tolocko D., Insel T.R. (1999). Localization of vasopressin (V1a) receptor binding and mRNA in the rhesus monkey brain. *J Neuroendocrinol* 11: 291–297

Young S.F., Smith J.L., Figueroa J.P., Rose J.C. (2003). Ontogeny and effect of cortisol on vasopressin 1b receptor expression in anterior pituitaries of fetal sheep. *Am J Physiol Regul Integr Comp Physiol* 284: 51–56

Zhao L., Brinton R.D. (2002). Vasopressin-induced cytoplasmic and nuclear calcium signalling in cultured cortical astrocytes. *Brain Res* 943: 117–131

Zhu X., Gilbert S., Birnbaumer M., Birnbaumer L. (1994). Dual signalling potential is common among Gs-coupled receptors and dependent on receptor density. *Mol Pharmacol* 46: 460–469

CHAPTER 5

PHARMACOLOGY OF THE VASOPRESSIN RECEPTORS

Jacques Hanoune

Institut Cochin, 22 Rue Méchain, 75014 Paris, France
Email: jacques.hanoune@inserm.fr

1. Introduction

As soon as the structure of vasopressin and oxytocin was known, several groups endeavoured to synthesize selective agonists and antagonists (see Manning and Sawyer, 1993, for the early literature). More recently pharmaceutical companies have invested quite a lot of effort in finding chemical compounds which could be administered orally, focusing on nonpeptide antagonists. The technique used to identify compounds of interest was the high throughput screening of thousands of small, nonpeptide molecules (defined as having a molecular weight inferior or equal to 500) belonging to a variety of chemical libraries. This has led to the discovery of an impressive number of nonpeptide vasopressin ligands, some of which are currently undergoing clinical trial at various phases of development. The term 'vaptan' was coined to officially name all the members of this new class of drugs (e.g. Relcovalpan for SR 49059, Tolvaptan for OPC-41061, Lixivaptan for VPA 985, Conivaptan for YM-087). The reader will find extensive information about the chemical and physiological characterization of those molecules in recent reviews by Thibonnier *et al.*, 2001, Serradeil-Le Gal *et al.*, 2002, Decaux *et al.*, 2008, Manning *et al.*, 2008 and Chini *et al.*, 2008. A short list of some of the currently available molecules is shown in Table 1 while the potential clinical use of vasopressin antagonists is shown in Table 2.

2. Radio-labelled Ligands

As the use of radio-labelled ligands was, and still is, instrumental in the pharmacological characterization of new compounds, we will briefly describe them before tackling the actual pharmacology of the various receptor isoforms.

Table 1. Some orally active nonpeptide vasopressin antagonists.

Name	Company	Chemical series
V1a receptor		
OPC-21268	Otsuka	Quinolinone derivative
SR-49059 (**Relcovaptan**)	Sanofi	Indoline derivative
YM-218	Yamanouchi	Benzazepine derivative
V1b receptor		
SSR-149415	Sanofi	Oxindole derivative
V2 receptor		
OPC-31260	Otsuka	Benzazepine derivative
OPC-41061 (**Tolvaptan**)	Otsuka	Benzazepine derivative
SR-121463	Sanofi	Oxindole derivative
VPA-985 (**Lixivaptan**)	Wyeth-Ayerst	Benzodiazepine derivative
WAY-140288	Wyeth-Ayerst	Benzodiazepine derivative
VP-343 and VP-339	Wakamoto	Quinoxaline derivative
VP-365	Wakamoto	Benzodiazepine derivative
FR-161282	Fujisawa	Benzodiazepine derivative
Mixed V1a/V2 receptor		
YM-087 (**Conivaptan**)	Yamanouchi	Benzazepine derivative
YM-471	Yamanouchi	Benzazepine derivative
JVT-605	Japan Tobacco	Thiazepine derivative
CL-385004	Wyeth-Ayerst	Benzodiazepine derivative

Tritiated arginine vasopressin (^{3}H AVP) first became available in 1977 providing an important molecule with specific radioactivity (60–80 Ci/mM), and we now have access to tritiated lysine vasopressin (LVP) and oxytocin (OT) as well. However, the use of such ligands is impaired by the fact that AVP is the natural endogenous hormone in most mammals and therefore they have relatively little selectivity for the various receptor isoforms. Furthermore, AVP can bind to the OT receptor with a very good affinity, only 2- to 5-fold less than for the vasopressin receptor.

Iodination of structural analogues of either vasopressin (I-OH-LVA) or oxytocin (I-OTA) (Fig. 1) has led to ligands endowed with better affinity and selectivity. In particular, I-OH-LVA has an affinity for the V1a receptor of 30pM in humans and 8pM in rats (Barberis et al., 1995). This compound is the ligand of choice for the characterization of the V1a receptor in many tissues. It can bind to the V1b receptor with an affinity of about 500pM.

Table 2. Potential clinical indications for vasopressin antagonists. CNS, central nervous system; SIADH, syndrome of inappropriate antidiuretic hormone.

V1a	V1b	Mixed V1a/V2	V2
Dysmenorrhoea	Anxiety, depression	Congestive heart failure	Congestive heart failure
Raynaud's disease	Cushing's syndrome	Hypertension	Liver cirrhosis
Hypertension		Brain oedema	Hyponatraemia
Brain oedema			Nephrotic syndrome
Motion sickness			Glaucoma
Oncology			Hypertension
CNS disorders			Diabetic nephropathy
			Meniere's disease
			SIADH

3. Pharmacology of the Vasopressin V1a Receptor

In addition to I-OH-LVA, another specific V1a ligand is $d(CH_2)_5(Tyr(Me)^2AVP$ or 'Manning compound' (Kruszinski et al., 1980). It is a cyclic antagonist with a high affinity and selectivity for the V1a receptor, compared with V1b and V2 receptors, and also with the oxytocin receptor. However, in 1991 Otsuka developed a quinolinone derivative, OTC-21268, as the first nonpeptide V1a antagonist

(Yamamura *et al.*, 1991). Two years later, Sanofi developed another potent nonpeptide antagonist, SR-49059 (Relcovaptan) for the V1a receptor (Serradeil-Le Gal *et al.*, 1993). This compound exerts a potent anti-vasopressin activity *in vitro* and has been tested in preclinical studies for the treatment of hypertension and dysmenorrhoea (Bossmar *et al.*, 1997; Brouard *et al.*, 2000; Steinwall *et al.*, 2004) but was abandoned due to evidence of liver toxicity. More recently, a benzazepine derivative, YM-218, has been developed by Yamanouchi (Tahara *et al.*, 2005). It is interesting to note that SR-49059 has been used functionally to rescue constitutively internalized V2 receptor (Bernier *et al.*, 2004; Wüller *et al.*, 2004; Bernier *et al.*, 2006) and V1a receptor (Hawtin, 2006) mutations by increasing their conformational stability. These pharmacological chaperones constitute a potential treatment for X-linked nephrogenic diabetes insipidus (Bernier *et al.*, 2006).

While exogenous arginine vasopressin has a plasma half-life of up to 24 minutes, the clinically useful V1a receptor agonist triglycyl-lysine vasopressin (terlipressin) has a prolonged duration of action of 6 hours. It behaves like a prodrug and is converted to lysine vasopressin in the circulation after the N-triglycyl residue is cleaved by endothelial peptidases. It is used clinically to restore vascular tone and to reduce bleeding due to oesophageal variceal haemorrhage (Kam *et al.*, 2004) and to induce natriuresis in patients with cirrhosis (Krag *et al.*, 2007; Martin-Llahi *et al.*, 2008). Ferring Pharmaceuticals has developed a new peptidergic agonist derivative, F-180, by the addition of a homoglutamine in position 4 of the arginine vasopressin molecule. It has a very good affinity for the human and bovine V1a receptor, but less so for the rat receptor (Andres *et al.*, 2002). It is long-acting and appears to be 18 times more potent than terlipressin and 4 times more than arginine vasopressin (Bernadich *et al.*, 1998).

4. Pharmacology of the Vasopressin V1b Receptor

Two good peptidergic V1b receptor agonist derivatives are available: d(D-3-Pal^2)AVP (Schwartz *et al.*, 1991) and d(Cha^4)AVP, the latter only selective for the human receptor (Derrick *et al.*, 2002). More recently, Pena *et al.* (2007) have demonstrated that d(Leu4, Lys8) vasopressin is a very good V1b selective agonist for the rat vasopressin receptor, which

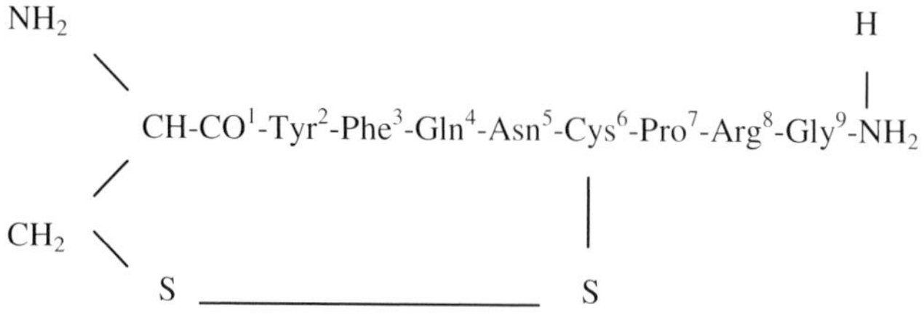

NH_2

\\

CH-CO^1-Tyr^2-Phe^3-Gln^4-Asn^5-Cys^6-Pro^7-Arg^8-Gly^9-NH$_2$

/   H

CH_2 \\ |

S ——————————— S

[^{3}H]AVP

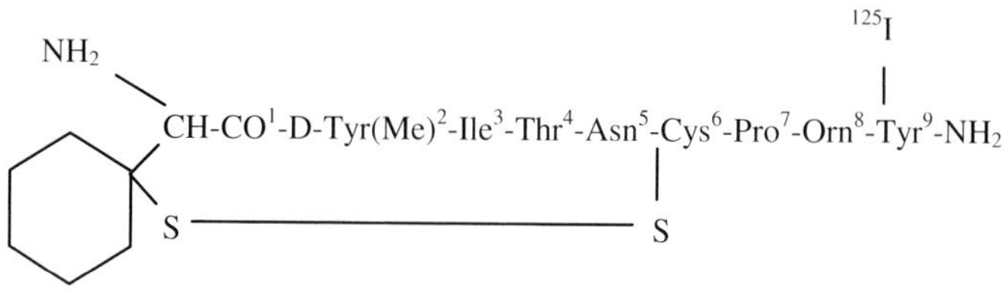

NH_2

\\ ^{125}I

CH-CO^1-D-Tyr(Me)^2-Ile^3-Thr^4-Asn^5-Cys^6-Pro^7-Orn^8-Tyr^9-NH$_2$

S ——————————— S

[^{125}I]-OH LVA

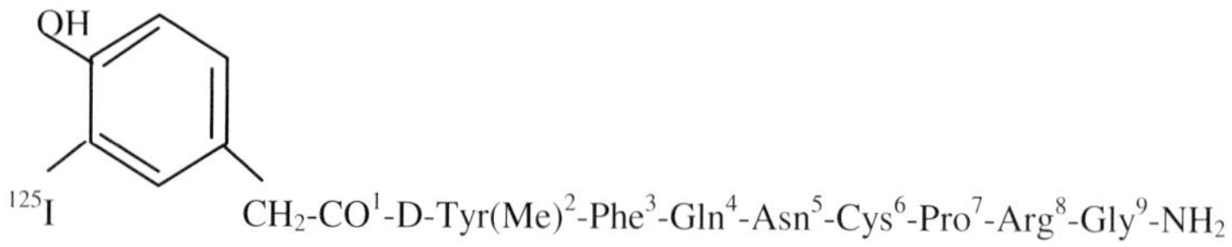

QH

^{125}I   CH$_2$-CO^1-D-Tyr(Me)^2-Phe^3-Gln^4-Asn^5-Cys^6-Pro^7-Arg^8-Gly^9-NH$_2$

[^{125}I]-OTA

Figure 1. Structure of the radioligands used to characterize the vasopressin receptors.

should be very useful in order to better delineate the potential clinical importance of the V1b receptor (Arban, 2007). Sanofi obtained the first non-peptidergic V1b antagonist, SSR-149415 (Serradeil-Le Gal et al.,

2002). It has been useful in demonstrating an axiogenic role for vasopressin via the V1b receptor (Griebel *et al.*, 2002; Serradeil-Le Gal *et al.*, 2005; Stemmelin *et al.*, 2005). It has recently been shown that SSR149415, in addition to its high potency for the human V1b receptor, also displays a significant antagonism for the human oxytocin receptor (Griffante *et al.*, 2005).

5. Pharmacology of the Vasopressin V2 Receptor

The structural analogue of AVP, desamino 8D arginine vasopressin, or desmopressin[R] (DDAVP) is a V2 agonist with very potent antidiuretic activity (Zaoral *et al.*, 1967) and it is used clinically in the treatment of central diabetes insipidus due to the lack of vasopressin. It has no affinity for V1a and oxytocin receptors and consequently does not induce vasoconstriction or uterine contraction. However it has a good affinity for the V1b receptor (Saito *et al.*, 1997) and can increase the level of circulating adrenocorticotrophic hormone (ACTH) in certain patients (Scott *et al.*, 1999). A modification of positions 3 and 4 of DDAVP has led to d(Thi3)VDAV, a very potent and selective V2 agonist in the rat (Ben Mimoun *et al.*, 2001), but unfortunately it is less selective in humans. Modification of the N-terminal part of vasopressin analogues with 2 aminoindane carboxylic acid markedly increases their affinity for the V2 receptor (Kowalczyk *et al.*, 2007).

Numerous selective orally active vasopressin V2 receptor antagonists have been produced by several pharmaceutical companies, in particular OPC-31260, OPC-41061 (Tolvaptan), VPA-985 (Lixivaptan) and SR 121463 (Satavaptan). The latter drug is highly selective in rats, cattle and humans and induces a massive diuresis in rats after oral or intravenous administration (Serradeil-Le Gal *et al.*, 1996). At present, it is one of the best compounds to characterize the V2 receptor (Serradeil-Le Gal, 2001). These vasopressin V2 antagonists, so-called 'aquaretics', are able to specifically promote water excretion without the well-known side effects of classical diuretic or saliuretic agents on urinary sodium or potassium loss. They have been tried in the treatment of cirrhosis, heart failure, and for the syndrome of inappropriate antidiuretic hormone secretion (SIADH). In addition, they might be of interest in other pathological conditions such as brain oedema or glaucoma (Lacherez *et al.*, 2000).

A completely different approach to obtain vasopressin antagonists has been developed by Purschke *et al.* (2006), based on aptamers and spiegelmers which are 3D nucleic structures that are capable of binding to target molecules. The compound NOX-F37 is able to bind and inhibit AVP with a good affinity and it increases diuresis in the rat. It apparently has a better affinity for the V2 receptor than for the V1a receptor.

Another potentially interesting alternative to classical vasopressin antagonists is the use of compounds such as the opioid agonist niravoline, which interacts with the κ-receptor at hypothalamic sites and subsequently inhibits vasopressin secretion (Bosch-Marcé *et al.*, 1999; Thibonnier *et al.*, 2001).

6. Mixed Vasopressin V1a/V2 Receptor Antagonists

This class of dual V1a and V2 receptor antagonists now includes several compounds, but only one, Conivaptan, (YM-087), has been tested in humans. It is assumed that blockade of both V1a and V2 receptors would achieve a decrease in arterial blood pressure by modifying both peripheral resistance and circulating blood volume. Similarly, it would improve the haemodynamic and fluid status in heart failure (Yatsu *et al.*, 2002), probably more efficiently than the use of pure V2 antagonists (Thibonnier, 2003; De Luca *et al.*, 2005; Goldsmith and Gheorghiade, 2005).

7. Inter-species and Inter-organ Variability

In all the pharmacological studies performed with the above mentioned compounds, a major restriction in reaching a firm conclusion as to their potential clinical use has been the relatively large variability in specificity, depending on the species used and on the organ studied. For example, DDAVP, a selective V2 agonist in the rat, is less so in humans. Likewise, F-180 is a good V1a agonist in humans and cattle but is not at all specific in the rat. SSR149415, a pure V1b antagonist in the rat, is probably a mixed V1b/oxytocin antagonist in humans. There are many such examples. A good and extensive discussion of these problems can be found in various publications (Andres *et al.*, 2004; Guillon *et al.*, 2004; 2006; Chini *et al.*, 2008).

Conversely, too great a receptor selectivity is not always ideal, as is the case in the treatment of congestive heart failure. Here, the use of a pure V2 antagonist might be less beneficial than that of a mixed one. In fact, and as is so often the case in pharmacology, the final clinical efficacy of a novel treatment using a vasopressin antagonist depends on many parameters, and the apparent selective effect on one type of receptor will be only one of them.

8. Conclusion

It is striking that in spite of several well defined, large, multicentre double-blind clinical trials, the current, therapeutic use of vasopressin antagonists is still limited to Conivaptan, which has been approved by the US Food and Drug Administration for the intravenous treatment of euvolemic and hypervolemic hyponatraemia, and to Mozavaptan which is only available in Japan for the treatment of the paraneoplastic syndrome of inappropriate antidiuretic hormone secretion. Tolvaptan, Lixivaptan and Satavaptan are currently in Phase III clinical trials. As noted by Decaux *et al.* (2008), insufficient clinical data are currently available to propose the use of vasopressin antagonists for other clinical disorders. One can hope that in the near future, the various potential pitfalls associated with the pharmacological use of those drugs should be sufficiently well circumscribed to warrant other uses.

J. Hanoune

Bibliography

Andres M., Trueba M., Guillon G. (2002). Pharmacological characterization of F-180: a selective human V1a vasopressin receptor agonist of high affinity. *Br J Pharmacol* 135: 1828–1836

Andres M., Pena A., Derick S., Raufaste D., Trojnar J., Wisniewski K., Trueba M., Serradeil-Le Gal C., Guillon G. (2004). Comparative pharmacology of bovine, human and rat vasopressin receptor isoforms. *Eur J Pharmacol* 501: 59–69

Arban R. (2007). V1b receptors: new probes for therapy. *Endocrinology* 148: 4133–4135

Barberis C., Balestre M.N., Jard S., Tribollet E., Arsenijevic Y., Dreiffuss J.J., Bankowski K., Manning M., Chan W.Y., Schlosser S.S., Holsboer F., Elands J. (1995). Characterization of a novel linear radioiodinated vasopressin antagonist: an excellent radioligand for vasopressin V1a receptor. *Neuroendocrinology* 62: 135–146

Ben Mimoun M., Derick S., Andres M., Guillon G., Wo N.C., Chazn W.Y.T., Stoev S., Cheng L.L.K., Manning M. (2001). Vasopressin V2 agonists in Martinez F. and Fehrentz J.A. (eds), Peptides, 589–590. EDK Editions, Paris.

Bernadich C., Bandi J.C., Melin P., Bosch J. (1998). Effects of F-180, a new selective vasoconstrictor peptide, compared with terlipressin and vasopressin on systemic and splanchnic hemodynamics in a rat model of portal hypertension. *Hepatology* 27: 351–356

Bernier V., Lagacé M., Lonergan M., Arthus M.F., Bichet D.G., Bouvier M. (2004). Functional rescue of the constitutively internalized V2 vasopressin receptor mutant R137H by the pharmacological chaperone action of SR49059. *Mol Endocrinol* 18: 2074–2084

Bernier V., Morello J.P., Zarruk A., Debrand N., Salahpour A., Lonergan M., Arthus M.F., Laperrière A., Brouard R., Bouvier M., Bichet D.G. (2006). Pharmacological chaperones as a potential treatment for X-linked nephrogenic diabetes insipidus. *J Am Soc Nephrol* 17: 232–243

Bosch-Marcé M., Poo J.L., Jimenez W., Bordas N., Leivas A. (1999). Comparison of two aquaretic drugs (niravoline and OPC-31260) in cirrhotic rats with ascites and water retention. *J Pharmacol Exp Ther* 289: 194–201

Bossmar T., Brouard R., Dobert A., Akermlund M. (1997). Effects of SR49059, an orally active V1a vasopressin receptor antagonist on vasopressin-induced uterine contraction. *B. J Obstet Gynaecol* 104: 471–477

Brouard R., Bossmar T., Fournie-Lloreet D., Chassard D., Akerlund M. (2000). Effect of SR49059, an orally active V1a vasopressin antagonist, in the prevention of dysmenorrhoea. *Br J Obstet Gyneaecol* 107: 614–619

Chini B., Manning M., Guillon G. (2008). Affinity and efficacy of selective agonists and antagonists for vasopressin and oxytocin receptors: an "easy guide" to receptor pharmacology. *Prog Brain Res* 170: 513–517

Decaux G., Soupart A., Vassart G. (2008). Non-peptide arginine vasopressin antagonists: the vaptans. *Lancet* 371: 1624–1632

De Luca L., Orlandi C., Udelson J.E., Fedele F., Gheorghiade M. (2005). Overview of vasopressin receptor antagonists in heart failure resulting in hospitalization. *Am J Cardiol* 96 Suppl 1: 24–33

Derick S., Cheng L.L., Voirol M.J., Stoev S., Giacomini M., Wo N.C., Szeto H.H., Ben Mimoun M., Andres M., Gaillard R.C., Guillon C., Manning M. (2002). (1-deamino-4-cyclohexylalanine) arginine vasopressin: a potent and specific agonist for vasopressin V1b receptor. *Endocrinology* 143: 4655–4664

Goldsmith S.R., Gheorghiade M. (2005). Vasopressin antagonism in heart failure. *J Am Coll Cardiol* 46: 1785–1791

Griebel G., Simiand J., Serradeil-Le Gal C., Wagnon J., Pascal M., Scatton B., Maffrand J.P., Soubrie P. (2002). Anxiolytic and antidepressant effects of the non-peptide vasopressin V1b receptor antagonist SSR 149415 suggest an innovative approach for the treatment of stress-related disorders. *Proc Nat Acad Sci USA* 99: 6376–6385

Griffante C., Green A., Curcuruto O., Haslam C.P., Dickinson B.A., Arban R. (2005). Selectivity of d(Cha4)AVP and SSR149415 at human vasopressin and oxytocin receptors: evidence that SSR149415 is a mixed vasopressin V1b/oxytocin receptor antagonist. *Br J Pharmacol* 146: 744–751

Guillon G., Derick S., Pena A., Cheng L.L., Stoev R., Seyer R., Morgat J.L., Berberis C., Serradeil-Le Gal C., Wagnon J., Manning M. (2004). The discovery of novel vasopressin V1b receptor ligands for pharmacological, functional and structural investigations. *J Neuroendocrinol* 16: 356–361

Guillon G., Pena A., Murat B., Derick S., Trueba M., Ventura M.A., Szeto H.H., Wo N., Stoev S., Cheng L.L., Manning M. (2006). Position 4 analogues of (deamino-Cys^1) arginine vasopressin exhibits striking species differences or human and rat V2/V1b receptor selectivity. *J Peptide Sci* 12: 190–198

Hawtin S.R. (2006). Pharmacological chaperone activity of SR49059 to functionally recover mis-folded mutations of the vasopressin V1a receptor. *J Biol Chem* 281: 14604–14614

Kam P.C.A., Williams S., Yoong F.F.Y. (2004). Vasopressin and terlipressin: pharmacology and its clinical relevance. *Anesthesia* 59: 993–1001

Kowalczyk W., Sobolewski D., Prahl A., Derdowska I., Borovickova L., Slaninova J., Lammek B. (2007). The effect of N-terminal part modification of arginine vasopressin analogues with 2-aminoindane -2-carboxylic acid: a highly potent V2 agonist. *J Med Chem* 50: 2926–2929

Krag A., Moller S., Henriksen J.H., Holstein-Rathlou N.H., Larsen F.S., Bendtsen F. (2007). Terlipressin improves renal function in patients with cirrhosis and ascites without hepatorenal syndrome. *Hepatology* 46: 1863–1871

Kruszynski M., Lammek B., Manning M., Setoi J., Haldar J., Sawyer W.H. (1980). (1-beta mercapto-beta, beta cyclopentamethylenepropionic acid), 2-(O-methyl) tyrosine) arginine-vasopressin and (1-beta-mercapto-beta, beta cyclopentamethylenepropionic acid) arginine vasopressin, two highly potent antagonists of the vasopressin response to arginine vasopressin. *J Med Chem* 23: 364–368

Lacherez F., Barbier A., Serradeil-Le Gal C., Elena P.P., Maffrand J.P., Le Fur G. (2000). Effect of SR121463, a selective non-peptide vasopressin V2 receptor antagonist, in a rabbit model of ocular hypertension. *J Ocul Pharmacol Ther* 16: 203–216

Manning M., Sawyer W.H. (1993). Design, synthesis and some use of receptor specific agonists and antagonists of vasopressin and oxytocin. *J Recept Res* 13: 195–214

Manning M., Stoev S., Chini B., Durroux T., Mouillac B., Guillon G. (2008). Peptide and non-peptide agonists and antagonists for the vasopressin V1a, V1B V2 and OT receptors: research tools and potential therapeutic agents. *Prog Brain Res* 170: 473–512

Martin-Llahi M., Pepin M.N., Guevara M., Diaz F., Torre A., Monescillo A., Soriano G., Terra C., Fabrega E., Arroyo V., Rodes J., Gines P. (2008). Terlipressin and albumin vs albumin in patients with cirrhosis and hepatorenal syndrome: a randomized study. *Gastroenterology* 134: 1352–1359

Pena A., Murat B., Trueba M., Venture M.A., Bertrand G., Chen L.L., Stoev S., Szeto H.H., Wo N., Brossard G., Serradeil-Le Gal C., Manning M., Guillon G. (2007). Pharmacological and physiological characterization of d(Leu4,Lys8) vasopressin, the first V1b-selective agonist for rat vasopressin/oxytocin receptors. *Endocrinology* 148: 4136–4146

Purschke W.G., Eulberg D., Buchner K., Vonhoff S., Klussmann S. (2006). An L-RNA-based aquaretic agent that inhibits vasopressin *in vivo*. *Proc Nat Acad Sci USA* 103: 5173–5178

Saito M., Tahara A., Sugimoto T. (1997). 1-deamino-8-D-arginine vasopressin (DDAVP) as an agonist on V1b vasopressin receptor. *Biochem Pharmacol* 212: 751–757

Scott L.V., Medback S., Dinan T.G. (1999). ACTH and cortisol release following intravenous desmopressin: a dose-response study. *Clin Endocrinol* 51: 653–658

Serradeil-Le Gal C., Wagnon J., Garcia C., Lacour C., Guiraudou P., Christophe B., Villanova G., Nisato D., Maffrand J.P., Le Fur G., Guillon G., Cantau B., Barberis C., Trueba M., Ala Y., Jard S. (1993). Biochemical and pharmacological properties of SR 49059, a new, potent, nonpeptide antagonist of rat and human vasopressin V1a receptors. *J Clin Invest* 92: 224–231

Serradeil-Le Gal C., Lacour C., Valette G., Garcia G., Foulon L., Galindo G., Bankir L., Pouzet B., Guillon G., Barberis C., Chicot D., Jard S., Vilain P., Garcia C., Marty E., Rufaste D., Bossard G., Nisato D., Maffrand J.P., Le Fur G. (1996). Characterization of SR 121463A, a highly potent and selective orally active vasopressin V2 receptor antagonist. *J Clin Invest* 98: 2729–2738

Serradeil-Le Gal C. (2001). An overview of SR 121463, a selective non-peptide vasopressin V2 receptor antagonist. *Cardiovascular Drugs Rev* 19: 201–214

Serradeil-Le Gal C., Wagnon J., Valette G., Garcia G., Pascal M., Maffrand J.P., Le Fur G. (2002). Non-peptide vasopressin receptor antagonists: development of selective and orally active V1a, V2 and V1b receptor ligands. *Prog Brain Res* 139: 197–210

Serradeil-Le Gal C., Wagnon J., Tonnerre B., Roux R., Garcia G., Griebel G., Aulombard A. (2005). An overview of SSR149415, a selective nonpeptide vasopressin V1b receptor antagonist for the treatment of stress-related disorders. *CNS Drug Rev* 11: 53–68

Steinwall M., Bossmar T., Gaud C., Akerlund M. (2004). Inhibitory effects of SR 49059 on oxytocin and vasopressin induced uterine contractions in non-pregnant women. *Acta Obstet Gynecol Scand* 83: 12–18

Stemmelin J., Ludovic L., Salome N., Griebel G. (2005). Evidence that the lateral septum is involved in the antidepressant-like effects of the vasopressin V1b receptor antagonist SSR 149415. *Neuropsychopharmacology* 30: 35–42

Tahara J., Tahara A., Kusayama T., Wada K., Ishii N., Taniguchi N., Suzuki T., Yatsu T., Uchida W., Shibasaki M. (2005). Effects of YM218, a nonpeptide vasopressin V1a receptor selective antagonist on human vasopressin and oxytocin receptors. *Pharmacol Res* 51: 275–281

Thibonnier M, Coles P, Thibonnier A & Shoham M (2001). The basic and clinical pharmacology of nonpeptide vasopressin receptor antagonists. *Ann. Rev. Pharmacol. Toxicol.*, 41, 175–202

Thibonnier M (2003). Vasopressin receptor antagonists in heart failure. *Curr. Op. Pharmacol.*, 3, 683–687

Wüller S, Wiesner B, Löffler A, Furkert J, Krause G, Hermosilla R, Schaefer M, Schülein R, Rosenthal W & Oksche A (2004). Pharmacochaperones post-translationally enhance cell surface expression by increasing conformational stability of wild-type and mutant vasopressin V2 receptors. *J. Biol. Chem.*, 279, 47254–47263

Yamamura Y, Ogawa H, Chihara T, kondo K, Onogawa T, Nakamura S, Mori T, Tominaga M & Yabuuchi Y (1991). OPC-21268, an orally effective, nonpeptide vasopressin V1 receptor antagonist. *Science*, 252, 572–574

Yatsu T, Kusayama T, Tomura Y, Arai Y, Aoki M, Tahara A, Wada K & Tsukada J (2002). Effect of conivaptan, a combined vasopressin V1a and V2 receptor antagonist, on vasopressin–induced cardiac and haemodynamic changes in anesthetised dogs. *Pharmacol. Res.*, 46, 375–381

Zaoral M, Kolc J & Storm F (1967). Synthesis of 1-deamino-8-D-aminobutyrine-vasopressin, 1-deamino-8-D-lysine vasopressin and 1-deamino-8-D-arginine vasopressin. *Coll. Czech Chem. Comm.*, 32, 1250–1257

CHAPTER 6

VASOPRESSIN AND ITS RENAL EFFECTS

John Laycock

Division of Neuroscience and Mental Health
Faculty of Medicine, Imperial College London
Charing Cross Campus, London W6 8RF
Email: j.laycock@imperial.ac.uk

1. Introduction

The principal physiological effect of vasopressin is without doubt its action in the collecting duct to stimulate water reabsorption, but it has other effects along the nephron which play an important contributory part, as well as other more discrete actions on specific transport mechanisms. In order to fully appreciate these various renal effects, it is useful to first consider the general structure of the kidney, its vasculature and its regulation, as well as the functions of the different parts of the renal unit, the nephron.

The main functions of the kidneys are generally a) to participate in the regulation of salt, water and acid-base balance, b) the reabsorption (conservation) of many molecules of metabolic use, such as glucose and amino acids, c) the general metabolism and excretion of numerous products both endogenous and exogenous (e.g. many drugs and toxins) and d) to act in its own right as an endocrine organ. Consequently, the kidneys clearly play an important part in wider aspects of animal physiology, such as in cardiovascular, respiratory and general metabolic regulation. Vasopressin is principally concerned with the renal control of water reabsorption, but it also plays a role in the regulation of salt and urea reabsorption, and in the fine control of renal blood flow to the kidneys. Before considering the various renal actions of vasopressin in any detail, it is useful to briefly consider the different sections of the nephrons which comprise the kidneys.

2. The Kidneys

Each human kidney comprises well over 1 million nephrons. A cross-section of the kidney clearly indicates an outer cortex and an inner medulla surrounded by a fibrous renal capsule, and these two distinguishable parts are associated with different sections of the nephrons (see Fig. 1). The initial part of the nephron is the renal corpuscle, or Bowman's capsule, which surrounds a network of capillaries called the glomerulus (also called the capillary tuft). Arterial blood reaches the glomerulus via an afferent arteriole and leaves it via an efferent arteriole. Many of these capsules are close to the outer surface of the renal cortex and are part of cortical nephrons, but some lie deeper within the kidney close to the medullary region, and for this reason their nephrons are called juxtamedullary. The endothelial cells of the glomerular capillaries a) are fenestrated, which makes them relatively permeable, b) are surrounded by a basement membrane containing negatively-charged glyoproteins and c) have foot-like projections from modified epithelial cells called podocytes, which are wrapped around the endothelial cells and the basement membrane. These three components form the inner wall of the capsule. The outer wall of the capsule consists of another layer of epithelial cells. The gap between the two walls of the capsule is called Bowman's space.

The net pressure in the glomerular capillaries is the major driving force for the process of ultrafiltration by which water and other small molecules and ions in the plasma are pushed through the endothelial cell-basement membrane-podocyte barrier. The cellular constituents, most of the proteins and other larger constituents remain in the blood, generally because of their size and charge. The blood then enters the efferent arterioles and the peritubular arteries, while the ultrafiltrate enters Bowman's space. Approximately 20% of the plasma reaching the kidneys is filtered at the glomeruli (i.e. a typical normal glomerular filtration rate of 125 ml/min from a plasma flow rate of 625 ml/min). From here the isotonic filtrate enters the next section of the renal nephron, called the proximal convoluted tubule.

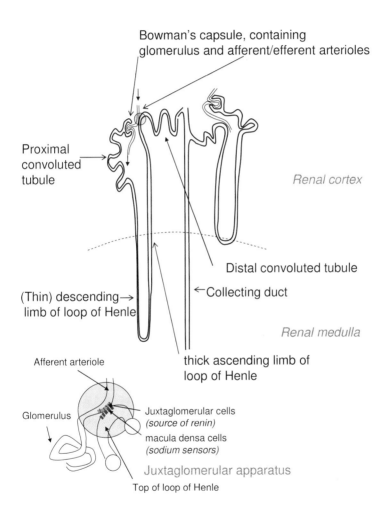

Figure 1. The outer cortical and inner medullary regions of the kidney, with examples of a cortical and a juxtamedullary nephron. The enlarged diagram in the bottom left-hand corner shows the area of contact between the top of the ascending limb of the loop of Henle and the afferent arteriole.

The proximal convoluted tubules (PCTs) lie in the cortical region of the kidney. If each nephron is approximately 50–60 mm long, then the PCT represents the first 20–25% of its length. From each glomerulus, the proximal tubule is composed of an initial segment (S1) which is very tightly convoluted and then becomes more gently undulating (segment 2, S2), before straightening as it passes into the medulla (segment 3, S3).The epithelial cells lining it have prominent brush borders, numerous mitrochondria and are linked together by tight junctions.

It is along the PCT that approximately two-thirds of the glomerular filtrate is reabsorbed back into the peritubular capillaries. Here, polar molecules such as glucose and amino acids, as well as ions, water and other molecules are transferred from tubular lumen to blood by means of a variety of transporters and channels in the apical (luminal) membrane (transcellular reabsorption), some of them by active or facilitated mechanisms, or across the tight junctions between the epithelial cells (paracellular reabsorption). Thus, for example, glucose entry into the PCT epithelial cell occurs via a luminal membrane carrier molecule which simultaneously binds sodium ions. This dual-molecule transport mechanism is driven by the maintenance of a sodium ion electrochemical concentration gradient across the luminal membrane, provided by the continuous energy-requiring activity of a sodium-potassium ATPase pump in the outer basolateral membrane. Similar mechanisms function for the transport of other essential molecules such as amino acids and lactate. The osmotically-driven movement of water across epithelial cell layers occurs through specific water channels called aquaporins. It is estimated that approximately 66% of the glomerular filtrate is reabsorbed by the time it reaches the next segment of the nephron, the loop of Henle. Secretion of some substances also occurs along the PCT by transcellular and paracellular processes. Water transport is determined solely by the osmotic gradient generated by solute (almost entirely Na) transport in the PCT, so the fluid entering the loop of Henle is still isotonic.

The loop of Henle passes deep down from the renal cortical into the medullary region of the kidney (the descending limb) and then turns and heads back up towards the cortex (the ascending limb). The more superficial, cortical, nephrons have short loops of Henle, some of which may not penetrate the medullary region at all. The juxtamedullary nephrons have longer loops which pass deep into the medullary region and some of them have thin loops which go as far down as the renal papillae. The structure of the loop of Henle differs along its length: the descending limb epithelial cells are thin and flattened, and contain few mitochondria, as are the cells after the hairpin bend in the lower part of the ascending limb. In contrast, the cells of the upper part of the ascending limb (the thick ascending limb) are more cuboidal, are rich in mitochondria and have a brush border, all reminiscent of the PCT and indicating the presence of active transport mechanisms.

The loop of Henle is the part of the nephron where the osmotic gradient necessary for the ultimate concentration of tubular fluid is established by a process called the countercurrent multiplier system. The thin descending limb is not engaged in any significant active transport of ions, but water in the tubular fluid can cross the epithelial cell layer via the tight junctions between the cells and enter the medullary interstitium in the presence of an appropriate osmotic gradient. The water can then enter the surrounding network of peritubular capillaries, resulting in a concentration of the tubular fluid. In addition, sodium, chloride and urea can move across the tight junctions from the interstitium into the tubular fluid in the presence of appropriate gradients, enhancing the concentration of the tubular fluid. Thus the osmolality of the tubular fluid reaches its maximal value at the bend of the loop. For the juxtaglomerular nephrons with the more deeply penetrating loops in the inner medulla, this osmolality can reach 1,200 $mOsmol.kg^{-1}$ in humans, and well over 3,000 $mOsmol.kg^{-1}$ in rats.

In contrast with the thin descending limb, the lower thin part of the ascending limb is impermeable to water and so the tubular fluid reaching the upper thick segment is hypertonic. The thick ascending limb is also impermeable to water, but here sodium, potassium and chloride ions are transported in a ratio of 1:1:2 (i.e. electroneutral) from the tubular fluid across the luminal membranes into the epithelial cells, and therefore the tubular fluid gets increasingly dilute as the fluid approaches the cortical region of the kidney. Indeed, the fluid which leaves the thick ascending limb of the loop of Henle and enters the next segment of the nephron, the distal convoluted tubule, is actually hypotonic, due mainly to the active reabsorption of sodium and chloride ions. Urea is now a major contributor to the tubular fluid osmolality because much of the sodium chloride has been actively pumped out of the nephron into the interstitium. The driving force for this process is the Na-K-ATPase pump in the basolateral membranes of the epithelial cells. The other consequence of this selective transport of ions in different parts of the loop of Henle, together with the varying permeability to water along its length, results in the generation of a large osmotic gradient within the interstitium, from the approximately isotonic cortical to the hypertonic inner medullary regions of the kidney. Thus the active transport of sodium chloride in the thick ascending limb from tubular fluid into the interstitium provides the osmotic gradient for the movement of water out of the tubular fluid in the thin descending limb. Because of the countercurrent flow of tubular fluid in the two limbs of the loop of Henle the consequence is an increasing osmolality from cortex to inner medulla which plays an essential role in the concentrating ability of the kidney along the final segment of the nephron, the collecting duct. Crucially, the osmolality of the medullary interstitium is considerably higher than that of the plasma. Vasopressin plays an important role in maintaining the countercurrent multiplication system in the loop of Henle.

In between the end of the thick ascending limb of the loop of Henle and the collecting duct is the distal convoluted tubule (DCT) which lies within the cortex of the kidney. A particular region at the terminal part of the ascending limb and the initial part of the DCT, called the macula densa, contains specialised sodium-sensing cells. These macula densa cells, because of the structural arrangement of the nephron (see Fig. 1) are in intimate contact with other specialised cells in the wall of the afferent arteriole as it approaches the glomerulus (the juxtaglomerular cells). The detection of a low sodium concentration in the tubular fluid approaching the beginning of the PCT by the macula densa cells results in the activation of the granular juxtaglomerular cells, which secrete the enzyme renin into the afferent arteriole. Renin catalyses the formation of the decapeptide angiotensin I from a circulating precursor protein angiotensinogen synthesised in the liver. Angiotensin I acts a precursor for the bioactive octapeptide hormone angiotensin II in the presence of angiotensin-converting enzyme (ACE). Angiotensin II is a potent vasoconstrictor which also stimulates the production of the mineralocorticoid hormone aldosterone (corticosterone in rodents) in the zona glomerulosa of the cortical region of the adrenal gland, which lies adjacent to the superior pole of the kidney. Aldosterone stimulates sodium reabsorption as well as potassium and hydrogen secretion in the DCT and cortical collecting duct. The interactions between vasopressin and the renin-angiotensin system are considered in more detail in Chapter 8. Like the ascending limb of the loop of Henle, the DCT is relatively impermeable to water.

While the DCT wall is composed of tubular cells similar to those lining the thick ascending limb, the collecting duct wall consists of two main cell types, each with specific functions, the principal and the intercalated cells. A number of DCTs from different nephrons in a kidney can connect to the same collecting duct via connecting tubules. The DCT extends into the initial cortical segment of the cortical collecting duct. The collecting ducts can be up to 20 mm long and they pass down from the cortical to the medullary region of the kidney to terminate in the renal papillae leading to the ureter. Of the 120 ml/min (typical glomerular filtration rate, GFR) normally entering the proximal convoluted tubules, about 12ml/min actually reaches the start of the collecting ducts. The collecting duct is the final concentrating segment of the nephron where, in the presence of circulating vasopressin and an osmotic gradient across the nephron, water is reabsorbed so that the amount of fluid usually excreted from the kidneys is in the region of 1 ml/min. In addition, the collecting duct is the final segment where sodium and urea reabsorption can take place, as well as the final regulation of renal acid-base balance, and these effects are also under hormonal control. There are two cell types in the collecting duct which are targets for vasopressin: the principal cells, which are mainly involved in water reabsorption, and the intercalated cells, which are important with regards to urea and hydrogen ion transport.

3. The Renal Actions of Vasopressin

a) *Glomerular filtration and renal blood flow*
As mentioned earlier, the principal physiological role of vasopressin is the regulation of renal water excretion. Vasopressin exerts its antidiuretic effect by stimulating water reabsorption in the collecting ducts. However, various other renal actions have been identified, such as effects on ion and urea transport, GFR and renal blood flow. The actions of vasopressin are covered section by section along the renal nephron.

Vasopressin was first identified as a hormone which might influence GFR many years ago (Dworkin *et al.*, 1983). A possible site of action is the mesangial (smooth muscle-like) cell, because cultures of these cells are associated with a vasopressin-induced decrease in glomerular ultrafiltration coefficient (Ausiello *et al.*, 1980). While the presence of V2 receptors in the glomerular region of the nephron has not been shown, there is evidence for the presence of V1 receptors (V1R).

The presence of vasopressin V1a receptor mRNA in the glomerulus by Terada *et al.* (1993) indicated the potential expression of this receptor in the vascular component of the initial part of the nephron. Indeed, the V1a receptor was suggested to mediate effects of vasopressin on renal blood flow, since stimulation is associated with a decreased medullary blood flow in anaesthetized renal-denervated rats (Nakanishi *et al.*, 1995). However, it is quite possible that the V1a receptor mRNA was actually in afferent or efferent arterioles, contaminating the glomerular extracts (see below). Autoradiographic localization of V1a receptors using a specific nonpeptide ligand indicated only sparse binding in the cortex (Serradeil-Le Gal *et al.*, 1996), while maximal binding was shown in the outer part of the inner medulla. Furthermore, in this study the labelling was mainly associated with medullary interstitial cells and the vasa recta vasculature. In addition to being present in the renal arcuate and intralobular arteries, the V1a receptors have been located on the microvasculature of the renal cortex and medulla, specifically on afferent and efferent arterioles, the glomerulus itself and vasa recta capillaries (Park *et al.*, 1997). Some V1R agonists, such as octapressin, produce a selective reduction in medullary blood flow in conscious rabbits (Evans *et al.*, 2000). Likewise, in anaesthetized rabbits the infusion of a V1R agonist reduces renal medullary, but not cortical, blood flow (Correia *et al.*, 2001) with no changes being observed in the juxtamedullary glomerular arterioles. This suggests that the vasoconstrictor effect was in the downstream vasculature.

On the other hand, there is evidence for a vasopressin-induced V1R-mediated decrease in GFR, with the reduction being greater in the outer cortical than the middle and inner cortical regions, which indicates a redistribution of intrarenal blood flow (Roald *et al.*, 2004). These authors conclude that this redistribution is likely to be due to an effect on afferent/efferent arterioles rather than an effect on medullary vasa recta vessels. Interestingly, the V1a receptor number appears to increase in afferent arterioles during establishment of hypertension in spontaneously hypertensive rats (Vagnes *et al.*, 2004). The Brattleboro rat with diabetes insipidus (DI) has also been used to examine whether vasopressin influences the GFR, and it would appear that following long-term infusion there is an increase which could be due to an alteration in tubuloglomerular feedback from the macula densa (Gellai *et al.*, 1984; Trinh-Trang-Tan *et al.*, 1984).

With regard to a possible effect of vasopressin on vasa recta blood flow, videomicroscopic imaging of the exposed renal medulla of anaesthetized rats showed that the polypeptide clearly decreased it in both ascending and descending limb regions (Zimmerhackl *et al.*, 1985). Furthermore, the effect was completely blocked with a V1R antagonist, which suggests a direct vascular effect of vasopressin. Further evidence for a direct V1a receptor effect on outer medullary descending vasa recta was provided by a study of diameter changes in isolated perfused tissue (Turner and Pallone, 1997). These authors also noted that the V2 receptor agonist DDAVP appeared to block the V1R-mediated vasoconstriction, suggesting a possible regulatory interaction by vasopressin.

Thus, vasopressin does appear to affect renal blood flow via V1 receptors, partly by an action on the GFR but also a likely effect on vasa recta blood flow.

Finally, it is interesting to note that vasopressin is likely to have an effect on urea transport in the vasa recta. Of the various urea transporter (UT) isoforms, the UTB isoforms are involved with urea transport across the outer medullary descending vasa recta (Pallone, 1994). Furthermore, expression of the UTB1 protein is downregulated by long-term treatment with a selective vasopressin V2 agonist (Trinh-Trang-Tan *et al.*, 2002) indicative of a vasopressin influence on urea transport in the vasa recta. While there is some evidence to suggest that the UTB transporter may also function as a water channel, it is unlikely to play a significant physiological role (Yang and Verkman, 2002).

b) *Vasopressin and the proximal tubule*
In their study of the microlocalization of vasopressin receptors along the rat nephron, Terada *et al.* (1993) identified small but nevertheless detectable signals for V1aR mRNA in proximal tubules, but not V2 receptor mRNA. However, they are present in LLC-PK1 cells (Jans *et al.*, 1989) which are derived from porcine kidneys and which have characteristics of the proximal tubule (Rabito, 1986). There is no evidence to date for any vasopressin-induced water transport either in the proximal tubule or the LLC-PK1 cell line. There are also reports that these cells have V1a receptors and that vasopressin induces intracellular calcium mobilization, an effect which is blocked by a V1 receptor antagonist (Burnatowska-Hledin and Spielman, 1987). Interestingly, vasopressin appears to increase amiloride-sensitive Na channel activity, with increased redistribution of the associated Apx(L) protein to the apical membrane (Raychowdhury *et al.*, 2004).

Thus vasopressin has no effect on proximal tubular water reabsorption, but may conceivably have a small effect on sodium reabsorption, presumably by a V1 receptor mediated action.

c) *Vasopressin and the loop of Henle*

Vasopressin exerts various effects on reabsorptive processes in the loop of Henle, thus playing an important role in regulating the countercurrent multiplier system which generates the progressive increase in osmolality from cortex down to medulla. Following the initial demonstration of vasopressin-sensitive adenyl cyclase along the ascending limb of the loop of Henle by Morel's group (Imbert *et al.*, 1975) various labelling and molecular studies have identified the vasopressin receptor associated with the loop of Henle as being the V2R (Ammar *et al.*, 1991; Ostrowski *et al.*, 1992; Terada *et al.*, 1993; Firsov *et al.*, 1994; Nonoguchi *et al.*, 1995). While some binding studies suggest the presence of V1R in the medullary thick ascending limb (Ammar *et al.*, 1992) others haven't been able to detect them (Ostrowski *et al.*, 1993). On the other hand, vasopressin does appear to stimulate inositol triphosphate production in this segment, which suggests a V1R-linked mechanism (Baudouin-Legros *et al.*, 1993). At present, the general consensus is that vasopressin exerts its main effects in the ascending limb via the V2 receptor but it is quite possible that, particularly at high circulating concentrations, it may have as yet unidentified effects via V1 (V1a) receptors.

As indicated earlier, the principal effect of vasopressin in the medullary thick ascending limb of the loop of Henle (TALH) is to stimulate the active reabsorption of sodium and chloride ions, first proposed by Rocha and Kokko (1973) and subsequently confirmed by others (Hall and Varney, 1980; Sasaki and Imai, 1980; Hubert *et al.*, 1981). There are various sites (ion channels or transporters) in the thick ascending limb cell which could be influenced by vasopressin and result in an increase in ion transport (see Knepper *et al.*, 1999). These would include the Na^+-K^+-$2Cl^-$ co-transporter in the apical (luminal) membrane, the Na^+-K^+-ATPase in the basolateral membrane, a basolateral membrane chloride channel, two apical membrane potassium channels and a Na^+-H^+ exchanger also in the apical membrane (Fig. 2). They are all involved in the transcellular transport of ions, but in addition, sodium ions move down the electrical gradient from lumen to basolateral spaces paracellularly.

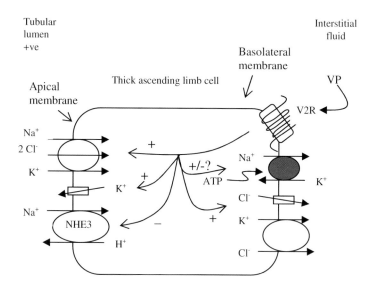

Figure 2. The ion transporter systems currently believed to be present in the thick ascending limb of loop of Henle cells some of which are influenced by vasopressin. V2R, vasopressin type 2 receptor; +, stimulation; −, inhibition; +/−, unclear overall effect.

Various studies have indicated that vasopressin stimulates the furosamide-sensitive Na^+-K^+-$2Cl^-$ (NK2Cl) cotransporter in the apical membrane of the TALH (Molony *et al.*, 1987; Sun *et al.*, 1991; Kim *et al.*, 1999) which would certainly lead to an increase in transcellular NaCl transport. Furthermore, expression of this cotransporter is dependent on Gsα-mediated hormone stimulation, probably resulting in long-term changes in cellular cAMP levels (Ecelbarger *et al.*, 1999). While there is evidence for passive water movement through this cotransporter in ciliary pigmented epithelial cells, this is not the case in the TALH (Hamann *et al.*, 2005). Interestingly, in apical Na^+-H^+ exchanger (NHE3) knockout mice, there is a downregulation in TALH NK2Cl activity and collecting duct aquaporin 2 expression, with a consequent impairment in fluid regulation despite an increase in circulating vasopressin concentration (Amlal *et al.*, 2003). Apart from anything else, these results support the general concept that collecting duct AQP2 regulation involves factors in addition to vasopressin.

There is still some controversy about whether vasopressin directly stimulates or inhibits the basolateral membrane Na-K-ATPase transporter. Charlton and Baylis (1990) showed a stimulatory effect while Fryckstedt and Aperia (1992) showed the opposite. At present this potential target effect remains unresolved. Vasopressin has also been shown to stimulate basolateral Cl transport via cAMP (Schlatter and Greger, 1985). Furthermore, it is likely to increase K transport out of the thick ascending limb cell across the apical membrane via two specific K channels (Wang, 1994). One of them has been cloned and has been shown to be phosphorylated by cAMP-dependent protein kinase A (Xu *et al.*, 1996), as well as other messengers such as protein kinase C. Abundance of this renal outer medullary potassium channel (ROMK) in the thick ascending limb is increased by the V2 receptor agonist dDAVP and by fluid restriction (Ecelbarger *et al.*, 2001b).

Vasopressin also reduces bicarbonate absorption in the medullary thick ascending limb by inhibiting the apical N+/H+ exchange (NHE3) pump (Good, 1990; Borensztein *et al.*, 1993) and not the NHE1 mechanism located in the basolateral membranes which is blocked by amiloride and nerve growth factor (Good *et al.*, 2004). Interestingly, aldosterone also inhibits the apical NHE3 exchanger via a non-genomic pathway (Good *et al.*, 2005). Vasopressin may also stimulate Ca and Mg transport in the loop of Henle (de Rouffignac *et al.*, 1983; Elalouf *et al.*, 1984) although this may well be isolated to the cortical, but not the medullary, thick ascending limb (Wittner *et al.*, 1988). The latter conclusion contrasts with the observation that the addition of vasopressin (1 mM) to the luminal perfusate of rat medullary thick ascending limb increased the intracellular Ca. At least some of the increase appeared to be due to release from intracellular stores (Burgess *et al.*, 1994).

Urea transport by means of specific urea transporter (UT) proteins also occurs in the loop of Henle, particularly in the thin descending limb. A role for vasopressin in stimulating the short UTA2 splice variant present in this segment of the nephron has been suggested since levels increase in Brattleboro DI rats following treatment with ddAVP (Wade et al., 2000). For further details, see the excellent reviews on urea transport by Knepper et al. (1999) and Sands (2003).

Before leaving the loop of Henle, it is worth noting that there is also some evidence to suggest that vasopressin at high (nM) concentrations might increase passive Cl permeability (Takahashi et al., 1995) in the thin ascending limb, which could increase the movement of NaCl out into the interstitial fluid.

d) Vasopressin and the distal convoluted yubule
The late part of the distal convoluted tubule merges with the beginning of the cortical collecting duct. The distal convoluted tubule is not generally permeable to water, even in the presence of vasopressin, although the neuropeptide may influence ion transport here. Electrophysiological and ion flux studies on a murine distal convoluted tubule cell line derived from transgenic mice expressing the simian virus 40 (mpkDCT cells) indicated that the V2 receptor agonist DDAVP stimulates chloride transport resulting in a net Cl absorption (Van Huyen et al., 2001). Transcellular calcium transport is also enhanced by DDAVP in these mpkDCT cells according to patch-clamp studies by Diepens et al., 2003). Vasopressin also stimulates Mg uptake in another immortalised mouse distal convoluted cell line, and this effect appears to be V2 receptor-cAMP mediated because protein kinase A (PKA) blockade inhibits the effect (Bapty et al., 1998). Of particular interest is the possibility that luminal vasopressin might have an effect on ion transport. Thus in the late distal tubule (early cortical collecting duct), luminally applied vasopressin stimulates K^+ secretion, an effect blocked by a V1 receptor antagonist (Amorim and Malnic, 2000). This process, perhaps not surprisingly, seems to be mediated by the activation of the phospholipase $C–Ca^{2+}$-protein kinase C (PKC) signalling pathway (Amorim et al., 2004).

e) *Vasopressin and the collecting duct*

The principal cells of the collecting duct are generally accepted to be the target sites for vasopressin's main physiological action, the reabsorption of water. However, vasopressin clearly has other important effects in this section of the nephron, specifically on urea and ion transport in the intercalating cells.

i) *Water transport*

In order to appreciate the role played by vasopressin on water transport in the principal cells of the collecting duct, it is useful to consider the various components which are believed to be involved in its mechanism of action. Here, we briefly consider the components directly relevant to the renal actions of vasopressin and the reader is directed to the chapter on vasopressin's mechanisms of action for greater detail (Chapter 4). The chief elements of the mechanism of action of vasopressin on water reabsorption in the collecting duct are shown in Fig. 3.

Receptors:

Under normal hydrated conditions vasopressin circulates in the plasma at a concentration of approximately 1–5 pg.ml^{-1} (1–5 pmol.l^{-1}) with maximal antidiuresis being obtained at a circulating concentration of the order of 12 pg.ml^{-1} (12 pmol.l^{-1}). It exerts its effects following its binding to one or other of its receptors on the plasma membranes of its target cells. V2 receptors have been identified in the kidneys, and so have V1a and V1b receptors. For more detail about vasopressin receptors, see Chapters 4 and 5. *In vivo*, for example in the anaesthetized water-loaded rat, the antidiuretic response to a single intravenous injection of vasopressin is elicited within a couple of minutes to reach its maximal effect some 3–5 minutes later.

That it is the V2 receptor which is involved in the vasopressin-induced renal reabsorption of water is indicated by linking the binding of a known V2 receptor agonist such as DDAVP to medullo-papillary membranes (Marchingo *et al.*, 1988) with its antidiuretic potency (Berde and Boissonas, 1968). The cloning of V2 receptors in rats (Lolait *et al.*, 1992) and humans (Birnbaumer *et al.*, 1992) was followed by the clear demonstration of V2 receptor mRNA along all sections of the collecting duct by reverse transcription polymerase chain reaction (RT-PCR) (Terada *et al.*, 1993; Firsov *et al.*, 1994) and by *in situ* hybridization histochemistry (Ostrowski *et al.*, 1993). Bouley *et al.* (2005b) suggest that once vasopressin has induced internalization of its V2 receptor, the receptor is delivered to lysosomes where it is degraded, hence the downregulation effect and the requirement for long-term new receptor protein synthesis.

While there is clear evidence for the location of V2 receptors along different segments of the nephron in addition to the collecting duct, the same is not the case for the V1 receptors. Indeed, early work suggestive of V1-receptor mediated renal effects was based on studies identifying increases in intracellular calcium ion concentration and/or inositol triphosphate production in toad bladder epithelial cells (Schlondorff and Satriano, 1985), cultured LLCK-PK1 cells (Burnatowska-Hledin and Spielman, 1987) and rabbit collecting duct cells (Burnatowska-Hledin and Spielman, 1989; Ando *et al.*, 1989). Indeed, a protein kinase C mediated autoregulation of vasopressin's action on increased water permeability via cyclic AMP had been proposed for toad bladder (Schlondorff and Levine, 1985), also suggestive of a V1 receptor effect. Furthermore, V1a receptor mRNA is clearly detected in different parts of the nephron including the various segments of the rat collecting duct (Terada *et al.*, 1993).

A recent study of vasopressin receptor distribution along mouse and human collecting ducts specifically locates V1a receptor mRNA in intercalated cells of the medullary collecting duct, but it is more generally distributed between principal and intercalated cells in the cortical collecting duct (Carmosino, *et al.*, 2006). In the same study, the V2 receptor mRNA is generally distributed along the whole collecting duct but, as expected, with higher expression in the medullary section. Furthermore, there is a complete overlap with AQP2 mRNA, indicative of its location to principal cells involved in water transport. While the V2 receptor is mainly located on the basolateral membranes of its target cells, there is also evidence for its existence on luminal (apical) membranes in terminal inner medullary collecting ducts (Nonoguchi *et al.*, 1995). Certainly, vasopressin in relatively high (10 nmol) concentrations added to the luminal surface of perfused rabbit cortical collecting ducts, while not having any direct effect on water transport, does appear to inhibit the water permeability increase induced by basolaterally applied (20 pmol) hormone (Ando *et al.*, 1991). It is quite possible that V1 receptors could mediate this indirectly inhibitory effect since they may be present on luminal membranes according to studies relating to effects of luminally applied vasopressin (e.g. Amorin and Malnic, 2000).

It is also worth appreciating that a dual angiotensin II/vasopressin receptor with separate AII and vasopressin binding domains has been identified by rat kidney cDNA library screening (Ruiz-Opazo *et al.*, 1995). This receptor may somehow be linked to salt and water metabolism since the hypertensive salt-sensitive Dahl rat appears to have a mutation of this dual AII/vasopressin receptor (Ruiz-Opazo *et al.*, 2002).

G proteins, G protein receptor kinases and β-arrestins:
The transmembrane vasopressin receptors are linked to well-established guanine nucleotide binding proteins (G proteins) and also to more recently identified G-protein-coupled receptor kinases (GRKs) and intracellular proteins called β-arrestins (1 and 2). Activation of the G proteins following binding of extracellular ligand results in the initiation of intracellular signalling pathways, mediating the actions associated with the hormone, such as the activation of enzymes (e.g. adenyl cyclase) or membrane channels. The GRKs can then rapidly phosphorylate the G proteins which results in their subsequent attachment to β-arrestins.

The inactivation and recycling of vasopressin receptors is an important part of the agonist-receptor-G protein signalling mechanism. The desensitization-resensitization process of the receptor after binding to its ligand is now believed to be induced by the β-arrestins (see Lefkowitz and Shenoy, 2005). Phosphorylation of the vasopressin-V2 receptor complex by a GRK promotes its binding to β-arrestin, which dephosphorylates it. Consequently, the β-arrestin acts as a docking protein by directing the receptor to its clathrin-mediated endocytic trafficking system. Thus the β-arrestin-V2 receptor is internalised into the endosomes and returned slowly to the plasma membrane, unlike the more rapid dissociation which can occur for instance when β-arrestin binds to a receptor such as the β-adrenergic receptor, allowing the more rapid release of this receptor back to the membrane (Oakley *et al.*, 1999). Indeed, it appears that different GRKs are linked to either the Gs-dependent or the β-arrestin-mediated pathways. Most of the phosphorylation of the V2 receptor and consequent recruitment of the slower β-arrestin signalling pathway appears to be mediated by GRKs 2 and 3, while phosphorylation by GRKs 5 and 6 may actually have different (qualitative) effects on the same pathway (Ren *et al.*, 2005).

Interestingly, recent work indicates that GRKs can function as dimers, and as such they may well represent the basic signalling unit (Bulenger *et al.*, 2005). The vasopressin receptors have been shown to exist as homo- and hetero-dimers in transfected human embryonic kidney cells (Terrillon *et al.*, 2003). The heterodimerization between V1a and V2 receptors in these transfected cells appears to promote their interaction with β-arrestin protein and their consequent recycling between plasma membrane and the internal endosomes (Terrillon *et al.*, 2004). Thus it is a likely conjecture to believe that agonist binding to a specific receptor results in heterodimerization (e.g. in kidney cells) and subsequent potential complex interactions between intracellular mechanisms.

Adenyl cyclases and phosphodiesterases:
Ligand binding to its specific receptor activates either a stimulatory (Gs) protein or an inhibitory (Gi) protein, the consequence of which is a configurational separation and displacement of the α and βγ subunits of the G protein. These subunits activate the membrane-bound enzymes which are associated with them. When vasopressin binds to a V2 receptor, its associated Gs protein is activated and consequently the α subunit binds to, and activates, the adjacent intracellular enzyme adenyl cyclase (AC). This enzyme then stimulates the conversion of adenosine

triphosphate (ATP) to cyclic adenosine monophosphate (cAMP) which acts as a second messenger within the cell. So far, up to nine different isomers of AC have been identified, of which four (AC 4, 5, 6 and 9) have been shown to exist in renal tissue with AC6 being the predominant isoform (Hanoune *et al.*, 1997). However, which of the ACs are influenced by vasopressin is still unclear.

Brattleboro rats lacking circulating vasopressin (BDI) appear to have reduced levels of mRNA for all four isoforms compared with normal rats (Shen *et al.*, 1997). However, treatment of BDI rats with the V2 agonist DDAVP increased the renal mRNA for AC5, 6 and 9 but decreased AC4 mRNA further (Shen *et al.*, 1998). In line with these findings, treatment of normal rats with a specific V2 receptor antagonist was associated with slight reductions in AC5, 6 and 9 but actually increased AC4 mRNA (Shen *et al.*, 1998). Thus the synthesis of renal cAMP production could involve any one of these isoforms, and vasopressin can influence all four. Indeed the AC5 and 6 isoforms, which are inhibited by calcium-calmodulin, are both present in the outer medullary collecting duct, where their mRNA has been located by RT-PCR (Chabardes *et al.*, 1996) and by *in situ* hybridization (Helies-Toussant *et al.*, (2000). At present, the general consensus is that the most predominant type, AC6, is the main form activated by vasopressin in the principal cells associated with water transport. To complicate matters, proteomic analysis of inner medullary collecting duct proteins in Brattleboro DI rats indicates that 72 hours of dDAVP treatment is associated with a downregulation of AC6 (van Balkom *et al.*, 2004). These authors have suggested that this down-regulation of AC6 may be linked to a long-term vasopressin escape phenomenon. This is particularly interesting because it is also believed that stimulation of AC6 is associated with a (presumably) PKA-dependent increase in intracellular calcium (Star *et al.*, 1988; Champagneulle *et al.*, 1993; Ecelberger *et al.*, 1996), which shows an oscillatory rhythm following vasopressin administration (Yip, 2002). The intracellular calcium release is associated with the activation of intracellular calcium channels (Chou *et al.*, 2000). Thus AC6, via PKA, may induce not only the reabsorption of water but also its own long-term regulation by negative feedback via a calcium-mediated mechanism. In addition, a number of other proteins are likely to be involved in the vasopressin escape phenomenon, as indicated recently in a study using combined proteomics and bioinformatics pathway analysis (Hoorn et al., 2005).

In contrast, another calmodulin-sensitive adenylyl cyclase, AC3, shown to be present in the rat renal collecting duct as well as AC6, is downregulated in inner medullary collecting ducts of long-term (7 day) DDAVP-treated BDI rats (Hoffert et al., 2005). Furthermore, calcium-calmodulin inhibitors block vasopressin-dependent cAMP accumulation. Calmodulin inhibition also blocks the vasopressin-induced increase in urea permeability in isolated collecting tubules (Hoffert et al., 2005). Therefore it would seem that calcium-calmodulin is involved in the stimulation of urea (and water) transport mechanisms as well as in their long-term regulation.

Thus the V2 receptor-G protein coupled AC, when activated, phosphorylates intracellular enzyme PKA which has three main effects in principal cells. First, it is associated with the rapid mobilization of the vasopressin-dependent water channel aquaporin 2 (AQP2) molecules from the storage intracellular vesicles (aggraphores) to the apical membrane where they are inserted. Second, it stimulates the longer-term synthesis of new AQP2 proteins. As a third action it is clear that receptor desensitization is induced so that the effect initiated by vasopressin binding to its receptor is limited. There is also the potential self-regulating Ca^{2+}-mediated negative feedback effect on its own production and/or activity (see above).

It now appears that the AC-mediated intracellular effects of vasopressin can actually be circumvented by the activation of different pathways. For instance, Bouley et al. (2000) showed that in rat kidney slices and LLC-PK1 cells nitric oxide donors and atrial natriuretic factor can mimic the effect of vasopressin on AQP2 trafficking from intracellular vesicle to plasma membrane by stimulating cyclic guanosine monophosphate (cGMP). More recently the same research group showed that sildanafil citrate (Viagra), a cGMP phosphodiesterase inhibitor, raises intracellular cGMP levels and this is associated with the insertion of AQP2 into the apical membranes of target cells (Bouley *et al.*, 2005a). Indeed, it would also appear that nitric oxide generation is stimulated by vasopressin via a V2 receptor mediated mechanism involving a mobilization of intracellular Ca^{2+}, which is at least partly associated with the phosphoinositide pathway (O'Connor and Cowley, 2007).

The phosphodiesterase (PDE) enzyme which inactivates cyclic AMP also exists as a number of different isoforms. Of the nine identified, PDE4 seems to be the one associated with the inner medullary collecting duct (IMCD) according to a study with cultured IMCD cells (Yamaki *et al.*, 1992). See also Chapter 4.

Protein kinases:
As mentioned above, the function of AC is to phosphorylate intracellular protein enzymes. For vasopressin working through its V2 receptor, this is PKA in the principal cells. The activation of PKA is associated with immediate and longer-term events which reflect the movement of aquaporin (specifically AQP2) from intracellular stores to the apical membranes of the principal cells, followed by their insertion into those membranes, the subsequent removal and recycling of AQP2 (trafficking), and the longer-term synthesis of new AQP2 molecules.

The immediate effect of vasopressin is to stimulate the movement of AQP2 from its intracellular storage vesicle to the apical membrane where it is inserted. When vasopressin is removed, the AQP2 molecules return to their intracellular vesicle storage sites (a process sometimes called the endocytotic component of the cycle). This process was initially, and aptly, named the shuttle hypothesis when first proposed (Wade *et al.*, 1981) and it has now been shown to occur in isolated perfused collecting ducts (Nielson *et al.*, 1995) and in treated rats (Marples *et al.*, 1995). These components of the AQP2 shuttle are clearly associated with AC, and presumably of PKA. Indeed, phosphorylation of specific amino acids in the AQP2 molecule by PKA has been shown to occur (see Chapter 4) but whether, and how, this influences the effectiveness of the molecule in allowing increased water permeability or to its own recycling is still unclear. For example, phosphorylation of

AQP2 serine 256 (S256) in transfected renal CD8 cells is probably relevant to the translocation of AQP2 through the Golgi, but this step seems to be independent of PKA (Procino *et al.*, 2003). More recent work using transfected MCDK-C7 cells with a mutation at S256 of AQP2, producing constitutively phosphorylated AQP2 (hence membrane-bound), indicates that blocking PKA with the inhibitor H-89 still allows redistribution to intracellular vesicles, as with forskolin-treated wild-type cells (Nejsum *et al.*, 2005). Finally, a variety of proteins, including cellubrevin, N-ethylmaleimide sensitive fusion protein (NSF) and soluble NSF attachment protein (SNAP), which are believed to be involved in vesicle targeting, have been identified in sections of rat IMCD and direct vasopressin-induced vesicle fusion events (Franki *et al.*, 1995). This is clearly an area of increasing investigation.

PKA-anchoring proteins (AKAPs) appear to play an important role in compartmentalizing PKA, and thus influence the signalling regulating the vasopressin-induced water reabsorption process (Klussmann and Rosenthal, 2001; Henn *et al.*, 2005). One such AKAP, the AKAP18d variant which is expressed in IMCD and is located within the same intracellular vesicles as PKA and AQP2, is directed likewise to the plasma membrane by vasopressin (Henn *et al.*, 2004).

The longer-term action of vasopressin is associated with the stimulation of transcription in the cell nucleus leading to increased AQP2 expression. Renal medullary AQP2 mRNA is increased in water-deprived rats (Ma *et al.*, 1994; Yamamoto *et al.*, 1995). The subcutaneous injection of vasopressin into rats is also associated with an increased expression of AQP2 mRNA, reaching a peak somewhere around 6 hours after injection (Terashima *et al.*, 1997). Interestingly, in the same study the V2 receptor mRNA decreased, reaching its nadir around 3 hours after the injection, but returning to basal levels by the time AQP2 mRNA was at its zenith, indicating an interesting time-frame divergence between V2 receptor and AQP2 expression. Increased vasopressin-induced AQP2-expression appears to be related to cAMP-mediated phosphorylation of a cAMP-response element binding (CREB) transcription factor and c-fos activation in transfected LLC-PK1 cells, the combination of which, via CRE and activator protein-1 (AP1) binding sites, is associated with activation of the AQP promoter region and increased AQP2 transcription (Yasui *et al.*, 1997). The involvement of the cyclic AMP response element (CRE) in the AQP gene promoter was also shown by Matsumura *et al.* (1997). Whether PKA has any bearing on the vasopressin induced increase in AQP2 gene expression and protein synthesis is presently uncertain.

Interestingly, it is clear that AQP2 protein degradation is also increased following vasopressin-stimulated AQP2 synthesis in immortalized murine collecting duct cells (Hasler *et al.*, 2002). The possibility that vasopressin might influence the degradation of AQP2 directly via a post-transcriptional mechanism that may involve a PKA-dependent negative feedback effect has recently been suggested (Hasler *et al.*, 2006).

Aquaporins:
In 1988, a 28 kDa polypeptide named channel-like integral protein (CHIP) was identified by Agre's group (Denker *et al.*, 1988). This molecule was later renamed aquaporin 1 (Agre *et al.*, 1993) after it had been shown to have the functional characteristic of a water channel in oocytes (Wright *et al.*, 1989). There are now at least ten mammalian aquaporin (AQP) isoforms so far identified, with seven of them expressed in mammalian kidneys in varying degrees of abundance (AQP1, 2, 3, 4, 6, 7 and 8). Most of them (AQP1, 2, 3, 4 and 7) are membrane-spanning molecules with six intramembranous regions having both NH_2 and COOH terminals located within the cytoplasm. AQP6 and 8 are located almost entirely in vesicles, while AQP2 is found in vesicles as well as in apical membranes. Some of the aquaporins function as tetramers across the bilipid membranes (e.g. AQP1, 2, 3) while AQP4 is believed to form larger oligomeric forms. There have been many reviews on the subject of aquaporins over the last 10 years (Chrispeels and Agre, 1994; Nielsen and Agre, 1995; Sabolic and Brown, 1995; King and Agre, 1996), and a more recent one specifically on renal aquaporins by Nielsen *et al.* (2002) is particularly recommended. Aquaporins are not only found in animal cells and micro-organisms but also in plant cell

membranes, where they are similarly involved in water and small neutral solute transport (Chaumont *et al.*, 2005).

AQP1 is the principal water channel found in proximal tubules, as well as in the descending thin limb of the loop of Henle (Nielsen *et al.*, 1993a). These segments of the renal nephron are highly permeable to water and function independently of vasopressin. AQP1 is present both in apical (luminal) and basolateral membranes. It is particularly important in the proximal tubule where most of the osmotically driven reabsorption of water takes place. The transepithelial water permeability of isolated perfused segments of thin descending limb of loop of Henle taken from AQP1 knockout (null) mice indicated that this channel is the principal water channel and plays an important part in the countercurrent concentrating mechanism in this segment (Chou *et al.*, 1999). Furthermore, AQP1 is also located in the endothelial cells of the descending vasa recta, the blood vessels which travel down through the medulla in parallel with the descending limbs (Nielsen *et al.*, 1995). AQP1 may also be a channel which allows carbon dioxide to traverse cell membranes and therefore could be relevant for bicarbonate handling (Cooper *et al.* 2002) although this view is controversial (Fang *et al.*, 2002).

AQP2 is the main aquaporin located in the apical membranes and intracellular vesicles of the collecting duct principal cells, and to a lesser extent in the distal connecting tubules (Nielsen *et al.*, 1993b). Some Immunostaining for AQP2 has also been shown in the basolateral membranes of principal cells in the inner medullary region of the collecting duct (Marples *et al.*, 1995). This aquaporin is the main water channel which is regulated by vasopressin and therefore requires special consideration (see below). In the kidneys, AQP3 and AQP4 are both located in the basolateral membranes of the principal cells of collecting ducts (Echevarria *et al.*, 1994; Ishibashi *et al.*, 1994; Ma *et al.*, 1994). These two channels appear to be necessary for getting water out of the principal cells and into the basolateral spaces. The role of AQP3 is somewhat complicated by the fact that it is not only a water channel but is also involved in renal glycerol and urea transport (Ishibashi *et al.*,

1994). AQP3 is localized chiefly in the cortical and medullary collecting ducts, with the greatest expression identified in the base of the inner medulla (Ecelberger *et al.*, 1995). Interestingly, vasopressin infusion into a Brattleboro DI rat results in increased expression not only of AQP2 but also AQP3 (but not AQP4) in cortical and medullary collecting ducts (Terris *et al.*, 1996). Deletion of the AQP3 gene in mice results in greatly increased fluid intake and urine excretion, which is only partially decreased by treatment with the V2 receptor agonist desamino-D-arginine vasopressin (Ma *et al.*, 2000).

Interestingly, these AQP3 null mice appear to lack AQP2 and AQP4 expression in the cortical connecting tubules and collecting ducts, which would contribute to the polyuria (Kim *et al.*, 2005). These authors also report a significant natriuresis in the mice which may be due, in part at least, to an observed decrease in the α-subunit of the Na-K-ATPase in the cortical collecting ducts. In contrast, there appears to be a compensatory increase in inner medullary AQP2 and AQP3, but not AQP4, expression in rats with streptozotocin-induced diabetes mellitus (Nejsum *et al.*, 2001). Immunocytochemistry locates renal AQP4 mainly in the proximal two-thirds of the inner medulla, with little or none being detected in the outer medullary or cortical collecting ducts (Terris *et al.*, 1995). Interestingly, studies on AQP4 knockout mice indicate that this water channel is indeed the main one responsible for water permeability in the inner medullary collecting duct, but the deletion of the gene is only associated with a mild loss of concentrating ability (Chou *et al.*, 1998) presumably because most water reabsorption takes place prior to this segment of the nephron.

Aquaporin 6 is located in the acid-regulating intercalated cells of the cortical and medullary collecting duct. In contrast with AQP1, 2, 3 and 4 this AQP is only located in vesicle membranes, and not in the plasma membranes of the cells (Yasui *et al.*, 1999a; 1999b). Furthermore, this AQP has minimal water channel function, but is mainly concerned with anion transport, particularly nitrate but also halides (Yasui *et al.*, 2002). It appears that the trafficking of AQP6 to vesicle membranes is due to its N-terminus (Beitz *et al.*, 2005).

AQP7 is located in various tissues including the kidneys where it is located in the apical membranes of proximal tubule (segment 3) cells along with AQP1 channels. This aquaporin acts not only as a water channel, but is also involved in glycerol and urea transport and as such is sometimes called an aquaglyceroporin (Ishibashi et al., 1994). AQP7 knockout mice show only a relatively small but significant decrease in proximal brush-border osmotic water permeability compared with wild-type controls, but the deficiency nevertheless contributes to the urinary concentrating deficiency which is observed in AQP1/AQP7 double knockout mice (Sohara et al., 2005). A more important physiological role for AQP7 may well be related to its glycerol-transporting function, particularly in adipocytes, and its relation to lipid metabolism (MacDougald and Burant, 2005).

Little is known about the role of AQP8 in the kidney, where immunochemistry locates it mainly intracellularly in proximal tubules and to a lesser extent in the cortical and medullary collecting ducts (Elkjaer et al., 2001). It is also present in other tissues such as testis, liver, heart, lungs and intestinal tract.

Vasopressin and the aquaporins:
Regarding vasopressin's stimulation of water reabsorption, AQP2 is the main aquaporin involved, located in the apical membranes and intracellular vesicles of the collecting duct principal cells and to a lesser extent in the distal connecting tubules (Nielsen et al., 1993b). Some immunostaining for AQP2 has also been shown in the basolateral membranes of principal cells in the inner medullary region of the collecting duct (Marples et al., 1995). This aquaporin is the main water channel which is regulated by vasopressin and therefore requires special consideration. With the use of phosphoproteomic analysis, two AQP2 phosphorylation sites have recently been identified on rat renal IMCD cells, which change state in response to acute administration of vasopressin (Hoffert et al., 2006). Vasopressin increased AQP2 monophosphorylation at S256 and diphosphorylation at pS256/261 whereas monophosphorylation at S261 decreased, indicating that both sites are implicated in vasopressin-induced AQP2 trafficking.

Interestingly, vasopressin may affect the AQP2 phosphorylation process via a mobilization of intracellular Ca^{2+} within IMCD cells, and this is associated with cAMP, but not PKA, activation (see Balasubramanian and Yip, 2008). This vasopressin-stimulated Ca^{2+} pathway may well contribute to the overall regulation of AQP2 trafficking and apical membrane insertion.

As mentioned above, AQP3 and 4 are involved in transporting water across the basolateral membranes, and AQP3 expression also appears to be vasopressin-sensitive.

Intracellular microtubule and microfilament networks:
Trafficking of the vesicles containing the AQP2 molecules from intracellular sites to the apical membrane appears to depend on the integrity of the microtubular network. Microtubules are intracellular polar structures which are anchored at one (negative) end called the organizing centre, and have free (positive) ends within the cytoplasm. It is likely that the organizing centres are located towards the apical membrane with the free ends directed inwards within the cytoplasm (Meads and Schroer, 1995). A protein complex composed of dynein-dynactin is associated with the attachment of intracellular vesicles to the microtubular structure, providing both attachment (dynein) and motor unit (dynactin) for moving the vesicle in the negative (apical membrane) direction. This contrasts with kinesin proteins, which move vesicles in the opposite direction and may be involved in the return of AQP2 to intracellular loci.

Disruption of microtubules in isolated rabbit cortical collecting tubules with nocodazole inhibited the increase in hydraulic conductivity by vasopressin or a cAMP analogue, but only when administered before the hormone, not after the effect had been induced (Phillips and Taylor, 1989). Similar results were obtained with the microtubule disrupting agent colcemid (Phillips and Taylor, 1992; Tajika *et al.*, 2005) and colchicine (Sabolic *et al.*, 1995). Likewise, disruption of microtubules with nocodazole inhibited the redistribution of AQP2 to apical membranes of principal cells in an isolated inner medullary collecting tubule preparation (Shaw and Marples, 2002). Interestingly, dynein and dynactin are located within the intracellular vesicles, together with AQP2 in collecting duct principal cells, implying that they could well be involved in the trafficking of the vesicles towards the apical membranes (Marples *et al.*, 1998).

F-actin microfilaments are also believed to play a role in the trafficking of intracellular vesicles containing AQP2 to the apical membrane, as indicated in the review by Noda and Sasaki (2005). Depolymerization of the actin cytoskeleton by cytochalasins is associated with an inhibition of vasopressin-induced water transport in toad bladder (Wade and Kachadorian, 1988; Franki *et al.*, 1992). However, vasopressin itself depolymerises F-actin in the apical region of rat IMCD segments (Simon *et al.*, 1993). The general belief is that the actin cytoskeleton matrix provides a barrier to the movement of vesicles in the subapical region of the cell and that its disruption (by depolymerization) is required to allow the vesicles to reach their target apical membrane.

So why do the cytochalasins inhibit vasopressin-induced water transport? Franki *et al.* (1992) have proposed that there are at least two pools of F-actin, one being the subapical pool blocking movement of vesicles which is depolymerised by vasopressin, the other being actin filaments which are necessary in promoting the movement of vesicles and which are depolymerised by the cytochalasins. Thus, if the cytochalasins block the formation of the actin filaments promoting movement of AQP2 vesicles, then even in the presence of vasopressin water transport will be inhibited.

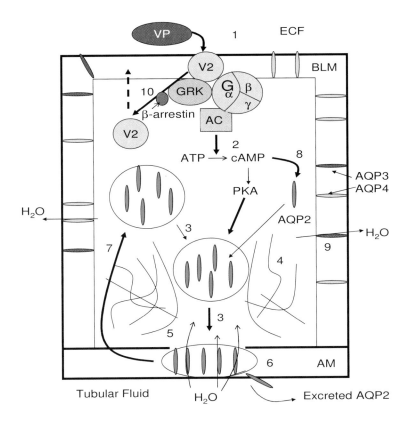

Figure 3. Proposed elements of the mechanism of action of vasopressin on water reabsorption in the principal cells of the collecting duct: 1. Vasopressin (VP) in the extracellular fluid (ECF) binds to its basolateral membrane (BLM)-bound V2 receptor and its associated G protein is activated. 2. The αs unit activates adenylyl cyclase (AC) resulting in cAMP formation from ATP; cAMP stimulates phosphorylation of protein kinase A (PKA). 3. PKA stimulates trafficking of intracellular vesicles containing AQP2 water channels to the apical membrane (AM). 4. This process involves a cAMP-dependent involvement of the microtubular (MT) network. 5. The probable depolymerization of the apically located actin mesh is also VP-cAMP dependent. 6. The AQP2 proteins are inserted into the AM and in the presence of a concentration gradient water transport into cell occurs. 7. The re-uptake of AQP2 back into vesicles is followed by migration back into a more central region of cell. 8. cAMP stimulates longer-term nuclear synthesis of new AQP2 molecules. 9. Water leaves cell across the BLMs via AQP3 and 4 (AQP3 may also be under vasopressin control to some extent). 10. Recycling of the V2 receptor involving GRK and β-arrestin. Chronic effects may include an escape mechanism from vasopressin's action on AQP2. See text for details.

Interestingly, non-muscle myosin II (a calcium-calmodulin-dependent protein) and its myosin light chain kinase, which could provide the motor for vesicle movement along the actin filaments, are stimulated by the V2 agonist DDAVP (Chou *et al.*, 2004). A recent paper by Riethmuller *et al.* (2008) disagrees with the concept that depolymerisation of actin results in aquaporin-containing vesicle translocation to the plasma membrane. Instead, using atomic force microscopy they provide evidence suggesting that this process is actually associated with a relaxation of actomyosin.

ii) *Urea transport*

Another role of vasopressin in the kidneys is to stimulate urea transport in the collecting duct. This polar molecule requires a specific transporter in order for it to cross cell membranes at the kind of rate measured, as indicated by a number of cell transport studies in the 1970s and 1980s (reviewed in Sands *et al.*, 1997; Sands, 1999). There are two urea transporter (UT) genes, both located on chromosome 18, associated with UTA and UTB proteins and their various isoforms. In the collecting duct, there are three UTA isoforms likely to play a role in urea transport, UTA1, UTA2 and UTA3 (Bagnasco *et al.*, 2000). A recent UTA promoter and beta-galactose reporter gene study indicates that UTA1 and UTA3 are colocalized with AQP2 in the IMCD principal cells (Fenton *et al.*, 2006). The main, but not exclusive, segment of the collecting duct associated with vasopressin-stimulated urea transport is the terminal section of the IMCD, and UTA1 and UTA3 are located in the apical membranes (in humans, Bagnasco *et al.*, 2001; in rats, Nielsen *et al.*, 1996). The mechanism is likely to involve a V2 receptor-initiated cAMP-PKA-dependent pathway culminating in rapid phosphorylation of UTA1, and maybe of UTA3 (Zhang *et al.*, 2002). The UTA1 urea transporter in initial IMCD sections is also stimulated by vasopressin as shown in streptozotocin-induced diabetic rats (Pech *et al.*, 2005). This effect of vasopressin on IMCD urea transport is rapid but there is also a longer-term effect. The latter possibly involves vasopressin effects on UTA1 (protein levels decrease) and UTA3 (protein levels increase). More detail is provided in Sands (2003).

Interestingly, angiotensin II, which does not affect basal urea permeability, enhances vasopressin-stimulated urea permeability through a PKC-mediated mechanism (Kato *et al.*, 2000). Furthermore, hyperosmolality also increases urea transport in terminal IMCD via a PKC-mediated mechanism, but this is independent of vasopressin (Star *et al.*, 1988).

iii) *Ion transport*
The reabsorption of sodium ions also occurs in the distal nephron along the distal convoluted tubule and cortical collecting duct under the influence of hormones, particularly aldosterone but also vasopressin. Sodium channels in the apical membranes convey sodium ions into the epithelial cells while a Na, K-ATPase pumps them out across the basolateral membranes. The presence of basolateral sodium channels also has to be considered as well as influences on sodium transport by actions influencing other ionic transport mechanisms.

Early studies in isolated perfused rat cortical collecting ducts indicated that vasopressin (10^{-10}M) stimulates a sustained net sodium reabsorption and potassium secretion (Tomita *et al.*, 1985). Vasopressin was also shown to have effects on anion transport in rat cortical collecting ducts, with an increased absorption of chloride and inhibition of bicarbonate secretion being indicated (Tomita *et al.*, 1986). Another study using rat IMCDs suggested that vasopressin stimulates net sodium absorption by a luminal (apical) effect, which appears to be V1 receptor-mediated (Kudo *et al.*, 1990).

In contrast, vasopressin appears to reversibly hyperpolarize the transepithelial voltage and decrease the transepithelial resistance in isolated perfused rat cortical collecting ducts, effects mimicked by cAMP agonists (suggestive of a V2 receptor mediated effect) and blocked by amiloride added to the luminal perfusate (Schafer and Troutman, 1990). These authors concluded that vasopressin increases sodium transport across the apical membranes of the principal cells via a cAMP-dependent mechanism involving amiloride-sensitive sodium channels. The amiloride-sensitive epithelial sodium channel (ENaC) comprises three homologous subunits (α, β and γ) (Canessa *et al.*, 1994). Interestingly, 5-day administration of DDAVP to Brattleboro rats and to normal Sprague Dawley rats, is associated with increased ENaC β and γ subunit mRNA in the renal cortex without any change in α subunit mRNA (Nicco *et al.*, 2001). These authors also showed that there was an associated long-term increased sodium (and water) reabsorption, implying that the effect of chronic vasopressin is to induce transcription of ENaC subunits.

The apical sodium channels in A6 epithelial cells are endocytosed in a similar manner to the AQP2 channels, and cAMP is also involved in this trafficking process (Butterworth *et al.*, 2001). Furthermore, cAMP increases the number of sodium channels inserted into the apical membranes in another renal cell line, Madin-Darby canine kidney (MDCK) cells (Morris and Schafer, 2002). More recently, the long-term effect of vasopressin on the ENaC has been shown to be more to do with an increase in the intracellular pool of the β and γ subunits than with an increased insertion of ENaC into the apical membranes (Sauter *et al.*, 2006). This might suggest that the long-term effect of vasopressin on increased sodium reabsorption is directed more to the basolateral Na-K-ATPase than to the apical ENaC channels. On this point, activation of the extracellular signal-regulated protein kinase 1 and 2 (ERK1/2) pathway is necessary for the vasopressin-induced (as well as basal and aldosterone-induced) increase in Na-K-ATPase activity associated with stimulated sodium transport in mouse cortical collecting ducts or cultured mpkCCDc14 mouse principal cells (Michlig *et al.*, 2004).

However, the effect of vasopressin on sodium transport may be species specific to some extent, since in rabbit cortical collecting duct the stimulatory effect appears to be trasnsient and followed by a sustained inhibition, with chloride transport affected similarly (Holt and Lechene, 1981). Breyer (1991a) showed that this inhibitory effect of vasopressin on apical sodium transport, which is also cAMP-dependent, could result from a simultaneous cAMP-mediated increase in the intracellular calcium ion concentration following the entry of this ion through the basolateral membrane (see also the review by Breyer, 1991b). A sodium–calcium exchange mechanism in the basolateral membrane could contribute to an increased calcium influx which could then inhibit luminal sodium absorption, as suggested by Breyer and Fredin (1996). This intracellular calcium signalling pathway may be relevant to interactive mechanisms involving other hormones. One vasopressin-induced transcription product VIP32 in mouse could be involved in the long-term downregulation of the ENaC, but this is purely speculative at this stage (Nicod *et al.*, 2002). Vasopressin increases not only the activity of sodium transport proteins but also their abundance as indicated by immunoblotting and immunohistochemistry studies on the $Na^+/K^+/2Cl^-$ co-transporter and epithelial sodium channel (Ecelbarger *et al.*, 2001a). Finally, it is useful to note that the decreased excretion of sodium seen in healthy individuals and patients with cranial DI given dDAVP infusions correlates with the decrease in water excretion and the increase in plasma osmolality and not with the fall in mean arterial blood pressure, suggesting that, as with other species, vasopressin exerts its antinatriuretic effect via a renal, not a haemodynamic, mechanism (Bankir *et al.*, 2005).

There is some evidence for a vasopressin-induced increase in potassium secretion in the cortical collecting duct, possibly secondary to the depolarization in the apical membrane brought about by the increased absorption of sodium ions (Schafer *et al.*, 1990) or by a direct effect on low-conductance potassium channels in the apical membrane (Cassola *et al.*, 1993). For a good review on potassium transport in the collecting duct, see Muto (2001).

Electrophysiological studies on rabbit cortical collecting duct have also indicated that luminally applied vasopressin might inhibit chloride conductance in the basolateral membrane, which is directly stimulated by basolaterally applied (bath) hormone (Narusa *et al.*, 1995). In a rat cortical collecting duct cell line, vasopressin stimulates a long-term transepithelial chloride secretion mediated by entry into the cells by a $Na^+/K^+/2Cl^-$ co-transporter in the baslateral membrane, as well as exit via a cystic fibrosis transmembrane regulator (CFTR) for chloride in the apical membrane, the latter showing increased transcription following vasopressin (Djelidi *et al.*, 1999). A DDAVP-induced increase in bi-directional chloride flux with net chloride absorption has also been observed in mouse cortical and medullary collecting duct cell lines (van Huyen *et al.*, 2001).

4. Conclusion

In summary, vasopressin plays a key role in regulating water reabsorption along the collecting duct, and plays a further role in the concentration of the tubular fluid by its actions on urea and sodium transport in different parts of the nephron. Other actions on renal function are also likely, such as effects on the renal vasculature and on distal nephron ion transport. Its renal actions are generally accepted to be via its V2 receptor and the activation of the AC second messenger system, but there are sufficient observations to indicate that the V1 receptor and the cellular location of both V1 and V2 receptors may play some role in influencing these effects. Finally, it has become clear that other, non-vasopressin-directed, mechanisms are clearly involved in the regulation of water and other transport processes. Furthermore, important interactions between vasopressin and other hormones are also likely to play a role.

Bibliography

Amlal H., Ledoussal C., Sheriff S., Shull G.E., Soleimani M. (2003). Downregulation of renal AQP2 water channel and NKCC2 in mice lacking the apical Na^+-H^+ exchanger NHE3. *J Physiol* 533: 511–522

Amorim J.B.O., Malnic G. (2000). V1 receptors in luminal action of vasopressin on distal K+ secretion. *Am J Physiol* 278: F809–F816

Amorim J.B., Musa-Aziz R., Mello-Aires M., Malnic G. (2004). Signalling path of the action of AVP on distal K+ secretion. *Kidney Int* 66: 696–704

Ausiello D.A., Kreisberg J.I., Roy C., Karnovsky M.J. (1980). Contraction of cultured rat glomerular cells of apparent mesangial origin after stimulation with angiotensin II and vasopressin. *J Clin Invest* 65: 754–760

Ando Y., Breyer M.D., Jacobson H.R. (1989). Dose-dependent heterogeneous actions of vasopressin in rabbit cortical collecting ducts. *Am J Physiol* 256: F556–F562

Ando Y., Tabei K., Asano Y. (1991). Luminal vasopressin modulates transport in the rabbit cortical collecting duct. *J Clin Invest* 88: 852–959

Bagnasco S.M., Peng T., Nakayama Y., Sands J.M. (2000). Differential expression of individual UTA urea transporter isoforms in rat kidney. *J Am Soc Nephrol* 11: 1980–1986

Bagnasco S.M., Peng T., Janech M.G., Karakashian A., Sands J.M. (2001). Cloning and characterization of the human urea transporter UT-A1 and mapping of the *Slc14a2* gene. *Am J Physiol* 281: F400–F406

Balasubramanian L., Sham J.S.K., Yip K.P. (2008). Calcium signalling in vasopressin-induced aquaporin-2 trafficking. *Pflugers Arch Eur J Physiol* 456: 747–754

Balkom van B.W.M., Hoffert J.D., Chou C-L., Knepper M.A. (2004). Proteomic analysis of long-term vasopressin action in the inner medullary collecting duct of the Brattleboro rat. *Am J Physiol* F216–F224

Bankir L., Fernandes S., Bardoux P., Bouby N., Bichet D.G. (2005). Vasopressin-V2 receptor stimulation reduces sodium excretion in healthy humans. *J Am Soc Nephrol* 16: 1920–1928

Bapty D.L.J., Ritchie B., Quamme G.A. (1998). Glucagon and arginine vasopressin stimulate Mg2+ uptake in mouse distal convoluted tubule cells. *Am J Physiol* 274: F328–F335

Berde B., Boissonnas R.A. (1968). Basic pharmacological properties of synthetic analogues and homologues of the neurohypophysial hormones, in *neurohypophysial hormones and similar polypeptides*. Handbook of Experimental Pharmacology vol. 23, pp. 802–870. Springer-Verlag

Birnbaumer M., Seibold A., Gilbert S., Ishido M., Barbaris C., Antaramian A., Brabet P., Rosenthal W. (1992). Molecular cloning of the receptor for human antidiuretic hormone. *Nature* 357: 333–335

Bouley R., Breton S., Sun T-X., McLaughlin M., Nsumu N.N., Lin H.Y., Ausiello D.A., Brown D. (2000). Nitric oxide and atrial natriuretic factor stimulate cGMP-dependent membrane insertion of aquaporin 2 in renal epithelial cells. *J Clin Invest* 106: 1115–1126

Bouley R., Pastor-Soler N., Cohen O., McLaughlin M., Breton S., Brown D. (2005a). Stimulation of AQP2 membrane insertion in renal epithelial cells *in vitro* and *in vivo* by the CGMP phosphodiesterase inhibitor sildenafil citrate (Viagra). *Am J Physiol* 288: F1103–F1112

Bouley R., Lin H.Y., Raychowdhury M.K., Marshansky V., Brown D., Ausiello D.A. (2005b). Downregulation of the vasopressin type 2 receptor after vasopressin-induced internalization: involvement of a lysosomal degradation pathway. *Am J Physiol* 288: C1390–1401

Breyer M.D. (1991a). Feedback inhibition of cyclic adenosine monophosphate-stimulated Na+ transport in the rabbit cortical collecting duct via Na(+)-dependent basolateral Ca++ entry. *J Clin Invest* 88: 1502–1510

Breyer M.D. (1991b). Regulation of water and salt transport in collecting duct through calcium-dependent signalling mechanisms. *Am J Physiol* 260: F1–F11

Breyer M.D., Fredin D. (1996). Effect of vasopressin on intracellular Na+ concentration in cortical collecting duct. *Kidney Int Suppl* 57: S57–S61

Bulenger S., Marullo S., Bouvier M. (2005). Emerging role of homo- and heterodimerization in G-protein-coupled receptor biosynthesis and maturation. *Trends in Pharm Sci* 26: 131–137

Burgess W.J., Balment R.J., Beck J.S. (1994). Effects of luminal vasopressin on intracellular calcium in microperfused rat medullary thick ascending limb. *Ren Physiol Biochem* 17: 1–9

Burnatowska-Hledin M.A., Spielman W.S. (1987). Vasopressin increases cytosolic free calcium in LLC-PK1 cells through a V1-receptor. *Am J Physiol* 253: F328–F332

Burnatowska-Hledin M.A., Spielman W.S. (1989). Vasopressin V1 receptors on principal cells of the rabbit cortical collecting tubule. Stimulation of cytosolic free calcium and inositol phosphate production via coupling to a pertussis toxin substrate. *J Clin Invest* 83: 84–89

Canessa C.M., Schild L., Buell G., Thorens B., Gautschi I., Horisberger J.D., Rossier B.C. (1994). Amiloride-sensitive epithelial Na$^+$ channel is made of three homologous subunits. *Nature* 367: 463–467

Carmosino M., Brooks H., Cai Q., Davis L.S., Opalenik S., Hao C-M., Breyer M. (2007). Axial heterogeneity of vasopressin receptor subtypes along the human and mouse collecting duct. *Am J Physiol Renal Physiol* 292: F351–360

Cassola A.C., Giebisch G., Wang W. (1993). Vasopressin increases density of apical low conductance K+ channels in rat CCD. *Am J Physiol* 264: F502–F509

Chabardes D., Firsov D., Aarab L.,Clabecq A., Bellanger A.C., Siaume-Perez S., Elalouf J.M. (1996). Localization of mRNAs encoding Ca^{2+}-inhibitable adenylyl cyclases along the renal tubule. Functional consequences for regulation of the cAMP content. *J Biol Chem* 271: 18264–19271

Chou C-L., Christensen B.M., Frische S., Vorum H., Desai R.A., Hoffert J.D., de Lanerolle P., Nielsen S., Knepper M.A. (2004). Non-muscle myosin II and myosin light chain kinase are downstream targets for vasopressin signalling in the renal collecting duct. *J Biol Chem* 279: 49026–49035

Correia A.G., Denton K.M., Evans R.G. (2001). Effects of activation of vasopressin –v1-receptors on regional kidney blood flow and glomerular arteriole diameters. *J Hypertension* 19: 649–657

de Rouffignac C. , Corman B., Roinel N. (1983). Stimulation by antidiuretic hormone of electrolyte tubular reabsorption in the rat kidney. *Am J Physiol* 244: F156–F164

Diepens R.J., den Dekker E., Bens M., Weidema A.F., Vanderwalle A., Bindels R.J., Hoenderop J.G. (2003). Characterization of a murine renal distal convoluted tubule cell line for the study of transcellular calcium transport. *Am J Physiol* 286: F483–489

Djelidi S., Fay M., Cluzeaud F., Thomas-Soumarmon A., Bonvalet J.P., Farman N., Biot-Chabaud M. (1999). Vasopressin stimulates long-term net chloride secretion in cortical collecting duct cells. *FEBS Lett* 460: 533–538

Dworkin L.D., Ishikara I., Brenner B.M. (1983). Hormonal modulation of glomerular function. *Am J Physiol* 244: F95–F104

Ecelbarger C.A., Yu S., Lee A.J., Weinstein L.S., Knepper M.A. (1999). Decreased renal Na-K-2Cl cotransporter abundance in mice with heterozygous disruption of the G(s)alpha gene. *Am J Physiol* 277: F235–244.

Ecelbarger C.A., Kim J.H., Wade J.R., Knepper M.A. (2001a). Regulation of the abundance of renal sodium transporters and channels by vasopressin. *Exp Neurol* 171: 227–234

Ecelbarger C.A., Kim J.H., Knepper M.A., Liu J., Tate M., Welling P.A., Wade J.R. (2001b). Regulation of potassium channel Kir 1.1 (ROMC) abundance in the thick ascending limb of Henle's loop. *J Am Soc Nephrol* 12: 10–18

Elalouf J.M., Roinel N., De Rouffignac C. (1984).. Effects of antidiuretic hormone on electrolyte reabsorption and secretion in distal tubules of rat kidney. *Pflügers Arch* 401: 167–173

Firsov D., Mandon B., Morel A., Merot J., Lemout S., Bellanger A-C., de Rouffignac C., Elalouf J-M., Buhler J-M. (1994). Molecular analysis of vasopressin receptors in the rat nephron. Evidence for alternative splicing of the V2 receptor. *Pflugers Arch* 429: 79–89

Franki N., Ding G., Gao Y., Hays R.M. (1992). Effect of cyctochalasin D on the actin cytoskeleton of the toad bladder epithelial cell. *Am J Physiol* 263: C995–C1000

Franki N., Macaluso F., Gao Y., Hays R.M. (1995). Vesicle fusion proteins in rat inner medullary collecting duct and amphibian bladder. *Am J Physiol* 268: C792–C797

Gellai M., Silverstein J.H., Hwang J.C., Larochelle F.T., Valtin H. (1984). Influence of vasopressin on renal haemodynamics in conscious Brattleboro rats. *Am J Physiol* 246: F819–F827

Good D.W., George T., Watts B.A.(2006). Nongenomic regulation by aldosterone of the epithelial NHE3 Na(+)/H(+) exchanger. *Am J Physiol* 290: C757–C763

Good D.W., Watts B.W., George T., Meyer J.W., Shull G.E. (2004). Transepithelial HCO$_3$- absorption is defective in renal thick ascending limbs from Na+/H+ exchanger NHE1 null mutant mice. *Am J Physiol* 287: F1244–F1249

Hall D.A., Varney D.M. (1980). Effect orf vasopressin on electrical potential difference and chloride transport in mouse medullary thick ascending limb of Henle's loop. *J Clin Invest* 66: 792-602

Hanoune J., Pouille Y., Tzavara E., Shen T., Lipskaya L., Miyamoto N., Suzuki Y., Defer N. (1997). Adenylyl cyclases: structure, regulation and function in an enzyme superfamily. *Mol Cell Endocrinol* 128: 179–194

Hamann S., Herrera-Perez J.J., Bundgaard M., Alvarez-Leefmans F.J., Zeuthen T. (2005). Water permeability of Na+-K+-2Cl- cotransporters in mammalian epithelial cells. *J Physiol* 568: 123–135

Hasler U., Mordasini D., Bens M., Bianchi M., Cluzeaud F., Rousselot M., Vandewalle A., Feraille E., Martin P-Y. (2002). Long-term regulation of aquaporin-2 expression in vasopressin-responsive renal collecting duct principal cells. *J Biol Chem* 277: 10379–10386

Hasler U., Nielsen S., Feraille E., Martin P-Y. (2006). Posttranscriptional control of aquaporin-2 abundance by vasopressin in renal collecting duct principal cells. *Am J Physiol* 290: F177–F187

Helies-Toussaint C., Aarab L., Gasc J.M., Verbavatz J.M., Chabardes D. (2000). Cellular localization of type 5 and type 6 ACs in collecting duct and regulation of cAMP synthesis. *Am J Physiol* 279: F185–F194

Henn V., Edemir B., Stefan E., Wiesner B., Lorenz D., Theilig F., Schmitt R., Vossebein L., Tamma G., Beyermann M., Krause E., Herberg F.W., Valenti G., Bachmann S., Rosenthal W., Klaussmann E. (2004). Identification of a novel A-kinase anchoring protein18 isoform and evidence for its role in the vasopressin-induced aquaporin-2 shuttle in renal principal cells. *J Biol. Chem* 279: 26654–26665

Henn V., Stefan E., Baillie G.S., Houslay M.D., Rosenthal W., Klaussmann E. (2005). Compartmentalized cAMP signalling regulates vasopressin-mediated water reabsorption by controlling aquaporin-2. *Biochem Soc Trans* 33: 1316–1318

Hoffert J.D, Chou C-L., Fenton R.A., Knepper M.A. (2005). Calmodulin is required for vasopressin-stimulated increase in cyclic AMP production in inner medullary collecting duct. *J Biol Chem* 280: 13624–13630

Hoffert J.D., Pisitkun T., Wang G., Shen R-F., Knepper M.A. (2006). Quantitative phosphoproteomics of vasopressin-sensitive renal cells: regulation of aquaporin-2 phosphorylation at two sites. *Proc Nat Acad Sci* 103: 7159–7164

Holt W.F., Lechene C. (1981). ADH-PGE2 interactions in cortical collecting tubule. 1. Depression of sodium transport. *Am J Physiol* 241: F452–460

Hoorn E.J., Hoffert J.D., Knepper M.A. (2005). Combined proteomics and pathways analysis of collecting duct reveals a protein regulatory network activated in vasopressin escape. *J Am Soc Nephrol* 16: 2852–2863

Imbert M., Chabardes D., Montegut M., Clique A., Morel F. (1975). Adenylate cyclase activity along the rabbit nephron as measured in single isolated segments. *Pflugers Arch* 354: 213–228

Jans D.A., Peters R., Zsigo J., Fahrenholz F. (1989). The adenylate cyclase-coupled vasopressin V2-receptor is highly laterally mobile in membranes of LLC-PK1 renal epithelial cells at physiological temperature. *EMBO* 8: 2481–2488

Kato A., Klein J.D., Zhang C., Sands J.M. (2000). Angiotensin increases vasopressin-stimulated facilitated urea permeability in rat terminal IMCDs. *Am J Physiol* 279: F835–F840

Kim G.H., Ecelbarger C.A., Mitchell C., Packer R.K., Wade J.B., Knepper M.A. (1999). Vasopressin increases Na-K-2Cl cotransporter expression in thick ascending limb of Henle's loop. *Am J Physiol* 276: F96–F103

Kim S.W., Gresz V., Rojek A., Wang W., Verkman A.S., Frokiaer J., Nielsen S. (2005). Decreased expression of AQP2 and AQP4 water channels and Na-K-ATPase in kidney collecting duct in AQP3 null mice. *Biol Cell* 97: 765–778

Klussmann E., Rosenthal W. (2001). Role and identification of protein kinase A anchoring proteins in vasopressin-mediated aquaporin-2 translocation. *Kidney Int* 60: 446–449

Knepper M.A., Kim G-L., Fernandez-Llama P., Ecelbarger C.A. (1999). Regulation of thick ascending limb transport by vasopressin. *J Am Soc Nephrol* 10: 628–634

Kudo L.H., van Baak A.A., Rocha A.S. (1990). Effect of vasopressin on sodium transport across inner medullary collecting duct. *Am J Physiol* 258: F1438–F1447

Lefkowitz R.J., Shenoy S.K. (2005). Transduction of receptor signals by β-arrestins. *Science* 308: 512–517

Lolait S.J., O'Carroll A-M., McBride O.W., Konig M., Morel A., Brownstein M.J. (1992). Cloning and characterization of a vasopressin V2 receptor and possible link to nephrogenic diabetes insipidus. *Nature* 357: 336–339

Ma T., Hasegawa H., Skach W.R., Frigeri A., Verkman A.S. (1994). Expression, functional analysis, and *in situ* hybridization of a cloned rat kidney collecting duct water channel. *Am J Physiol* 266: C139–C197

Ma T., Song Y., Yang B., Gillespie A., Carlson E.J., Epstein C.J., Verkman A.S. (2000). Nephrogenic diabetes insipidus in mice lacking aquaporin-3 water channels. *Proc Nat Acad Sci USA* 97: 4386–4391

Marchingo A.J., Abrahams J.M., Woodcock E.A., Smith A.I., Mendelsohn F.A.O., Johnston C.I. (1988). Properties of [3H]-desamino-8D-arginine vasopressin as a radioligand for vasopressin. *Endocrinology* 122: 1328–1336

Marples D., Schroer T.A., Ahrens N., Taylor A., Knepper L.A., Nielsen S. (1998). Dynein and dynactin colocalize with AQP2 water channels in intracellular vesicles from kidney collecting duct. *Am J Physiol* 274: F384–F394

Matsumura Y., Uchida S., Rai T., Sasaki S., Marumo F. (1997). Transcriptional regulation of aquaporin-2 water channel gene by cAMP. *J Am Soc Nephrol* 8: 861–867

Meads T., Schroer T.A. (1995). Polarity and nucleation of microtubules in polarized epithelial cells. *Cell Motil Cytoskeleton* 32: 273–288

Michlig S., Mercier A., Doucet A., Schild L., Horisberger J.D., Rossier B.C., Firsov D. (2004). ERK1/2 controls Na,K-ATPase activity and transepithelial sodium transport in the principal cell of the cortical collecting duct of the mouse kidney. *J Biol Chem* 279: 51002–51012

Muto S. (2001). Potassium transport in the mammalian collecting duct. *Physiol Rev* 81: 85–116

Narusa M., Yoshitomi K., Hanaoka K., Imai M., Kurokawa K. (1995). Electrophysiological study of luminal and basolateral vasopressin in rabbit cortical collecting duct. *Am J Physiol* 268: F20–F29

Nejsum L.N., Zelenina M., Aperia A., Frokiaer J., Nielsen S. (2005). Bidirectional regulation of AQP2 trafficking and recycling: involvement of AQP2-S256 phosphorylation. *Am J Physiol* 288: F980–988

Nicod M., Michlig S., Flahaut M., Salinas M., Fowler S., Jaeger N., Horisberger J.D., Rossier B.C., Firsov D. (2002). A novel vasopressin-induced transcript promotes MAP kinase activation and ENaC downregulation. *EMBO* 21: 5109–5117

Nicco C., Wittner M., Distefano A., Jounier S., Bankir L., Bouby N. (2001). Chronic exposure to vasopressin upregulates ENaC and sodium transport in the rat renal collecting duct and lung. *Hypertension* 38: 1143–1149

Nielsen S., Terris J., Smith C.P., Hediger M.A., Ecelbarger C.A., Knepper M.A. (1996). Cellular and subcellular localization of the vasopressin-regulated urea transporter in rat kidney. *Proc Nat Acad Sci* 93: 5495–5500

Nonoguchi H., Owada A., Kobayashi N., Takayama M., Terada Y., Koike J., Ujile K., Marumo F., Sakai T., Tomita K. (1995). Immunohistochemical localization of V2 vasopressin receptor along the nephron and functional role of luminal V2 receptor in terminal inner medullary collecting ducts. *J Clin Invest* 96: 1768–1778

Oakley R.H., Laporte S.A., Holt J.A., Barak L.S., Caron M.G. (1999). Association of b-arrestin with G protein-coupled receptors during clathrin-mediated endocytosis dictates the profile of receptor resensitization. *J Biol Chem* 274: 32248–32257

O'Connor P.M., Cowley A.W. Jr. (2007). Vasopressin-induced nitric oxide production in rat inner medullary collecting duct is dependent on V2 receptor activation of the phosphoinositide pathway. *Am J Physiol Renal Physiol* 293: F526–F532

Ostrowski N.L., Young III W.S, Knepper M.A., Lolait S.J. (1993). Expression of vasopressin V1a and V2 receptor messenger ribonucleic acid in the liver and kidney of embryonic, developing and adult rats. *Endocrinology* 133: 1849–1859

Pech V., Klein J.D., Kozlowski S.D., Wall S.M., Sands J.M. (2005). Vasopressin increases urea permeability in the initial IMCD from diabetic rats. *Am J Physiol* 289: F531–F535

Phillips M.E., Taylor A. (1989). Effect of nocodazole on the water permeability response to vasopressin in rabbit collecting tubules perfused *in vitro*. *J Physiol* 411: 529–544

Phillips M.E., Taylor A. (1992). Effect of cocemid on the water permeability response to vasopressin in isolated perfused rabbit collecting tubules. *J Physiol* 456: 591–608

Procino G., Carmosino M., Marin O., Brunati A.M., Contri A., Pinna L.A., Mannucci R., Nielsen S., Kwon T.H., Svelto M., Valenti G. (2003). Ser-256 phosphorylation dynamics of aquaporin 2 during maturation from the ER to the vesicular compartment in renal cells. *FASEB J* 17: 1886–1888

Rabito C. (1986). Occluding junctions in a renal cell line (LLC-PK1) with characteristics of proximal tubular cells. *Am J Physiol* 250: F734–F743

Raychowdhury M.K., Ibarra C., Damiano A., Jackson G.R. Jr, Smith P.R., McLaughlin M., Prat A.G., Ausiello D.A, Lader A.S., Cantiello H.F. (2004). Characterization of Na+-permeable cation channels in LLC-PK1 renal epithelial cells. *J Biol Chem* 270: 20137–20146

Reashima Y., Kondo K., Mizuno Y., Iwasaki Y., Oiso Y. (1998). Influence of acute elevation of plasma AVP level on rat vasopressin V2 receptor and aquaporin-2 RNA expression. *J Mol Endocrinol* 20: 281–285

Ren X-R., Reiter E., Ahn S., Kim J., Chen W. Lefkowitz R.J. (2005). Different G protein-coupled receptor kinases govern G protein and b-arrestin-mediated signalling of V2 vasopressin receptor. *Proc Nat Acad Sci* 102: 1448–1453

Riethmuller C., Oberleithner H., Wilhelmi M., Franz J., Schlatter E., Klokkers J., Edemir B. (2008). Translocation of aquaporin-containing vesicles to the plasma membrane is facilitated by actomyosin relaxation. *Biophys J* 94: 671–678

Ruiz-Opazo N., Akimoto K., Herrera V.L. (1995). Identification of a novel dual angiotensin II/vasopressin receptor on the basis of molecular recognition theory. *Nature Med* 10: 1074–1081

Ruiz-Opazo N., Lopez L.V., Herrera V.L. (2002). The dual AngII/AVP receptor gene N119S/C163R variant exhibits sodium-induced dysfunction and cosegregates with salt-sensitive hypertension in the Dahl salt-sensitive hypertensive model. *Mol Med* 8: 24–32

Sabolic I., Katsura T., Verbavatz J.M., Brown D. (1995). The AQP2 water channel: effect of vasopressin treatment, microtubule disruption and distribution in neonatal rats. *J Membr Biol* 145: 107–108

Sands J.M. (1999). Regulation of renal urea transporters. *J Am Soc Nephrol* 10: 635–646

Sands J.M. (2003). Molecular mechanisms of urea transport. *J Membr Biol* 191: 149–163

Sands J.M., Timmer R.T., Gunn R.B. (1997). Urea transporters in kidney and erythrocytes. *Am J Physiol* 273: F321–F339

Sauter D., Fernandes S., Goncalves-Mendes N., Boulkroun S., Bankir L., Loffing J., Bouby N. (2006). Long-term effects of vasopressin on the sub-cellular localization of ENaC in the renal collecting system. *Kidney Int* 69: 1024–1032

Schafer J.A., Troutman S.L. (1990). cAMP mediates the increase in apical membrane Na+ conductance produced in rat CCD by vasopressin. *Am J Physiol* 259: F823–31

Schafer J.A., Troutman S.L., Schlatter E. (1990). Vasopressin and mineralocorticoid increase apical membrane driving forcecfir K+ secretion in rat CCD. *Am J Physiol* 258: F199–F210

Schlondorff D., Levine S.D. (1985). Inhibition of vasopressin-stimulated water flow in toad bladder by phorbol myrstate acetate, dioctanoylglycerol, and RHC-80267. *J Clin. Invest* 76: 1071–1078

Schlondorff D., Satriano J.A. (1985). Interactions of vasopressin, cAMP, and prostaglandins in toad urinary bladder. *Am J Physiol* 248: F454–F458

Serradeil-Le Gal C., Raufaste D., Marty E., Garcia C., Maffrand J.P., Le Fur G. (1996). Autoradiographic localization of vasopressin V1a receptors in the rat kidney using [3H]-SR 49059. *Kidney Int* 50: 499–505

Shaw S., Marples D. (2002). A rat kidney tubule suspension for the study of vasopressin-induced shuttling of AQP2 water channels. *Am J Physiol* 283: F1160–F1166

Simon H., Gao Y., Franki N., Hays R.M. (1993). Vasopressin depolymerises apical F-actin in rat inner medullary collecting duct. *Am J Physiol* 265: C757–C762

Star R.A., Nonoguchi H., Balaban R., Knepper M.A. (1988). Calcium and cyclic adenosine monophosphateas second messengers for vasopressin in the rat inner medullary collecting duct. *J Clin Invest* 81: 1879–1888

Tajika Y., Matsuzaki T., Suzuki T., Ablimit A., Aoki T., Hagiwara H., Kuwahara M., Sasaki S., Takata K. (2005). Differential regulation of AQP2 trafficking in endosomes by microtubules and actin filaments. *Histochem Cell. Biol* 124: 1–12

Terada Y., Tomita K., Nonoguchi H., Yang T. (1993). Different localization and regulation of two types of vasopressin receptor messenger RNA in microdissected rat nephron segments using reverse transcription polymerase chain reaction. *J Clin. Invest* 92: 2339–2345

Tomita K., Pisano J.J., Knepper M.A. (1985). Control of sodium and potassium transport in the cortical collecting duct of the rat. Effects of bradykinin, vasopressin, and deoxycorticosterone. *J Clin Invest* 76: 132–136

Tomita K., Pisano J.J., Burg M.B., Knepper M.A. (1986). Effects of vasopressin and bradykinin on anion transport by the rat cortical collecting duct. Evidence for an electroneutral sodium chloride transport pathway. *J Clin Invest* 77: 136–141

Terrillon S., Barberis C., Bouvier M. (2004). Heterodimerization of V1a and V2 vasopressin receptors determines the interaction with b-arrestin and their trafficking patterns. *Proc Nat Acad Sci* 101: 1548–1553

Terrillon S., Durroux T., Mouillac B., Breit A., Ayoub M.A., Taulan M., Jockers R., Barberis C., Bouvier M(2003). Oxytocin and vasopressin V1a and V2 receptors form constitutive homo- and heterodimers during biosynthesis. *Mol Endocrinol* 17: 677–691

Trinh-Trang-Tan, M.M., Bouby N., Doute M., Bankir L. (1984). Effect of long- and short-term antidiuretic hormone availability on internephron heterogeneity in the adult rat. *Am J Physiol* 246: F879–F888

Trinh-Trang-Tan M.M, Lasbennes F., Gane P., Roudier N., Ripoche P., Cartron J.P. Bailly P. (2002). UT-B1 proteins in rat: tissue distribution and regulation by antidiuretic hormone in kidney. *Am J Physiol* 283: F912–F922

Turner M.R., Pallone T.L. (2003). Vasopressin constricts outer medullary descending vasa recta from rat kidneys. *Am J Physiol* 272: F147–F151

Van Huyen J.P., Bens M., Teulon J., Vandewalle A. (2001). Vasopressin-stimulated chloride transport in transimmortalized mouse cell lines derived from the distal convoluted tubule and cortical and inner medullary collecting ducts. *Nephrol Dial Transplant* 16: 238–245

Wade J.B., Stetson D.L., Lewis S.A. (1981). ADH action: evidence for a membrane shuttle mechanism. *Ann NY Acad Sci* 372: 106–117

Wade J.B., Kachadorian W.A. (1988). Cytochalasin B inhibition of toad bladder apical membrane responses to ADH. *Am J Physiol* 255: C526–C530

Wade J.B., Lee A.J., Liu J., Ecelbarger C.A., Mitchell C., Bradford A.D., Terris J., Kim G.H., Knepper M.A. (2000). UTA2: a 55kDa urea transporter protein in thin descending limb of Henle's loop whose abundance is regulated by vasopressin. *Am J Physiol* 278: F52–F62

Wittner M., di Stefano A., Wangemann P., Nitschke R., Greger R., Bailly C., Amiel C., Roinel N., de Rouffignac (1988). Differential effects of ADH on sodium, potassium, calcium and magnesium transport in cortical and medullary thick ascending limbs of mouse nephron. *Pflugers Arch* 412: 516–523

Yamamoto T., Sasaki K., Fushimi K., Kawasaki E., Yaoita E., Oota K., Hirata F., Marumo F., Kihara I. (1995). Localization and expression of a collecting duct water channel, aquaporin, in hydrated and dehydrated rats. *Exp Nephrol* 3: 193–201

Yang B., Verkman A.S. (2002). Analysis of double knockout mice lacking aquaporin-1 4F and UT-B; evidence for UT-B facilitated water transport in erythrocytes. *J Biol Chem* 277: 36782–36786

Yasui M., Zelanin S.M., Celsi G., Aperia A. (1997). Adenylate cyclase-coupled vasopressin receptor activates AQP2 promoter via a dual effect on CRE and AP1 elements. *Am J Physiol* 272: F443–F450

Zhang C., Sands J.M., Klein J.D. (2002). Vasopressin rapidly increases the phosphorylation of the UT-A1 urea transporter activity in rat IMCDs through PKA. *Am J Physiol* 282: F85–F90

CHAPTER 7

VASOPRESSIN AND THE CARDIOVASCULAR SYSTEM

John Laycock

Division of Neuroscience and Mental Health
Faculty of Medicine, Imperial College London
Charing Cross Campus, London W6 8RF
Email: j.laycock@imperial.ac.uk

1. Introduction

As mentioned in Chapter 1, vasopressin received its name following the pioneering work of Oliver and Schafer in 1898 which demonstrated the increase in arterial blood pressure in a dog following the injection of a pituitary extract. Attention on its vasopressor effect faded over the following years, particularly after Verney's demonstration in 1947 that the hormone exerts a powerful and physiologically relevant effect on urinary concentration at which time it came to be known as the antidiuretic hormone (ADH). However, interest in its vascular activities was rekindled following a number of studies on the vasoconstriction induced by topical application of the hormone on arterial sections. Particularly interesting is the absence of any obvious association between the clearly powerful pressor effect that vasopressin can exert and its involvement in hypertension – but there are possible explanations

The principal focus on the cardiovascular effects of vasopressin has been the peripheral actions of the hormone, but in addition it is important to appreciate that parvocellular vasopressinergic fibres from the paraventricular nuclei to other parts of the brain may also play a role. Furthermore, the recent discovery that dendritically released vasopressin may reach many other parts of the brain via the extracellular or cerebrospinal fluids and that vasopressin receptors are found in many central areas not targeted by vasopressinergic neurones suggests that this neuropeptide may have more far-reaching influences on the cardiovascular system that hitherto suspected, including effects on certain behaviours of potential relevance.

2. Vasopressin and Its Vasoconstrictor Effect

Vasopressin is now accepted as being an extremely powerful arterial and arteriolar vasoconstrictor which also has a lesser effect on veins and venules. As far back as the mid 1960s work was already being carried out to show the effect of early vasopressin analogues on vascular smooth muscle Altura *et al.*, 1965). Further *in vitro* studies measuring the change in diameter of isolated vascular rings following application of various endogenous molecules indicated that the neurohypophysial hormone was the most powerful of all known bioactive vasoconstrictor molecules, including angiotensin II (Altura, 1973). Only the more recently identified endothelin would seem to be a more powerful vasoconstrictor. In a review by Altura and Altura in 1977 the authors state: 'neurohypophyseal peptide hormones appear to be able to contract and relax vascular smooth muscle, the exact type of response being dependent on species, vascular bed, and region within a vascular bed. Receptors that subserve both contraction and relaxation may exist on different blood vessels within a species, with a preponderance of receptors that subserve contraction being present in most blood vessels'. This, and a similar statement by the same authors referring to the marked effect of various factors, including gender and sex hormones on neurohypophyseal peptide-induced contractions of vascular smooth muscle are quite prescient.

More recently, the technique of inserting a viewing window into the dorsal skinfold of conscious Syrian hamsters has shown that vasopressin produces a significantly greater vasoconstriction and reduction in blood flow in large arterioles than noradrenaline (norepinephrine), both giving similar pressor responses (Friesenecker *et al.*, 2006), which provides further evidence that the neurohypophysial hormone influences more than just peripheral vasoconstriction.

At around the same time as the earlier *in vitro* work, some studies were being published demonstrating clear pressor activity for infused vasopressin in anaesthetized and conscious animals. The advent of the Brattleboro rat with hereditary hypothalamic diabetes insipidus (BDI) due to the absence of circulating vasopressin, first identified by Valtin and colleagues in the early 1960s (Valtin *et al.*, 1962), provided an excellent experimental model for further studies on the cardiovascular role of vasopressin. While it was apparent that the BDI rat had a normal arterial blood pressure, it became equally clear that when subjected to volume depletion the blood pressure could not be restored or maintained as effectively as in normal control animals. Thus haemorrhage was shown to produce a significant marked attenuation in the recovery of the arterial blood pressure in anaesthetized BDI rats compared with normal controls (Laycock *et al.*, 1979). This effect was associated with an inability to effectively increase the total peripheral resistance, indicating a loss of vasoconstriction (Chapman *et al.*, 1986). Blockade of V1a receptors in the control (Long Evans parent strain) rats attenuated the recovery of the arterial blood pressure so that it was comparable to that seen in the BDI animals. Furthermore, the greater the loss of blood the lower the survival rate of the BDI rats was compared with the normal controls. Likewise, circulating vasopressin is necessary in order to ensure that blood pressure is maintained during dehydration in rats, and the effect is clearly due to V1 receptor mediated activity since administration of the V2 receptor agonist desamino 8D-arginine vasopressin (DDAVP) to dehydrated BDI rats was only capable of restoring fluid balance and not the blood pressure (Woods and Johnston, 1981).

Around the same time, a number of other studies confirmed the important vasoconstrictor role of vasopressin under these special volume depletion conditions (Cowley *et al.*, 1980; Aisenbrey *et al.*, 1981; Andrews and Brenner, 1981; Liard *et al.*, 1982; Pang, 1983; Schwartz and Reid, 1981, 1983; Szczepanska-Sadowska, 1972). The advent of specific vasopressin receptor agonists has provided further evidence of the V1 receptor-mediated sustained increase in arterial blood pressure, compared with the general lack of a pressor effect of similarly infused vasopressin (Cowley *et al.*, 1994; see Fig. 1). Hypertension is also induced following chronic infusion of a V1 receptor agonist into the intrarenal medullary interstitium of conscious rats (Szczepanska-Sadowska *et al.*, 1994), an effect not seen following vasopressin infusions for the same length of time (Cowley *et al.*, 1998). Interestingly, the nonpeptide V1a receptor antagonist SR-49059 blocks not only the vasopressin-induced increase in intracellular free calcium ion concentration (which presumably would result in subsequent smooth muscle contraction), but also the proliferation of human vascular smooth muscle cells (Serradeil-Le Gal *et al.*, 1992). A recent study of genetically modified mice lacking V1a receptors has interestingly shown that basal arterial blood pressure is significantly lower than that of wild-strain controls (Oikawa *et al.*, 2007).

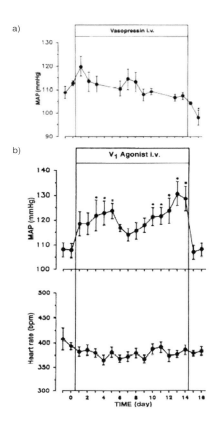

Figure 1. The effect in rats of intravenous infusion of a) arginine vasopressin on the mean arterial blood pressure (MAP) and b) of saline plus V1 receptor agonist on MAP and heart rate. *Significant difference from the two pre-treatment days (P < 0.05) (amended from Cowley *et al.*, 1994).

An additional enhancing effect of vasopressin's vasoconstrictor activity by a V1 receptor-mediated inhibition of interleukin-1β-stimulated nitric oxide and cGMP production has also been proposed following studies on cultured vascular smooth muscle cells (Kusano *et al.*, 1997).

Finally, in addition to the direct constrictor effect of vasopressin on vascular smooth muscle, there is an indirect effect mediated by catecholamines. This potentiation, described in Chapter 8 is also mediated by V1a receptors.

Despite the clearly powerful vasoconstrictor effect on isolated tissues such as aortic rings and arterial strips, and the potentially important role of vasopressin in maintaining arterial blood pressure, particularly under conditions of volume depletion, its clinical relevance regarding an involvement in the development of essential hypertension is controversial (see below). Certainly, it doesn't appear to be a major causal factor. This may be for a variety of reasons, including equally powerful compensatory mechanisms, a direct vasodilatory effect, a differential effect in various vascular beds, as well as a probable gender effect.

3. Compensatory Mechanisms

a) *The central nervous system*
One early seminal study, clearly showing the relatively small pressor effect of vasopressin infusions into conscious catheterised dogs, also demonstrated the powerful attenuating influence of an intact baroreceptor system and of the central nervous system (CNS) (Cowley *et al.*, 1974). Cowley's group showed that while the increase in arterial blood pressure was only manifest when vasopressin was infused in supra-physiological concentrations (relative to its maximal antidiuretic activity), section of the baroreceptor pathway resulted in an increased sensitivity to the same infusion doses of vasopressin. Furthermore the pressor sensitivity was further enhanced when cervical connection was disrupted. The enhanced baroreceptor response is greater with vasopressin than with other vasoactive molecules such as angiotensin II or noradrenaline.

Later, Cowley's group showed in a preliminary report that vasopressin appeared to actually enhance baroreceptor sensitivity directly (Cowley *et al.*, 1982), but this was not followed up. Certainly, stepwise decreases of carotid sinus pressure induced in anaesthetised neurohypophysectomised dogs showed that the subsequent increase in aortic pressure was greater in the presence of increased exogenous concentrations of vasopressin.

When the carotid sinus pressure was increased above the equilibrium point (between 60 and 105 mmHg), vasopressin induced a buffering reduction by decreasing heart rate and lowering cardiac output (Cowley *et al.*, 1984). This effect is likely to be mediated by both a reduction in sympathetic cardiac activity and an increase in vagal parasympathetic activity to the heart.

In a later study on conscious rats, vasopressin-induced increases in arterial blood pressure were potently reflex-buffered not only by decreases in heart rate (similar to angiotensin II), but also by reduced vasoconstriction as indicated by total peripheral resistance, indicating species differences in response (Webb *et al.*, 1986). Brizzee and Walker (1990) also showed enhanced cardiac baroreceptor reflex activity with vasopressin infusions compared with phenylethrine in response to increases in arterial blood pressure. Interestingly, while Ebert and Cowley (1992) were unable to show any alteration in either cardiac or baroreceptor reflexes in humans in response to physiological levels of vasopressin, higher levels of vasopressin (plasma concentrations of approximately 35 pg/ml) did appear to enhance the baroreceptor-mediated sympathetic reflex following nitroprusside-induced vasodilatation compared with a similar pressor dose of phenylethrine.

b) *Cellular mechanisms*

The action of a hormone is rapidly diminished by desensitization of the target cell to that hormone, and this is certainly the case for the vasoconstrictor effect of vasopressin. The rapid desensitization of cultured vascular smooth muscle in the presence of vasopressin was studied by Caramelo *et al.* (1991). Clearly, the binding of vasopressin to its receptor was an important feature, as was protein kinase C (PKC) activation. The cellular pathways involved in the process of downregulating the effects of vasopressin are considered in more detail in Chapter 4.

4. V2 Receptor-Mediated Vasodilatory Effect

Once specific agonists for different types of vasopressin receptor became available, various studies were performed to examine the more precise actions of vasopressin. Of particular interest was the finding that vasopressin has a vasodilatory effect which is mediated by V2 receptors and which is independent of the kidneys (Liard, 1988). Furthermore, this effect appears to be the result of local nitric oxide production because it is absent in the presence of N (G)-nitro-L-arginine methyl ester (L-NAME), an inhibitor of nitric oxide synthase (Liard, 1994). These vascular receptors would seem to be on the endothelial cells, which are the source of nitric oxide. Certainly, human lung microvascular endothelial cells but not umbilical vein endothelial cells have been shown to express vasopressin V2 receptors (Kaufman et al., 2000). Other endothelial cells, for example in the bovine cerebral vasculature, appear to respond to vasopressin stimulation by enhancing Na-K-Cl cotransporter activity via V1a receptors (O'Donnell et al., 2005). It would appear that the V2-mediated endothelium-dependent relaxation of human saphenous vein rings has to be 'unmasked' since it is only detectable in the presence of a V1 receptor antagonist (Aldasoro et al., 1997).

5. Direct Cardiac Effects

Vasopressin has various potential actions on the heart all of which would have effects on cardiac function, either acutely or chronically: a) coronary vessel constriction, b) contraction of cardiomyocytes and c) stimulation of cardiomyocyte growth and proliferation. It is worth remembering that vasopression expression has been identified in heart tissue, so that locally-mediated effects are quite possible, in addition to the effects of vasopressin in the general circulation.

a) *Coronary vasoconstriction*
It has been known for many years that vasopressin exerts its constrictor effect on the coronary circulation and that the effect is mediated by V1a receptors. By decreasing oxygen delivery to heart muscle, vasopressin can indirectly exert negative chronotropic and inotropic effects. For example, perfused isolated rat hearts respond to vasopressin by decreased coronary flow and oxygen consumption, and other measures of cardiac function, and a V1 receptor antagonist abolishes these effects (Boyle and Segal, 1986). The vasopressin-induced increase in intracellular free calcium ion concentration in cultured rat vascular smooth muscle cells is blocked by a V1 receptor antagonist (Matsui et al., 1992). In isolated perfused guinea pig hearts, the vasopressin-related increase in coronary vascular resistance is more pronounced with

constant coronary flow than with constant perfusion pressure, the former being associated with a greater increase in cardiac oxygen consumption (Graf *et al.*, 1997).

Coronary vasoconstriction mediated by V1a receptors has also been shown in anaesthetized goats (Fernandez *et al.*, 1998). Furthermore, the nonpeptide V1a/V2 receptor antagonist YM471 inhibits binding of vasopressin to V1a receptors on human coronary artery smooth muscle cells and prevents the accumulation of intracellular free calcium ions (Tahara *et al.*, 2002). Interestingly, the V1a receptor vasopressin agonist terlipressin had a coronary vasoconstrictor effect in isolated human erythrocyte-perfused rabbit hearts, which was less than that of vasopressin, while it only produced a significant decrease in myocardial performance at high (nM) intracoronary rates of infusion compared with vasopressin that produced an effect at much lower (pM) levels (Ouattara *et al.*, 2005). However, the effects of both terlipressin and vasopressin were almost entirely abolished by a V1a receptor antagonist.

b) *Cardiomyocyte contraction*
In addition to the likely effect of coronary artery vasoconstriction on heart function, it is possible that vasopressin might have a direct effect on heart muscle contraction. This possibility was suggested by a study of vasopressin on isolated, perfused, paced rat hearts under constant coronary flow (Walker *et al.*, 1988). The results of this study indicated that vasopressin has a direct positive inotropic effect, the increased contractions being blocked by V1, but not V2, receptor antagonists. Another study using cultured rat vascular smooth muscle cells showed a dose-dependent increase in contractility with vasopressin and this was associated with increased protein kinase C activity (Caramelo *et al.*, 1989). In contrast, the study by Matsui *et al.* (1992) examined the effect of vasopressin on cultured chick embryo ventricular cardiomyocytes, and concluded that vasopressin may have a direct negative inotropic effect which is blocked by a nonpeptide V1 receptor antagonist, perhaps indicative of species or other differences.

c) *Cardiomyocyte growth and proliferation (mitogenesis and hypertrophy)*
Cloned rat H9c2 embryonic ventricular myocytes respond to vasopressin by undergoing hypertrophy and this effect is PKC-dependent (Brostrom *et al.*, 2000). Protein kinase C-dependent protein synthesis was also

increased in rat neonatal cardiomyocytes by vasopressin, and this effect was blocked by a V1a, but not a V2, receptor antagonist (Nakamura *et al.*, 2000). Interestingly, vasopressin appears to inhibit the platelet-derived growth factor (PDGF)-mediated mitogenesis of rat embryonic H9c2 myocytes (Brostrom *et al.*, 2002). Indeed, in the presence of PDGF, vasopressin did not stimulate hypertrophy in these cells. On the other hand, vasopressin increases atrial natriuretic peptide (ANP) mRNA and protein expression, measures of cardiomyocyte hypertrophy, in primary cultures of neonatal mouse ventricular myocytes in a dose- and time-dependent manner (Hiroyama *et al.*, 2007). The hypertrophic effect is blocked by a V1a receptor antagonist and is absent in cardiomyocytes obtained from V1a receptor knockout mice. One transcription factor that may be involved in vasopressin-induced cardiomyocyte hypertrophy (rat H9c2 cells) is the cardiomyocyte-specific marker GATA-4 (Sharma *et al.*, 2007).

It is possible that vasopressin, via its V2 receptors, increases P19C16 stem-cell differentiation into contracting cells displaying GATA-4 which suggests that it may well play a role in early heart maturation (Gutkowska *et al.*, 2007. A role for vasopressin in stem-cell-derived cardiomyocyte genesis mediated by both V1a and V2 receptors was also shown in another paper by the same group (Gassanov *et al.* 2007). The V2 receptor-mediated effect appears to be linked to stimulation of endothelial nitric oxide synthase. V2 receptor expression is high in newborn (Days 1–5) compared with adult rats, when it is barely detected, in contrast with V1 receptor expression.

6. Central Cardiovascular Effects

Parvocellular axons project from the hypothalamic paraventricular nucleus (PVN) to other parts of the CNS, particularly to areas in or near the brainstem, such as the nucleus tractus solitarius and the dorsal nucleus of the vagus. From the nerve terminals of these axons, vasopressin acts as a neurotransmitter or neuromodulator. It has always seemed likely that the central release of vasopressin (and oxytocin) has some involvement with cardiovascular regulation. There are other projections of parvocellular neurones, to the forebrain (limbic areas) and spinal cord. Furthermore, it is clear that there are also projections (e.g.

catecholaminergic) from the brainstem (e.g. nucleus tractus solitarius) and other parts of the brain to the hypothalamic nuclei (Sawchenko and Swanson, 1982) implying that neuropeptide release is itself influenced by neuronal input from the cardiovascular and other regulatory structures located there. However, relatively little is known about the role of centrally released vasopressin on cardiovascular regulation or of the central pathways mediating sensory input from peripheral tissues. It is important to appreciate that innervation of brain areas with vasopressinergic fibres is relatively sparse, given the more widespread distribution of its receptors. It is therefore sensible to consider the possibility that vasopressin may reach many of its receptors not as a neurotransmitter/neuromodulator but as a hormone, transported by cerebrospinal fluid, for example.

Most studies to date indicate the presence of V1 receptors in various parts of the brain following intracerebroventricular (icv) administration of labelled vasopressin. For example, vasopressin binding sites with similar affinity to other V1 receptor-associated tissues such as hepatocytes and vascular smooth muscle were shown to be present in the amygdala, olfactory bulb and hippocampus by Barberis and Audigier (1985). Furthermore, autoradiographic studies by Lawrence *et al.*, (1988) indicated binding in brain areas, including the hypothalamus (supraoptic, paraventricular and suprachiasmatic nuclei), the hippocampus and the amygdala. Similarly, vasopressin V1a receptors were localized in several limbic structures such as the amygdala and bed nucleus of the stria terminalis, hypothalamic nuclei (suprachiasmatic and dorsal tuberalis) and in the nucleus tractus solitarius (Tribollet *et al.*, 1988).

While studies of vasopressin distribution in the brain have generally failed to show the presence of V2 receptors, one report on a vasopressin-induced antinociceptive effect in the conscious rat indicates that the action, in the periaqueductal gray, is blocked by a V2 receptor, and not a V1 receptor, antagonist (Yang *et al.*, 2006). It is interesting to note that the dual angiotensin II/vasopressin receptor, first identified in rat kidney (see Chapter 5), as well as the other novel vasopressin-activated calcium-mobilizing receptor (VACM-1) are both widely expressed in the rat CNS, and it has been suggested that they may well mediate vasopressin V2-like responses by neurones lacking the 'pure' V2 receptor (Hurbin *et al.*, 2000).

Vasopressin injected icv into anaesthetized rats (normal Sprague Dawley and vasopressin-deficient Brattleboro strains) produced rapid dose-related increases in mean arterial blood pressure (Pittman *et al.*, 1982). Another study using anaesthetized dogs showed that icv-administered vasopressin, at the (high) rate of 200 mU/min for 60 minutes, had no significant effect on arterial blood pressure or heart rate (Thomas *et al.*, 1987). Hypertonic saline-perfused icv produced an increase in vasopressin concentration in the cerebrospinal fluid and an increase in blood pressure which could be blocked by pre-treatment with a V1 antagonist (Morris *et al.*, 1986). An antipyretic effect in rats associated with icv vasopressin also indicates a V1 receptor-mediated effect since it can be blocked by a V1 antagonist (Naylor *et al.*, 1987). Dose-dependent increases in blood pressure were also shown with icv injections of vasopressin in conscious rats (Unger *et al.*, 1986).

The nucleus tractus solitarius is another area of the brain, closely linked to cardiovascular regulation, which has been shown to respond to vasopressin by an increase in mean arterial pressure following its injection into the region in conscious rats (King and Pang, 1987). The icv injection of vasopressin in conscious rabbits is also associated with an increase in arterial blood pressure (Martin *et al.*, 1985). A similar rise in blood pressure was observed in anaesthetized rabbits following the microinjection of vasopressin into the nucleus tractus solitarius, in the same study. Another study concluded that the increased blood pressure produced by icv vasopressin injections in anaesthetized rats could be at least partly mediated by V1 receptors in the nucleus tractus solitarius/vagal area (Pitman and Franklin, 1985).

V1 receptors in the rat nucleus tractus solitarius were also shown to be present in a study on brain slices by Raggenbass *et al.* (1989). Vasopressin also had a V1 receptor mediated pressor effect when vasopressin was infused icv into conscious dogs (Noszczyk *et al.*, 1993). The pressor effects observed in these various studies are generally accompanied by an increased heart rate (Martin *et al.*, 1985; Pitman and Franklin, 1985; Unger *et al.*, 1986; Noszczyk *et al.*, 1993), although a decrease (Morris *et al.*, 1986) or no effect (King and Pang, 1987) have also been reported. A review covering aspects of vasopressin and central cardiovascular regulation was published by Szczepanska-Sadowska (1996).

Hasser *et al.* (1997) reviewed the stimulatory effect of vasopressin on the sympathetic-mediated inhibitory baroreflex in response to increases in blood pressure, concluding that the area postrema is the most likely region to contain V1 receptors relevant to this action. That central V1 receptors are involved in the sympathetic and vagal baroreflex responses to increases in blood pressure has recently been shown in studies on V1a receptor knockout mice (Oikawa *et al.*, 2007).

There is little doubt that vasopressin has central effects. It is highly probable that some of those effects impinge on cardiovascular regulation. Thus its overall involvement in the regulation of blood pressure is almost certainly a balance between the central and peripheral actions it exerts. What is of current interest is a) the source of vasopressin and b) how it reaches its central receptors. Discussion of these points is provided in Chapter 11.

7. Cardiovascular Interactions with Other Hormones

Vasopressin has various interactions with other systems, endocrine or otherwise, which may be quite subtle. These interactions are covered in more detail in Chapter 8. Vasopressin, in addition to its direct effects on the vasculature and the heart described more fully in the sections above, can also influence cardiovascular function through its interactions with these other hormones and control systems. Amongst these are the renin-angiotensin-aldosterone system, the autonomic (particularly sympathetic) nervous system and the catecholamines, and gonadal steroids.

8. Vasopressin, the Kidneys and Arterial Blood Pressure

The original belief that vasopressin might exert an influence on cardiovascular regulation was partly linked to the likely consequences of its renal effects. Thus, if vasopressin increases water reabsorption, specifically from the collecting ducts via the V2 receptor-cAMP-aquaporin 2 pathway, then a chronic consequence would be the expansion of the circulating fluid volume which might be reflected in an increase in arterial blood pressure. A study of the pressor effects of vasopressin in anaesthetized Brattleboro DI rats chronically pretreated with the V2 agonist DDAVP indicated that the lower dose of vasopressin used (but not higher doses) had a significantly greater pressor effect than in control animals (Laycock, 1994), although there was no effect on basal blood pressure. In contrast, the chronic intravenous infusion of the V2 receptor agonist DDAVP into rats has been associated with a significant increase in blood pressure in uninephrectomized rats (Fernandes *et al.*, 2002). However, there is little evidence for a raised basal arterial blood pressure following the chronic intramedullary infusion of vasopressin as opposed to the infusion of a V1 receptor agonist which is clearly pressor (Cowley *et al.*, 1998), but this could at least partly be accounted for by the alternative actions of vasopressin acting via its endothelial V2 receptors as discussed earlier. Indeed, local effects of vasopressin on the renal circulation are interesting. For example, in microdissected vascular segments of cortical and medullary regions of rat kidney, only V1a receptor mRNA and protein were found, suggesting that any V2 receptor-mediated modulating effect on renal blood flow is indirect (Park *et al.*, 1997). The influence of vasopressin on local renal blood flow regulation is considered briefly in Chapter 6.

The dual angiotensin II/vasopressin receptor mentioned elsewhere (and in Chapter 4) could be linked to renal salt retention in hypertensive Dahl rats (Ruiz-Opazo *et al.*, 2002). Furthermore, Dahl salt-sensitive rats have a reduced nitric oxide synthase activity in the renal medulla, which makes them prone to the hypertensive effect of subpressor infusions of vasopressin, compared with control rats (Yuan and Cowley, 2001). This is particularly interesting since vasopressin itself appears to induce nitric oxide synthesis in the rat inner medullary collecting duct via V2 receptors, involving a phosphoinositide and calcium-mediated pathway rather than the usual cAMP intracellular system (O'Connor and Cowley, 2007).

There is currently little evidence for a V2 receptor-mediated pressor effect of vasopressin involving the kidneys, even long-term, in contrast with the V1 receptor-mediated pressor effect associated with its vasoconstrictor activity and its potential central effects. However, V2 receptor stimulation within the kidneys may well have a subtle influence not just on intrarenal blood flow, but also on systemic blood pressure.

9. Vasopressin and Cardiovascular Development

The synthesis and release of neurohypophysial vasopressin is already occurring by Week 15 in human fetuses (Schubert *et al.*, 1981) and judging by the presence of the hormone in fetal blood samples, which is measurable by Day 14 in fetal rats (Sinding *et al.*, 1980), and at least by Day 110 in ovine fetuses (Wintour *et al.*, 1982). Fetal blood pressure is generally much lower than that of adults in all these species, and while they do not seem to be related it is still unclear whether fetal plasma vasopressin has any physiological regulatory influence on it.

Immediately after birth, the circulating vasopressin concentration is high relative to adults under normal conditions of fluid balance, and tends to be higher following normal vaginal than in caesarean deliveries (Rees *et al.*, 1980). Circulating levels were also higher in sick babies (e.g. with respiratory distress syndrome), suggesting that the vasopressin is released as part of the stress response at this stage of life, particularly since there is no clear correlation with plasma or urine osmolalities at this age. The same early studies showed that within 24 hours of birth the circulating levels fall and remain low during the first week of life, followed by a slight rise thereafter. The neonatal kidney appears to be relatively unresponsive to vasopressin and it takes some weeks before maximal concentrating ability is achieved. The arterial blood pressure is also low at birth and for some time afterwards, only reaching approximate adult values (systolic and diastolic) in early adolescence. One study showed that conscious young (35–42 days old) male Brattleboro (BDI) rats lacking circulating vasopressin had significantly lower mean arterial blood pressure than their normal Long Evans (LE) counterparts. Furthermore, the administration of a V1 receptor antagonist produced a significantly reduced blood pressure in the normal LE controls only (Obika and Laycock, 1989a). While there are various other differences between young BDI and LE rats, it is interesting to note that pressor sensitivity to vasopressin seems to be reduced in young BDI rats compared with their LE counterparts, contrary to the situation found in adult animals of these two strains (Obika and Laycock, 1989b). Whether vasopressin has any role in the development of arterial blood pressure during early development remains unclear.

10. Vasopressin and Haemostasis

The process of repairing vascular walls, for instance following haemorrhage, involves a series of reactions, including platelet aggregation, binding to the damaged tissue and the coagulation of blood through the activation of clotting cascades. Both the vascular endothelium and platelets are involved in the process, and vasopressin can influence both components.

Studies indicating the presence and, indeed transport, of vasopressin in platelets in the circulation (Nussey *et al.*, 1986a) lead to the intriguing prospect of this hormone being delivered and released directly to a site of tissue (vascular wall) injury. Such a release could then be relevant for a localised vasoconstriction of the vascular smooth muscle via V1a receptors, as described earlier. However, vasopressin can have a number of other effects.

First, circulating vasopressin can induce calcium-dependent platelet aggregation (Haslam and Rosson, 1972) by binding to V1 receptors which in turn is associated with activation of phospholipase C and formation of intracellular 1,2 diacylglycerol and inositol triphosphate (Siess *et al.* 1986).

Second, vasopressin can influence platelet aggregation and adhesion to the endothelial lining by stimulating the release of von Willbrand factor (vWF). The V2 receptor agonist desmopressin is associated with the release of vWF (Nussey *et al.*, 1986b) and it is now generally accepted that vasopressin acts on endothelial cell V2 receptors, inducing an increased cAMP activity. This is associated with the release of vWF and tissue plasminogen activator, as well as the synthesis of the vasodilator nitric oxide (see Kaufmann and Vischer, 2003). Platelets also store vWF in their α-granules so its release will further promote platelet aggregation and adhesion, as well as protecting factor VIII:C from enzymatic degradation by binding to it in the circulation forming a vWF-Factor VIII:C complex (see Fig. 2).

Back in 1977, the vasopressin V2 receptor analogue DDAVP was shown to be associated with an increase in plasma clotting Factor VIII levels in patients with von Willbrand's disease and mild haemophilia (Manucci *et al.*, 1977). The precise mechanism of action of vasopressin regarding increased Factor VIII:C levels in the blood remains to be elucidated although much of this effect is probably related to the protection given to it by its binding to vWF in the circulation.

Thus, vasopressin is involved in the overall process of haemostasis and vascular repair by actions on the endothelial and smooth muscle cells, as well as having effects on platelets.

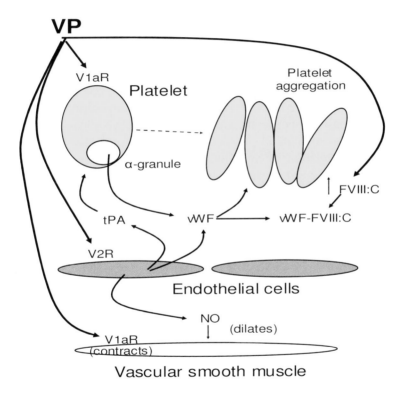

Figure 2. The actions of vasopressin on the vasculature (endothelial and smooth muscle cells) and platelets, acting through V1aR and V2R receptors. tPA, tissue platelet activator; FVIII:C, Factor VIII:C; vWF-FVIII:C, vWF-Factor VIII:C complex; NO, Nitric Oxide; vWF, von Willebrand Factor. Note that platelets are also a source of vasopressin.

11. Vasopressin and Hypertension

It is generally accepted that a raised circulating vasopressin concentration, even if present chronically, is not associated with a hypertensive state, as indicated by patients with the syndrome of inappropriate antidiuretic hormone, SIADH. Likewise, diabetes insipidus, whether in humans or animal models such as the Brattleboro rat, is not associated with hypotension. However, an early study by Cowley and colleagues did indicate that the plasma vasopressin concentration was raised in patients with moderate essential hypertension, and they concluded that vasopressin could be exerting a direct influence on extra- and intra-vascular volumes by renal and systemic vasoconstriction (Cowley et al., 1981). A more recent study has also found that vasopressin levels are raised in hypertensive subjects, particularly those with low renin concentrations, compared with controls (Zhang et al., 1999). Considering that one might expect a raised blood pressure to exert an inhibitory effect on vasopressin release, this relationship between circulating neurohypophysial hormone concentrations and blood pressure is perhaps surprising. Interestingly, electrical stimulation of an afferent renal nerve is associated with a pressor response which can be at least partially blocked by the administration of a vasopressin antibody, and is associated with an increase in the plasma vasopressin concentration (Caverson and Ciriello, 1987) Since the kidneys are likely to be causally related to hypertension, any direct link between the kidneys and the neurohypophysial system is of potential interest.

There is evidence in support of vasopressin being involved in the development of other forms of raised blood pressure, such as renovascular (e.g. two-kidney one clip Goldblatt hypertensive rat) and deoxycorticosterone acetate (DOCA)-salt loaded hypertension. There are many studies of these, and other experimental (e.g. Dahl rat strain, salt-induced), hypertensive states and while the general view is that vasopressin is involved through vascular and/or renal mechanisms (Share and Crofton, 1984; Burrell et al., 1994; Grillo et al., 1999; Yu et al., 2001; Brooks et al., 2006) or indeed central effects (Liang et al., 1997), this view is nevertheless controversial (Rabito et al., 1981; Matsuguchi et al., 1981; Burrell et al., 1997) and any causal relationship with essential hypertension is unclear. Indeed, the explanation is likely to be related to the fact that vasopressin is such a powerful vasoconstrictor that equally powerful compensatory mechanisms have evolved ensuring that it is normally preventing from producing potentially harmful hypertension.

Perhaps the use of vasopressin V1 antagonists will one day be shown to be beneficial in certain forms of hypertension. More interest is currently being shown in the individual V1 and V2 receptor-mediated effects on the heart and/or the vascular system, as discussed in earlier sections of this chapter. See also Chapter 12 for a consideration of clinical aspects of vasopressin.

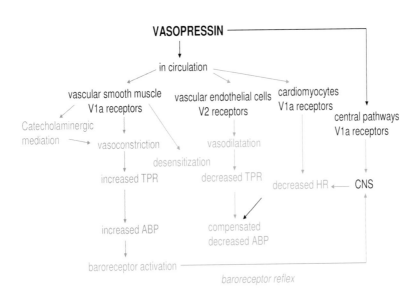

Figure 3. The main pathway for the vasopressin-induced increase in arterial blood pressure (in blue) and the various pathways which are likely to be activated in consequence, and which would contribute to the compensatory restoration of the blood pressure (in red). ABP, arterial blood pressure; HR, heart rate; TPR, total peripheral resistance.

12. Conclusion

It is certainly now agreed that vasopressin exerts a number of different effects, both directly and indirectly, on the cardiovascular system, and it is quite likely that the overall V1 receptor mediated pressor effect is counterbalanced by a variety of compensating mechanisms which prevent the development of a form of endocrine hypertension as indicated in Figure 3.

Bibliography

Aisenbrey G.A., Handelman W.A., Arnold P., Manning M., Schrier R.W. (1981). Vascular effects of arginine vasopressin during fluid deprivation in the rat. *J Clin Invest* 67: 961–968

Aldasoro M., Medina P., Vila J.M.., Otero E., Martinez-Leon J.B., lluch S. (1997). Endothelium-dependent relaxation of human saphenous veins in response to vasopressin and desmopressin. *J Vasc Surg* 25: 696–703

Altura B.M., Hershey S.G., Zweifach B.W. (1965). Effects of a synthetic analogue of vasopressin on vasdcular smooth muscle. *Proc Soc Exp Biol Med* 119: 258–261

Altura B.M. (1973). Selective microvascular constrictor actions of some neurohypophyseal peptides. *Eur J Pharmacol* 24: 49–60

Altura B.M., Altura B.T. (1977). Vascular smooth muscle and neurohypophyeal hormones. *Fed Proc* 36: 1853–1860

Andrews C.E., Brenner R.M. (1981). Relative contributions of arginine vasopressin and angiotensin II to maintenance of systemic blood pressure in the anaesthetized water-deprived rat. *Circ Res* 48: 254–258

Barbaris C., Audigier S. (1985). Vasopressin and oxytocin receptors in the central nervous system of the rat. *Ann Endocrinol (Paris)* 46: 35–39

Bernhart M.I., Chen S., Lusher J.M. (1983). DDAVP: does the drug have a direct effect on the vessel wall? *Throm Res* 31: 239–253

Boyle W.A., Segal L.D. (1986). Direct cardiac effects of vasopressin and their reversal by a vascular antagonist. *Am J Physiol* 251: H734–H741

Brizzee B.L., Walker B.R. (1990). Vasopressinergic augmentation of cardiac baroreceptor reflex in conscious rats. *Am J Physiol* 258: R860–R868

Brooks V.L., Freeman K.L., Yue Q. (2006). Time course of synergistic interaction between DOCA and salt on blood pressure: roles of vasopressin and hepatic osmoreceptors. *Am J Physiol Regul Comp Physiol* 291: R1825–R1834

Brostrom M.A., Reilly B.A., Wilson F.J., Brostrom C.O. (2000). Vasopressin-induced hypertrophy in H9c2 heart-derived myocytes. *Int J Biochem Cell Biol* 32: 993–1006

Brostrom M.A., Meiners S., Brostrom C.O. (2002). Functional receptor for platelet-derived growth factor in rat embryonic heart-derived myocytes: role of sequestered Ca_2^+ stores in receptor signalling and antagonism by arginine vasopressin. *J Cell Biochem* 84: 736–749

Burrell L.M., Phillips P.A., Stephenson J.M., Risvanis J., Rolls K.A., Johnston C.I. (1994). Blood pressure-lowering effect of an orally active vasopressin V1 receptor antagonist in mineralocorticoid hypertension in the rat. *Hypertension* 23: 737–743

Burrell L.M., Risvanis J., Phillips P.A., Naitoh M., Johnston C.I. (1997). Chronic vasopressin antagonism in two-kidney, one clip renovascular hypertension. *Clin Exp Hypertens* 19: 981–991

Caramelo C., Tsai P., Okada K., Brinner V.A., Schrier R.W. (1991). Mechanisms of rapid desensitization to arginine vasopressin in vascular smooth muscle cells. *Am J Physiol* 260: F46–F52

Caramelo C., Okada K., Tsai P., Schrier R.W. (1989). Phorbol esters and arginine vasopressin in vascular smooth muscle cell activation. *Am J Physiol* 256: F875–F881

Caverson M.M., Ciriello J. (1987). Effect of stimulation of afferent renal nerves on plasma levels of vasopressin. *Am J Physiol* 252: R80–R807

Chapman J.T., Hreash F., Laycock J.F., Walter S.J. (1986). The cardiovascular effects of vasopressin after haemorrhage in anaesthetized rats. *J Physiol* 375: 421–434

Cowley A.W. Jr, Cushman W.C., Quillen E.W. Jr, Skelton M.M., Langford H. (1981). Vasopressin elevation in essential hypertension and increased responsiveness to sodium intake. *Hypertension* 3: I93–100

Cowley A.W., Merrill D., Quillen D.W., Skelton M.M. (1982). Vasopressin enhancement of carotid baroreceptor reflex sensitivity. *Fed Proc* 41: 1116

Cowley A.W., Merrill D., Osborn J., Barber B.J. (1984). Influence of vasopressin and angiotensin on baroreflexes in the dog. *Circ Res* 54: 163–172

Cowley A.W., Monos E., Guyton A.C. (1974). Interaction of vasopressin and the baroreceptor reflex system in the regulation of arterial blood pressure in the dog. *Circ Res* 34: 505–514

Cowley A.W., Skelton M.M., Kurth T.M. (1998). Effects of long-term vasopressin receptor stimulation on medullary blood flow and arterial pressure. *Am J Physiol* 275: R1420–R1424

Cowley A.W., Switzer S.J. Guinn M.M. (1980). Evidence and quantification of the vasopressin arterial pressure control system in the dog. *Circ Res* 46: 58-67

Cowley A.W., Szczepanska-Sadowska E., Stepniakowski K., Mattson D. (1994). Chronic intravenous administration of V1 arginine vasopressin agonist results in sustained hypertension. *Am J Physiol* 267: H751–H756

Ebert T.J., Cowley A.W. (1992). Baroreflex modulation of sympathetic outflow during physiological increases of vasopressin in humans. *Am J Physiol* 262: H1372–H1376

Fernandez N., Garcia J.L., Garcia-Villalon A.L., Monge L., Gomez B., Dieguez G. (1998). Coronary vasoconstriction produced by vasopressin in anesthetized goats. Role of vasopressin V1 and V2 receptors and nitric oxide. *Eur J Pharmacol* 342: 225–233

Fernandes S., Bruneval P., Hagege A., Heudes D., Ghostine S., Bouby N. (2002). Chronic V2 vasopressin receptor stimulation increases basal blood pressure and exacerbates deoxycorticosterone acetate-salt hypertension. *Endocrinology* 143: 2759–2766

Friesenecker B.E., Tsai A.G., Martini J., Ulmer H., Wenzel V., Hasibeder W.R., Intaglietta M., Dunser M.W. (2006). Arteriolar vasoconstrictive response: comparing the effects of arginine vasopressin and norepinephrine. *Crit Care* 10: R75

Gassanov N., Jankowski M., Danalache B., Wang D., Grygorczyk R., Hoppe U.C., Gutkowska J. (2007). Arginine vasopressin-mediated cardiac differentiation. Insights into the role of its receptors and nitric oxide signalling. *J Biol Chem* 282: 11255–11265

Graf B.M., Fischer B., Eike M., Bosnjak Z.J., Stowe D.F. (1997). Differential effects of arginine vasopressin on isolated guinea pig heart function during perfusion at constant flow and constant pressure. *J Cardiovasc Pharmacol* 29: 1–7

Grillo C.A., Saravia F., Ferrini M., Piroli G., Roig P., Garcia S.I., de Kloet E.R. De Nicola A.F. (1998). Increased expression of magnocellular vasopressin mRNA in rats with deoxycorticosterone-acetate induced salt appetite. *Neuroendocrinology* 68: 105–115

Gutkowska J., Miszkurka M., Danalache B., Gassanov N., Wang D., Jankowski M. (2007). Functional arginine-vasopressin system in early heart maturation. *Am J Physiol Heart Circ Physiol* 293: H2262–H2270

Haslam R.J ., Rosson G.M. (1972). Aggregation of human platelets by vasopressin. *Am J Physiol* 223: 958–967

Hasser E.M., Bishop V.S., Hay M. (1997). Interactions between vasopressin and baroreflex control of the sympathetic nervous system. *Clin Exp Pharmacol Physiol* 24: 102–108

Hiroyama M., Wang S., Aoyagi T., Oikawa R., Sanbe A., Takeo S., Tanoue A. (2007). Vasopressin promotes cardiomyocyte hypertrophy via the vasopressin V1a receptor in neonatal mice. *Eur J Pharmacol* 559: 89–97

Hurbin A., Orcel H., Ferraz C., Moos F.C., Rabie A. (2000). Expression of the genes encoding the vasopressin-activated calcium-mobilizing receptor and the dual angiotensin II/vasopressin receptor in the rat central nervous system. *J Neuroendocrinol* 12: 677–684

Kaufmann J.E., Oksche A., Wollheim C.B., Gunther G., Rosenthal W., Vischer U.M. (2000). Vasopressin-induced von Willebrand factor secretion from endothelial cells involves V2 receptors and cAMP. *J Clin Invest* 106: 107–116

Kaufman J.E., Vischer U.M. (2003). Cellular mechanisms of the hemostatic effects of desmopressin (DDAVP). *J Thromb Haemost* 1: 682–689

King K.A., Pang C.C. (1987). Cardiovascular effects of injections of vasopressin into the nucleus tractus solitarius in conscious rats. *Br J Pharmacol* 90: 531–536

Kusano E., Tian S., Umino T., Tetsuka T., Ando Y., Asano Y. (1997). Arginine vasopressin inhibits interleukin-1b-stimulated nitric oxide and cyclic guanosine monophosphate production via the V1 receptor in cultured rat vascular smooth muscle cells. *J Hypertension* 15: 627–632

Lawrence J.A., Poulin P., Lawrence D., Lederis K. (1988). [3H]arginine vasopressin binding to rat brain: a homogenate and autoradiographic study. *Brain Res* 446: 212–218

Laycock J.F. (1994). Desamino-8D-arginine vasopressin treatment of Brattleboro rats: effect on sensitivity to pressor hormones. *Eur J Pharmacol* 271: 193–199

Laycock J.F., Penn W., Shirley D.G., Walter S.J. (1979). The role of vasopressin in blood pressure regulation immediately following acute haemorrhage in the rat. *J Physiol* 296: 267–275

Liang J., Toba K., Ouchi Y., Nagano K., Akishita M., Kozaki K., Ishikawa M., Eto M., Orimo H. (1997). Central vasopressin is required for the complete development of deoxycorticosterone-salt hypertension in rats with hereditary diabetes insipidus. *J Auton. Nerv Syst* 62: 33–39

Liard J.F. (1988). Effects of a specific antifiuretic agonist on cardiac output and its distribution in intasct and anephric dogs. *Clin Sci* 74: 293–299

Liard J.F. (1994). L-NAME antagonizes vasopressin V2-induced vasodilatation in dogs. *Am J Physiol* 266: H99–H106

Liard J.F., Deriaz O., Schelling P., Thibonnier M. (1982). Cardiac output distribution during vasopressin infusion or dehydration in conscious dogs. *Am J Physiol* 243: H663–H669

Mannucci P.M., Ruggeri Z.M., Pareti F.I., Capitanio A. (1977). 1-deamino-8-D-arginine vasopressin: a new pharmacological approach to the management of haemophilia and von Willebrands' diseases. *Lancet* 8017: 869–872

Martin S.M., Malkinson T.J., Veale W.L., Pittman Q.J. (1985). The action of centrally administered arginine vasopressin on blood pressure in the conscious rabbit. *Brain Res* 348: 137–145

Mattson P.F., Skelton M.M., Cowley A.W. Jr. (1997). Localization of the vasopressin V1a and V2 receptors within the renal cortical and medullary circulation. *Am J Physiol* 273: R243–R251

Matsui H., Kohmoto O., Hirata Y., Serizawa T. (1992). Effects of a nonpeptide vasopressin antagonist (OPC-21268) on cytosolic Ca_2^+ concentration in vascular and cardiac myocytes. *Hypertension* 19: 730–733

Matsuguchi H., Sxchmid P.G., van Orden D.,Mark A.L (1981). Does vasopressin contribute to salt-induced hypertension in the Dahl strain? *Hypertension* 3: 174–181

Morris M., Sain L.E., Schumacher S.J. (1986). Involvement of central vasopressin receptors in the control of blood pressure. *Neuroendocrinol* 43: 625–628

Nakamura Y., Haneda T., Osaki J., Miyata S. Kikuchi K. (2000). Hypertrophic growth of cultured neonatal rat heart cells mediated by vasopressin V1a receptor. *Eur J Pharmacol* 391: 39–48

Naylor A.M., Gubitz G.J., Dinarello C.A., Veale W.L. (1987). Central effects of vasopressin and 1-desamino-8D-arginine vasopressin (DDAVP) on interleukin-1 fever in the rat. *Brain Res* 401: 173–177

Noszczyk B., Lon S., Szczepanska-Sadowska E. (1993). Central cardiovascular effects of AVP and AVP analogs with V1, V2 and 'V3' agonistic or antagonistic properties in conscious dog. *Brain Res* 610: 115–126

Nussey S.S., Ang V.T., Bevan D.H., Jenkins J.S. (1986a). Human platelet arginine vasopressin. *Clin Endocrinol* 24: 427–433

Nussey S.S., Bevan D.H., Ang V.T., Jenkins J.S. (1986b). Effects of arginine vasopressin (AVP) infusions on circulating concentrations of platelet aVP, factor VIII:C and von Willebrand factor. *Thromb Haemost* 55: 34–36

Obika L.F.O., Laycock J.F. (1989a). Vasopressin V1-receptor blockade lowers arterial blood pressure in young conscious Long Evans rats. *Quart J Exp Physiol* 74: 371–374

Obika L.F.O., Laycock J.F. (1989b). Haemodynamic responses to vasopressin in anaesthetized young and adult Brattleboro rats. *Clin Sci* 76: 667–671

O'Connor P.M. Cowley A.W. Jr. (2007). Vasopressin-induced nitric oxide production in rat inner medullary collecting duct is dependent on V2 receptor activation of the phosphoinositide pathway. *Am J Physiol Renal Physiol* 293: F526–F532

O'Donnell M.E., Duong V., Suvatne J., Foroutan S., Johnson D.M. (2005). Arginine vasopressin stimulation of cerebral microvascular endothelial cell Na-K-Cl cotransporter is V1 receptor and [Ca] dependent. *Am J Physiol* 289: C283–C292

Oikawa R., Nasa Y., Ishii R., Kuwaki T., Tanoue A., Tsujimoto G., Takeo S. (2007). Vasopressin V1a recptor enhances baroreflex via central component of the reflex arc. *Eur J Pharmacol* 558: 144–150

Oliver G., Schafer E.A. (1895). On the physiological action of extracts of pituitary body and certain other glandular organs: preliminary communication. *J Physiol* 18: 277–279

Ouattara A., Landi M., Le Manach Y., Lecomte P., Leguen M., Boccara G., Coriat P., Riou B. (2005). Comparative cardiac effects'of terlipressin, vasopressin and norepinephrine on an isolated perfused rabbit heart. *Anesthesiology* 102: 85–92

Pang C.C.Y. (1983). Effect of vasopressin antagonist and saralasin on regional blood flow following haemorrhage. *Am J Physiol* 245, H749–H755

Pittman Q.J., Franklin L.G. (1985). Vasopressin antagonist in nucleus tractus solitarius/vagal area reduces pressor and tachycardia responses to paraventyricular nucleus stimulation in rats. *Neurosci Lett* 56: 155–160

Pittman Q.J., Lawrence D., McLean L. (1982). Central effects of arginine vasopressin on blood pressure in rats. *Endocrinology* 110: 1058–1060

Rabito S.F., Carretero O.A., Scicli A.G. (1981). Evidence against a role of vasopressin in the maintenance of high blood pressure in mineralocorticoid and renovascular hypertension. *Hypertension* 3: 34–38

Raggenbass M., Tribollet E., Dubois-Dauphin M., Dreifuss J.J. (1989). Vasopressin receptors of the vasopressor (V1) type in the nucleus of the solitary tract of the rat mediate direct neuronal excitation. *J Neurosci* 9: 3929–3936

Rocha e Silva M., Rosenberg M. (1969). The release of vasopressin in response to haemorrhage and its role in the mechanism of blood pressure regulation. *J Physiol* 202: 537–557

Ruiz-Opazo N., Lopez L.V., Herrera V.L. (2002). The dual AngII/AVP receptor gene N119S/C163R variant exhibits sodium-induced dysfunction and cosegregates with salt-sensitive hypertension in the Dahl salt-sensitive hypertensive model. *Mol Med* 8: 24–32

Sawchenko P.E., Swanson L.W. (1982). The organisation of noradrenergic pathways from the brainstem to the paraventricular and supraoptic nucleus in the rat. *Brain Res Rev* 4: 275–325

Schubert F., George J.M., Rao M.B. (1981). Vasopressin and oxytocin content of human fetal brain at different stages of gestation. *Brain Res* 213: 111–117

Schwartz J., Reid J. (1981). Effect of vasopressin blockade on blood pressure regulation during haemorrhage in conscious dogs. *Endocrinol* 109: 1778–1780

Schwartz J., Reid J. (1983). Role of vasopressin in blood pressure regulation in conscious water-deprived dogs. *Am J Physiol* 244: R74–R77

Serradeil-Le Gal C., Herbert J.M., Delisee C., Schaeffer P., Raufaste D., Garcia C., Dol F., Marty E., Maffrand J.P., Le Fur G. (1992). Effect of SR-49059, a vasopressin V1a antagonist, on human vascular smooth muscle cells. *Am J Physiol* 268: H404–H410

Share L., Crofton J.T. (1984). The role of vasopressin in hypertension. *Fed Proc* 43: 103–106

Sharma A., Masri J., Jo O.D., Bernath A., Martin J., Funk A., Gera J. (2007). Protein Kinase C regulates internal initiation of translation of the GATA-4 mRNA following vasopressin-induced hypertrophy of cardiac myocytes. *J Biol Chem* 282: 9505–9516

Siess W., Stifel M., Binder H., Weber P.C. (1986). Activation of V1-receptors by vasopressin stimulates inositol phospholipids hydrolysis and arachidonate metabolism in human platelets. *Biochem J* 233: 83–91

Sinding C., Robinson A.G., Seif S.M., Schmid P.G. (1980). Neurohypophysial peptides in the developing rat fetus. *Brain Res* 195: 177–186

Szczepanska-Sadowska E. (1972). The activity of the hypothalamo-hypophysial antidiuretic system in conscious dogs. *Pflugers Arch* 335: 139–146

Szczepanska-Sadowska E. (1996). Interaction of vasopressin and angiotensin II in central control of blood pressure and thirst. *Reg Pept* 66: 65–71

Szczepanska-Sadowska E., Stepniakowski K., Skelton M.M., Cowley A.W. (1994). Prolonged stimulation of intrarenal V1 vasopressin receptors results in sustained hypertension. *Am J Physiol* 267, R1217–R1225

Tahara A., Tsukada J., Tomura Y., Wada K-I., Kusayama T., Ishii N., Yatsu T., Uchida W., Taniguchi N., Tanaka A. (2002). Effect of YM471, a nonpeptide AVP receptor antagonist, on human coronary artery smooth muscle cells. *Peptides* 23: 1809–1816

Thomas G.R, Thibodeaux H., Margolius H.S., Webb J.G., Privitera P.J. (1987). Afferent vagal stimulation, vasopressin, and nitroprusside alter cerebrospinal fluid kinin. *Am J Physiol* 253: R136–R141

Tribollet E., Barbaris C., Jard S., Dubois-Dauphin M., Dreifuss J.J. (1988). Localization and pharmacological characterization of high affinity binding sites for vasopressin and oxytocin in the rat brain by light microscopic autoradiography. *Brain Res* 442: 105–118

Unger T., Rohmeiss P., Demmert G., Luft F.C., Ganten D., Lang R.E. (1986). Differential actions of neuronal and hormonal vasopressin on blood pressure and baroreceptor reflex sensitivity in rats. *Cardiovasc Pharmacol* 8 Supp l: S81–86

Verney E.B. (1947) The antidiuretic hormone and the factors which determine its release. *Proc Roy Soc Med B* 135: 25–106

Walker B.R., Childs M.E, Adams E.M. (1988). Direct cardiac effects of vasopressin: role of V1- and V2-vasopressinergic mechanisms. *Am J Physiol* 255: H261–H265

Webb R.L., Osborn J.W., Cowley A.W. (1986). Cardiovascular actions of vasopressin: baroreflex modulation in the conscious rat. *Am J Physiol* 251: H1244–H1251

Wintour E.M., Congiu M., Hardy K.J., Hennessy D.P. (1982). Regulation of urine osmolality in fetal sheep. *Quart J Exp Physio,* 67: 427–435

Woods R., Johnston C.I. (1983). Contribution of vasopressin to the maintenance of blood pressure during dehydration. *Am J Physiol* 245: F615–F621

Yang J., Chen J., Liu W., Song C., Lin B. (2006). Through V2, not V1 receptor relating to endogenous opiate peptides, arginine vasopressin in periaqueductal gray regulates antinociception in the rat. *Reg Pept* 137: 156–161

Yu M., Gopalakrishnan V., McNeill J.R. (2001). Role of endothelin and vasopressin in DOCA-salt hypertension. *Br J Pharmacol* 132: 1447–1254

Yuan B., Cowley A.W. Jr. (2001). Evidence that reduced renal medullary nitric oxide synthase activity of Dahl S rats enables small elevations of arginine vasopressin to produce sustained hypertension. *Hypertension* 37: 524–528

Zhang X., Hense H-W., Riegger G.A.J., Schunkert H. (1999). Association of arginine vasopressin and arterial blood pressure in a population-based sample. *J Hypertension* 17: 319–324

CHAPTER 8

VASOPRESSIN AND ITS INTERACTIONS WITH OTHER HORMONES AND CONTROL SYSTEMS

John Laycock

Division of Neuroscience and Mental Health
Faculty of Medicine, Imperial College London
Charing Cross campus, London W6 8RF
Email: j.laycock@imperial.ac.uk

1. Introduction

The various actions and mechanisms of action of vasopressin on the different physiological systems of the body are increasingly being ever more clearly defined. At the same time, so has our overall appreciation of the complexity of the fine control of these systems grown. This is partly because we increasingly understand that many different factors can influence a particular physiological function, but also because we are beginning to define how the various factors and control systems interact with each other. In this chapter some of these interactions between vasopressin and other control systems, mainly hormonal, are considered, the focus being on some of its specific target organs and tissues such as the kidneys and the cardiovascular system. Clearly there are potential interactions at various levels, including the hormone release stage and the action at the target tissue. A comprehensive review of all possible interactions would be beyond the scope of this book.

2. Vasopressin Interactions

a) *The renin-angiotensin system*

There are two renin-angiotensin systems (RAS) in the body, one peripheral and the other central. The peripheral system involves the renal production of the enzyme renin and its proteolytic action on a circulating precursor, angiotensinogen synthesised in the liver, producing the bioactive octapeptide angiotensin II (ATII). Since ATII does not readily cross the blood-brain barrier but, when injected intracerebroventricularly, has clear central effects such as increasing blood pressure, it became clear that a central system involving ATII synthesis in the brain was also present. However, the two systems do not function independently of each other, and peripherally produced ATII has central effects by acting on angiotensin (AT) receptors in the circumventricular organs (CVOs), which have permeable (fenestrated) capillaries and lie outside the blood-brain barrier. These CVOs include the median eminence at the base of the hypothalamus, the subfornical organ and the organum vasculosum of the lamina terminalis (OVLT). Angiotensin II can be further modified by enzymes to smaller peptides such as the septapeptide ATIII and the hexapeptide ATIV (see von Bohlen and Albrecht, 2006). The CVOs are also those areas of the brain associated with osmosensitive cells (the osmoreceptors), responsive to changes in the circulating plasma osmolality (particularly sodium ion concentration).

The interactions between the RAS and vasopressin have been the subject of study for a number of years, and the general consensus is that the interactions occur at a number of sites, including the kidneys (peripheral system) and the brain (central system). Furthermore, the interactions could provide a negative feedback regulation between the RAS and vasopressin which both operate on physiological systems such as blood pressure regulation and fluid balance, and which include renal and central actions (Fig. 1). For example, both ATII and vasopressin are pressor hormones which act peripherally on the vasculature to constrict arterioles and arteries through AT1 and V1 receptors respectively, but both molecules also act as neurotransmitters (or neuromodulators) centrally, e.g. to increase blood pressure through autonomic nerve pathways. Certainly, areas of the brain involved in the regulation of various physiological functions such as cardiovascular regulation, thirst and certain behaviours are innervated by vasopressinergic and/or angiotensinergic fibres. Thus parvocellular vasopressinergic projections from the paraventricular nuclei terminate in central areas, including the limbic system (e.g. hippocampus involved in memory), and the midbrain (e.g. the nucleus tractus solitarius, involved in cardiovascular regulation), as well as the spinal cord (Zimmerman et al., 1984).

The interaction between vasopressin and renin has also been studied. For example, there is good evidence that a peripheral increase in circulating vasopressin is associated with decreased plasma renin activity in conscious dogs and it appears to be associated with a V1 receptor-mediated action (Schwartz and Reid, 1986). This appears to occur following activation of the baroreceptor reflex and consequent decreased sympathetic activity in the renal nerves. Despite the apparent lack of any detected change in arterial blood pressure, total baroreceptor denervation prevented the vasopressin-induced decrease in plasma renin activity (Gregory et al., 1988). Confirmation of a V1 receptor-mediated effect by vasopressin on renin production (decreased granular renin expression/glomerulus) has recently been provided from studies using V1aR-deficient (V1aR$^{-/-}$) mice, which have reduced plasma renin and AII levels compared with wild-type controls (Aoyagi et al., 2008).

The evidence for an angiotensinergic innervation of hypothalamic vasopressinergic neurones is lacking. However, the recent review on the neuroendocrine regulation of water balance by Antunes-Rodriguez et al. (2004) includes a description of some of the various ways these two systems interact at the level of the brain. For example, intracerebroventricular injections of ATII are associated with increased vasopressin release (Mahon et al., 1995) and ATII stimulates vasopressin mRNA expression in hypothalamic paraventricular neurones (Dawson et al., 1998). Indeed, the pressor effect of centrally administered ATII appears to be mediated by centrally released vasopressin acting on V1 receptors (Lon et al., 1996).

In contrast some of the earlier *in vivo* studies failed to show any significant increase in vasopressin release following peripheral ATII administration (Shade and Share, 1975; Henrich *et al.*, 1986). The presence of AT receptors in various regions of the mammalian brain has been detected, including the paraventricular and supraoptic nuclei (in sheep, McKinley *et al.*, 1986; in rabbit, Mendelsohn *et al.*, 1988; and in humans, McKinley *et al.*, 1987). Thus it is quite possible that locally produced ATII has an effect on neurones in these hypothalamic nuclei. Indeed, ATII applied to supraoptic neuronal slice preparations potentiates the excitatory postsynaptic inputs, an effect suppressed by the AT1 receptor antagonist losartan (Ozaki *et al.*, 2004), suggestive of a potential direct effect. A central interaction between the two polypeptides in the regulation of arterial blood pressure has been proposed by Lon *et al.* (1996), since V1 receptor blockade appears to inhibit not only the pressor effect of icv administered vasopressin but also that of ATII. In addition, losartan the AT1R antagonist, appears to block the pressor (and to a large extent the dipsogenic) effect of vasopressin injected into the lateral preoptic area as effectively as a V1 receptor antagonist in conscious rats (Abrao Saad *et al.*, 2004). Thus, the central interactions between vasopressin and ATII are clearly diverse and require further studies in order to elucidate their physiological significance.

In addition to the likelihood of central interactions between the vasopressin and ATII systems, there are peripheral interactions between them as well. The peripheral effect of vasopressin on renin release has generally been shown to be inhibitory (Vander, 1968; Burrag *et al.*, 1967; Khokhar *et al.*, 1976), but there have also been occasional reports of a lack of effect, for instance in isolated perfused rat kidney (Hofbauer *et al.*, 1976). The inhibitory effect of ATII on renin release in sheep is at least partly due to a centrally mediated action via ATII receptors, since it can be blocked by the ATII receptor inhibitor losartan (McKinley *et al.*, 2001). Bilateral renal nerve section results in the loss of most of this inhibition, suggesting that the effect of AII involves a reduction in renal sympathetic nerve activity (Fig. 1).

An intriguing ATII/vasopressin dual receptor has been identified in renal tissue and elsewhere, and certainly the two hormones are likely to have an interaction on sodium and water transport in the kidneys quite possibly at least in part through this intriguing receptor (see Chapter 3). In the general circulation, there may also be interactions between vasopressin and AII (as with other vasoactive hormones), for instance in the vasculature. A recent study on human arterial rings indicated that the addition of low-dose (100 pg/ml) vasopressin to the application of ATII abolished the tachyphylaxis observed with repeated applications of the latter peptide, and indeed produced enhanced responses, indicating synergism between the polypeptides (Hidaka *et al.*, 2005).

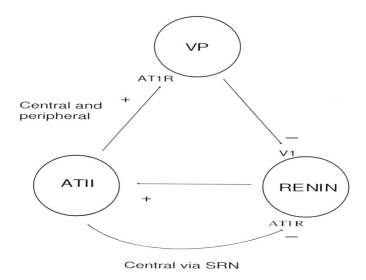

Figure1. The principal (central and peripheral) interactions between vasopressin (VP), renin and angiotensin II (ATII). The stimulatory effect of peripheral ATII on VP release is via AT1 receptors (AT1R) in circumventricular organs such as the subfornical organ. The central effect of ATII on peripheral renin release is believed to be mediated by the sympathetic renal nerves (SRN). + indicates stimulation/synthesis, – inhibition.

b) *Prostaglandins*

The principal prostaglandin synthesized in the kidney is PGE2, which acts as an attenuator of the renal vasoconstrictor effects of vasopressin, ATII and catecholamines by dilating the glomerular microcirculation and the vasa recta. However, it also appears that PGE2 can have a direct vasoconstrictor effect, as well as stimulating renin production, resulting in an increase in ATII production. The vasoconstrictor response to ATII is presumably kept in check by the PGE2-induced attenuation of its action.

It also has various effects on salt and water balance, but studies in general point to similar divergences to those seen regarding the vasculature. The general consensus is that PGE2 directly inhibits salt absorption in perfused collecting ducts, as well as potently inhibiting vasopressin-stimulated water absorption. In addition, it is possible that it has a direct stimulatory effect on basal water absorption. The likely explanation for these diverse, sometimes apparently opposite, effects, is the presence of a number of different PGE2 receptors. In the kidneys, the two main PGE2 receptors found in the collecting ducts are EP1 and EP3. EP1 receptors are linked to the intracellular calcium signalling pathway involving inositol triphosphate and diacylglycerol synthesis, and are present in increasing amounts descending from cortical, through medullary to papillary sections. Activation of these receptors is generally associated with the inhibition of sodium and water reabsorption. EP3 receptors (many spliced variants) are associated with decreased cAMP generation, and although they are found in high density in cortical and medullary collecting duct sections (as well as thick ascending limb of loop of Henle) a clear physiological role for PGE2 stimulation of these receptors is unclear. For a review on PGE2, its receptors and its functions in the kidney, see Breyer and Breyer (2000).

Of other more recent studies, Zelenina *et al.* (2000) have shown that PGE2 added to vasopressin-stimulated rat inner medullary slices reverses the translocation of aquaporin 2 to apical membranes, that it stimulates sodium reabsorption in MDCK (C7 subclone) principal cells (Wegmann and Nusing, 2003). Also, prostaglandins (e.g. PGE2), along with nitric oxide, may be involved in the escape phenomenon which occurs when water loading is accompanied by vasopressin V2 receptor agonist DDAVP treatment (Murase *et al.*, 2003). Indeed, other prostaglandins could be involved, since *in situ* hybridization indicates that PGF2α receptor mRNA is localized in the cortical collecting duct in rabbit kidney (basolateral membranes), and that its activation inhibits the vasopressin-stimulated increase in water permeability (Hebert *et al.*, 2005). Finally, one recent paper implicates PGE2 in downregulating a V1 receptor-mediated vasopressin-induced contraction of renal medullary interstitial cells (Hughes and Kohan, 2006), an effect which might have some bearing on its transport actions. Thus, the involvement of prostaglandins in the actions of vasopressin on salt and water transport is still not completely understood.

c) *Nitric oxide*
The short-lived free radical nitric oxide (NO) is produced in various parts of the kidney (and elsewhere) by the enzymatic action of NO synthases (NOS) on L-arginine, where they are likely to have disparate effects on the vasculature and specific locations along the nephron. In addition to the direct effects of NO generated within renal cells, it is quite likely that paracrine effects can also occur because of the high diffusibility of the molecule, the latter effect being somewhat restricted by the very short half-life of a few seconds. A recent *in situ* hybridization study examining the distribution of the three NOS isoforms (inducible iNOS, endothelial eNOS and neuronal nNOS) along the nephron in wild-type healthy mice only identified low basal levels of nNOS expression in macula densa and similarly low levels of eNOS in vascular endothelial cells, with no iNOS in either cortical, medullary or papillary epithelial cells unless stimulated with lipopolysaccharide (Holmqvist *et al.*, 2005). It is quite likely that other stimuli also increase iNOS expression in the tubular epithelial segments. However, other studies indicate that the eNOS and nNOS isoforms are also present. For instance, eNOS expression in the outer medulla increases with water restriction and vasopressin increases nNOS in the outer medulla and papilla in Brattleboro rats (Martin *et al.*, 2002). Proteomic analysis has

also indicated that DDAVP treatment to Brattleboro rats increases the expression of iNOS (van Balkom *et al.*, 2004).

Generation of NO within renal cells is believed to result in the activation of the cyclic GMP signalling pathway which, apart from other intracellular effects, is associated with a decreased cAMP activity. In this way, it is possible that NO influences vasopressin-induced activities such as its stimulation of water and solute transport in collecting duct cells. Indeed, many studies suggest that NO inhibits vasopressin-stimulated water transport (e.g. Garcia *et al.*, 1996). On the other hand, vasopressin may also influence the generation of NO in inner medullary collecting duct (IMCD) cells via intracellular calcium ion mobilization (Mori *et al.*, 2002) suggestive of a V1 receptor-mediated mechanism. Whilst research to date implicates the production of NO in the regulation of salt and water balance and a possible influence on the actions of vasopressin, controversy still reigns regarding the precise physiological roles of NO (see Ortiz and Garvin, 2002; 2003).

Interestingly, the expression of NO and cyclooxygenase-2 (COX-2) in the renal macula densa cells, both stimulators of renin production by the adjacent juxtaglomerular cells, is decreased in V1aR-deficient mice compared with wild-type mice (Aoyagi *et al.*, 2008). In the latter animals the V1aR is co-localised with nNOS and COX-2.

d) *Oxytocin*

Vasopressin and oxytocin (OT) are both neurohypophysial nonapeptides with a similar structure consisting of a ring of six amino acids, including two cysteines linked by a disulphide bridge forming one cystine, and a three amino acid side chain (see Chapter 2). The two polypeptides differ by just two of the amino acids; consequently it is not surprising that both hormones have a certain degree of ligand capability for each other's receptors. Since specific V2R antagonists can induce a further diuresis in Brattleboro rats lacking circulating vasopressin a possible explanation is that the effect is caused by the blocking of a V2-mediated antidiuretic action by OT (Serradeil-Le-Gal *et al.*, 1995). Indeed, Chou *et al.* (1995) also concluded that OT exerts its antidiuretic effect (at high physiological concentrations) by an action on V2 receptors. The dose-response curve for OT in an IMCD cell preparation was to the right of the VP curve. A more recent study also using Brattleboro DI rats showed that a high dose intraperitoneal infusion of OT produced a marked antidiuresis, which was completely reversed by a highly specific nonpeptide V2R antagonist (Pouzet *et al.*, 2001). However, another study indicated that OT and vasopressin stimulate cAMP accumulation in human glomerular epithelial cells via different receptors (Spath *et al.*, 1996) and this conclusion was also reached in a study using a rat IMCD cell line, also showing that the same intracellular pool of cAMP was used by both OT and V2 receptor systems (Wargent *et al.*, 1999). Thus it is still unclear whether OT, when present in high circulating concentrations, exerts its antidiuretic effect purely via V2 receptors, or whether OT receptors are also involved.

Furthermore, it is also possible that OT activates vasopressin V1 receptors, for instance in producing vasoconstriction in isolated perfused rat kidneys — an effect which is blocked by a selective V1a antagonist (Loichot *et al.*, 2001). Whether the latter effect is of physiological relevance during parturition or lactation is purely speculative at this stage.

Of current interest is the likelihood that OT receptors can exist as oligomers, either of more than one OT receptor (homodimers) or in conjunction with vasopressin V1 and/or V2 receptors (heterodimers), as demonstrated by coimmunoprecipitation studies involving antibody exposure to intact transfected human embryonic kidney cells (Terrillon *et al.*, 2003; Devost and Zingg, 2004). The existence of such complex receptor formations would certainly go some way to explaining existing discrepancies, particularly if they were tissue (and species) specific.

Finally, OT and vasopressin are each released not only from their respective nerve terminals but also from their respective hypothalamic dendrites. So far the effects shown are essentially autocrine on their own release (see Ludwig and Leng, 2006), but it is likely that they can also influence each other's neuronal activities and release patterns. If this is the case, then cross-talk between the different neurones has many implications regarding interaction between the two polypeptides and their influence over each other's actions.

e) *Natriuretic peptides*

Of the various natriuretic peptides, the best known is probably atrial natriuretic peptide (ANP) which, as its name suggests, is associated mainly, but not solely, with the cardiomyocytes of the atria, where it is released into the general circulation. The others are brain natriuretic peptide (BNP), C-type peptide and urodilatin. Brain natriuretic peptide is not only associated with the brain, where it acts as a neurotransmitter (as does ANP), but also with the cardiomyocytes of the heart, while C-type peptide is found particularly in endothelial cells and urodilatin in the kidneys. The two main polypeptides, ANP and BNP, have similar structures, and both are associated with an increased renal sodium excretion, vasodilatation, a reduction in extracellular fluid volume (ECFV) and decreased arterial blood pressure. The principal stimuli for their release from the atria are an increase in ECFV (more specifically the blood volume) and an increase in arterial blood pressure, which would be associated with a stretch of the cardiomyocytes. Since an increased arterial blood pressure would normally be associated with the inhibition of vasopressin release, any direct interaction between the cardiac natriuretic peptides and vasopressin might appear to be unlikely. However, the increase in circulating ANP associated with volume expansion can be blocked by lesions of the median eminence, and it has been suggested that this could indicate the involvement of one or more of the posterior pituitary polypeptides such as vasopressin (Antunes-Rodrigues *et al.*, 1991). An indirect relationship, with raised natriuretic peptides and vasopressin, certainly exists in chronic heart failure (see Kalra *et al.*, 2001). In this condition, circulating vasopressin levels are raised probably as a consequence of the decreased arterial blood pressure detected by high-pressure baroreceptors. Vasopressin increases AQP2 expression (Nielsen *et al.*, 1997) and consequently stimulates renal water reabsorption, which results in mild expansion of the ECFV. This volume expansion is linked with the enhanced atrial distention and hyponatraemia associated with this condition and consequently ANP (and BNP) are also raised as a compensatory mechanism (Zimmerman *et al.*, 1987).

On the other hand, various studies in the 1980s indicated that ANP, whether administered peripherally or centrally, in either *in vivo* or *in vitro* preparations, inhibits vasopressin secretion (see Gutkowska *et al.*, 1997). Thus the two peptide systems do interact with each other by direct and indirect mechanisms.

f) *Adrenomedullin*

Adrenomedullin, a polypeptide originally extracted from human phaeochromocytoma and since then found in peripheral tissues such as adrenal medulla, heart (ventricles), lung and kidney, is highly expressed in the endothelial cells of the vasculature and is also found centrally, particularly in the hypothalamic supraoptic and paraventricular nuclei (see Hinson *et al.*, 2000). It is still unclear where the adrenomedullin in the general circulation originates from under normal conditions, but endothelial cells must be one likely possibility. One important action of adrenomedullin is to decrease arterial blood pressure by producing an NO-mediated vasodilatation which is associated with a fall in total peripheral resistance. Interestingly, an early study of the effect of centrally (intracerebroventricular, icv) administered adrenomedullin to conscious rats reduced the increases in plasma vasopressin induced by either intraperitoneal injection of hypertonic saline (osmolar stimulus) or polyethylene glycol (hyovolaemic stimulus), indicative of a direct influence on vasopressin release (Yokoi *et al.*, 1996). Adrenomedullin immunoreactivity and gene expression are both present in neurones located in the hypothalamic supraoptic and paraventricular nuclei. The icv administration of this polypeptide produces a marked reduction in the proto-oncogene c-fos mRNA (which is expressed in neurones in response to direct stimulation by growth factors and neurotransmitters) mainly in the oxytocic, not the vasopressinergic neurones in rat (Ueta *et al.*, 2000).

Centrally administered adrenomedullin stimulates the oxytocinergic neurones and consequently raises the circulating concentration of oxytocin, but not vasopressin (Hashimoto *et al.*, 2005). Furthermore, intravenous adrenomedullin in human subjects had no influence at all on the ATII-induced increase in circulating vasopressin levels (Petrie *et al.*, 2001). In contrast, intravenous administration of adrenomedullin to sheep subsequently subjected to a haemorrhage showed a significant potentiation of the hypovolaemia-induced release of vasopressin, an effect not observed in pregnant animals (Charles *et al.*, 2001). One possible explanation might be that there is a species difference relevant to the action of adrenomedullin on vasopressin release. However, more recently, another study has implicated centrally administered adrenomedullin in the dose-dependent release of vasopressin in rats (Taylor *et al.*, 2005), so other factors could be relevant.

Another related molecule called intermedin/adrenomedullin-2 has also been shown to stimulate vasopressin secretion when it is administered icv in a dose-dependent manner (Taylor and Samson, 2005).

At present, it would appear that adrenomedullin interacts with vasopressin at the point of release, but the precise direction of this effect remains unclear.

g) *Catecholamines and the sympathetic nervous system*
Ever since Bartelstone and Nasmyth (1965) first showed that vasopressin potentiates the effect of catecholamines on aortic strips, various studies have examined the interactions between the neurohypophysial hormone and catecholamines, particularly noradrenaline, on the cardiovascular system. The effect of vasopressin may be due partly to a presynaptic facilitation of sympathetic activity, according to studies in the pithed rat (Streefkerk *et al.*, 2002) and in humans (Streefkerk *et al.*, 2004). In the latter study a subpressor infusion of vasopressin significantly increased the (sympathetic-mediated) forearm blood flow response to lower body negative pressure, but had no effect on the baseline forearm blood flow. However, a postsynaptic mechanism is also likely since vasopressin enhances the constrictor effect of noradrenaline on human saphenous vein and mesenteric artery rings, an effect blocked by the addition of a

V1 receptor antagonist (Medina *et al.*, 1997, 1998). A similar finding was obtained with human renal arteries (Segarra *et al.*, 2002).

In contrast, various studies have indicated that the sympathetic nervous system exerts an inhibitory influence on the peripheral actions of vasopressin. For example, noradrenaline appears to inhibit vasopressin-stimulated transepithelial sodium transport across frog skin, an effect involving $\alpha 2$ adrenoceptors (Gudme *et al.*, 2001). Furthermore, dopamine and noradrenaline inhibit water transport in the rat IMCD via $\alpha 2$ adrenoceptors (Edwards and Brooks, 2001). The use of 6-hydroxydopamine (6-OHD) which destroys sympathetic nerve fibres has been another technique used to examine this interaction. For example, in anaesthetized rats treated with this drug, the pressor effect of exogenous vasopressin was significantly enhanced (Laycock and Lightman, 1989), indicating that the sympathetic nervous system normally dampens down its constrictor action. In Brattleboro rats lacking vasopressin, this increased sensitivity to vasopressin and to other pressor hormones is further enhanced (Laycock and Lightman, 1989). Indeed, an increased sensitivity to pressor hormones including vasopressin and noradrenaline is also seen in patients with diabetes insipidus, compared with normal controls (Williams *et al.*, 1988).

A more recent conscious rat study, also using intravenously administered 6-OHD, has shown that the release of vasopressin (and oxytocin) is attenuated, but only by hypotensive, not hyperosmolar, stimuli, suggesting that the peripheral sympathetic nervous system somehow influences the hypothalamo-neurohypophysial system (Stocker *et al.*, 2006). The central administration of noradrenaline increases blood pressure through an action at least partly due to a stimulation of vasopressin release since the effect can be blocked by a vasopressin antagonist (Manning's compound, see Chapter 4) (Pelosi *et al.*, 2006). On the other hand microdialytic application of vasopressin to rat supraoptic nucleus, mimicking dendritically released neuropeptide, increases noradrenaline release from the nucleus (Yamashita *et al.*, 2001).

The interaction between vasopressin and the baroreceptor reflex (baroreflex) is also a subject of much interest. Generally, it seems that vasopressin enhances the cardiac and vascular components of the reflex probably through not only the sympathetic but also the parasympathetic systems (i.e. enhanced bradycardia and vasodilation) through an action which is V1a receptor-mediated and in the nucleus tractus solitarius/vagal area (see also Chapter 7).

It is likely that vasopressin and the sympathetic nervous system, together with the catecholamines, do interact, and it is probable that the interactions are both peripheral and central. Currently, there is much interest in the potential use of vasopressin instead of, or in combination with, catecholamines (e.g. adrenaline) in various clinical conditions such as septic shock, ventricular fibrillation and cardiac arrest. Even in the clinical context, a greater understanding of the interactions between them is likely to be of benefit to the patient. Certainly, a recent study indicates the benefits of using combinations of vasopressin and a catecholamine in a variety of clinical situations (Jochberger *et al.*, 2005).

h) *Gonadal steroids*
Over the last thirty or so years, various gender differences have been described for vasopressin, for example regarding its vascular and renal actions, and more recently its involvement in directing social/aggressive behaviours. At least some of these differences relate directly to its peripheral interactions with the gonadal steroids. Of the two types of oestrogen receptor (ER), the one mainly detected in the kidney is the α form, with the β form generally undetectable, at least in mouse (Couse *et al.*, 1997) and rat (Wells *et al.*, 2005). In contrast, ERβ has been detected in human collecting duct while the ERα form only appears to be in interstitial cells (Taylor and Al Azzawi, 2000). Androgen receptors are also expressed in the rat renal collecting duct (Boulkroun *et al.*, 2005). In the vasculature both isoforms have been localized in the heart (myocardium only) and main vessels (aorta, carotid, coronary and inferior vena cava) in humans (Taylor and Al-Azzawi, 2000). In mice, it is mostly the ERα isoform which can be detected in the main blood vessels and heart, with slight detectable levels of ERβ in the heart only

(Couse *et al.*, 1997). According to one report, vascular smooth muscle and endothelial cells in aorta and other vessels express ERβ while Erα is the predominant form expressed in uterine vessels (Andersson *et al.*, 2001). Oestrogen receptors (Erα) have also been located in neurones projecting to the supraoptic nucleus from various parts of the brain, including the organum vasculosum of the lamina terminalis and the medial preoptic nucleus in rats (Voisin *et al.*, 1997) while ERβ mRNA is expressed in the oxytocin and vasopressin neurones of the supraoptic and paraventricular nuclei (Hrabovszky *et al.*, 1998).

Progestin receptors are also located in vasopressin-producing cells projecting to the bed nucleus of the stria terminalis and amygdale (Auger and De Vries, 2002). These vasopressinergic neurones also express oestrogen (Axelson and Leeuwen, 1990) and androgen (Zhou *et al.*, 1994) receptors. Thus the gonadal steroids can have an influence on vasopressin release, directly or indirectly, by actions in the hypothalamus or in projecting areas of the brain. It is becoming clear that the actions of steroids on vasopressinergic neurones are likely to involve not only genomic but also non-genomic effects. For example, the progesterone-binding membrane protein 25-Dx is co-expressed with vasopressin in paraventricular, supraoptic and suprachiasmatic neurones (Meffre *et al.*, 2005).

Despite evidence that renal salt and water handling in males and females of various species (including humans) differs, and that the actions of vasopressin on the kidneys are influenced by gonadal steroids, the precise nature and physiological significance of these influences is unclear. An early study by Share's group investigating the antidiuretic effect of vasopressin in anaesthetized male rats, and female rats on different days of the oestrous cycle, showed that non-oestrous females had a reduced response to an intravenous infusion of the polypeptide compared with the male and oestrous rats, although this difference was abolished when a higher, maximally antidiuretic, dose was infused (Toba *et al.*, 1991). An *in vitro* study using papillary collecting duct cells also showed a greater density of vasopressin V2 receptors and a greater vasopressin-stimulated increase in cAMP accumulation in male than in female rat preparations (Wang *et al.*, 1993).

Water deprivation is associated with a greater antidiuresis in male than in female rats, although plasma vasopressin levels are higher in the latter animals despite comparable plasma osmolalities, and gonadectomy decreases urine flow in female but not male animals (Wang *et al.*, 1996). Orchidectomy decreases renal sensitivity to vasopressin while testosterone treatment to female rats increases renal sensitivity to the hormone (Pavo *et al.*, 1995). A more recent study on conscious female rats during the oestrous cycle found that similar vasopressin infusions had a greater antidiuretic effect on pro-oestrus and dioestrus day 1, compared with oestrus, but with the highest dose, which produced an antidiuresis on all days of the cycle, there were no significant differences between the days (Hartley and Forsling, 2002).

Regarding the cardiovascular system, there is also evidence to support the view that the gonadal steroids interact with vasopressin in the peripheral tissues. For example, early studies showed that the pressor responses to vasopressin are generally greater in conscious male rats than in female animals (Crofton *et al.*, 1986). Furthermore, the responses vary on different days of the oestrous cycle, such that rats in oestrus (low circulating oestrogen and progesterone) have similar pressor responses to males (Crofton *et al.*, 1988), suggesting that these gonadal steroids tend to attenuate the action of vasopressin on vascular tissue. Likewise, haemorrhage in female rats is associated with a depressed pressor effect, particularly in prooestrus when steroid levels are at their highest, compared with males (Crofton and Share, 1990). The blood pressure recovery, again compared with males, is also significantly impaired in pro-oestrous rats (Iyengar and Laycock, 1993), a difference which is not apparent in Brattleboro rats lacking vasopressin (Morrissey *et al.*, 1996). In contrast, *in vitro* studies on isolated rat aortic rings also indicate effects of gonadal steroids on their contractile responsiveness to vasopressin, but here contractions were greater in females (all days of cycle) than in males (Stallone *et al.*, 1991). The endothelium has been implicated, and vasopressin appears to induce a greater nitric oxide (NO) synthesis in male than in female rat aortic rings from this source (Stallone, 1993). Indeed, loss of the androgenic influence on NO production in rats with testicular feminisation (TFm) due to an androgen receptor defect, results in an enhanced contractile response of aortic rings to vasopressin similar to that seen in females in contrast to normal male rats, the response being inhibited by an NO synthase inhibitor in the TFm and female rats only (Stallone *et al.*, 2001). However, this only partly accounts for the sexually dimorphic response observed in response to vasopressin in aortic and mesenteric tissues. Another component appears to be the stimulation of cyclooxygenase (COX2) and thromboxane A2 vasoconstrictor activity by oestrogen, which potentiates the action of vasopressin on female rat aortic rings (Li and Stallone, 2005).

There are also sexually dimorphic differences in behavioural responses to vasopressin (and oxytocin) in animals, but this will be considered in the chapter devoted to central effects (Chapter 10).

Interactions between vasopressin and the gonadal steroids, whether central or peripheral, are certainty not featured in some recent reviews discussing the cardiovascular effects of sex steroids (Turgeon *et al.*, 2006), nor even in reviews on cardiovascular endocrinology (Baxter *et al.*, 2003), and so they remain in the realm of vasopressin (and/or maybe gonadal steroid) aficionados, at least for the time being.

i) *The hypothalamo-pituitary-adrenal axis*
There is a clear relationship between vasopressin and the glucocorticoids since the former is a releasing hormone for corticotrophin (ACTH) from the anterior pituitary, resulting in glucocorticoid synthesis and release from the adrenal cortex. This involvement in the hypothalamo-pituitary-adrenal stress pathway is important and will be considered elsewhere (see Chapter 9).

In addition, there are possible interactions at the level of peripheral tissues. One recent study indicates that vasopressin can stimulate 11β-hydroxysteroid dehydrogenase type 2 expression in human kidney epithelial cells, as do natural and synthetic glucocorticoids (Rubis *et al.*, 2006). Vasopressin could therefore play a protective role by enhancing the conversion of the bioactive glucocorticoid cortisol to the inactive cortisone in the kidney, decreasing its potential for binding to mineralocorticoid receptors.

j) *The hypothalamo-pituitary-thyroid axis*

Hypo- and hyper-thyroid disorders are associated with alterations in water balance which may at least partly be consequences of altered vasopressin secretion. The water retention of hypothyroidism has been linked to the syndrome of inappropriate ADH (SIADH) and there is some evidence to suggest a stimulatory role for thyrotrophin releasing hormone (TRH) on vasopressin release when injected intravenously (iv) into rabbits (Weitzman *et al.*, 1979), although others have not found any effect. A more recent study indicated that daily iv TRH injections were associated with decreased hypothalamic and neurohypophysial vasopressin content, and a small but significant increase in plasma concentration in normally hydrated rats, in contrast with findings made in dehydrated animals in which the pituitary vasopressin content increased (Ciosek, 2002). Thus at present there is little substantiated evidence for an important interaction between vasopressin and the thyroidal axis.

k) *Other anterior pituitary hormones*

In addition to its relationship with the pituitary-adrenal axis (see above, and Chapter 9), there have been occasional reports of vasopressin interactions with other adenohypophysial hormones such as luteinizing hormone (LH), prolactin and growth hormone.

i) *Luteinizing hormone and follicle stimulating hormone*

While there is little work that has been done to examine any role for vasopressin in follicle stimulating hormone (FSH) release, it is not unlikely that there is some influence similar to that shown for LH.

An early indication that vasopressin might be involved in the reproductive axis inhibition by certain stressors was provided by the observation that a subcutaneous injection of histamine was only associated with a reduction in circulating LH levels in normal rats and not in Brattleboro rats lacking vasopressin (Cover *et al.*, 1991). Since then, it has become clear that the vasopressin component of the hypothalamic influence on the anterior pituitary is part of the influence on the gonadotrophin inhibition, which is part of the response to stress. Furthermore, vasopressin has been implicated in the timing of the LH surge in female rats. Rats with suprachiasmatic lesions do not have an LH surge or ovulate, even with oestradiol treatment. However, vasopressin microdialysed into the medial preoptic area in oestrogen-replaced ovariectomised rats with suprachiasmatic lesions did induce transient but significant LH surges at specific times during the light-dark cycle (Palm *et al.*, 1999). This would be in agreement with the knowledge that there are vasopressinergic fibres which project from the suprachiasmatic nucleus to the preoptic nucleus, the latter being involved in the control of LH release. Indeed, there is a certain time window during pro-oestrus, when the vasopressin exerts its circadian effect (Palm *et al.*, 2001), and its action is mediated by V1a receptors in the preoptic area (Kalamatianos *et al.*, 2004).

ii) *Prolactin*

In female rats during pro-oestrus, there is a prolactin surge initiated by oestradiol concomitant with those of LH and FSH. Again, there is evidence that the suprachiasmatic nucleus is involved in the circadian regulation of the prolactin surge but, unlike the LH surge, it is the afternoon decrease in vasopressin which is associated with it (Palm *et al.*, 2001). These authors suggest that prolactin release is controlled by the combination of two actions: on the one hand, an inhibitory effect of vasopressin from the suprachiasmatic nucleus, possibly at least in part via dopamine release on the prolactin surge (effect blocked by the dopamine antagonist domperidone); on the other hand, a separate stimulatory effect from the suprachiasmatic nucleus, via putative prolactin stimulating factors. An additional relationship between the neurohypophysial system and prolactin is suggested by the intriguing possibility that copeptin, the glycopeptide released with vasopressin, may be a prolactin releasing factor, at least in carp (Flores *et al.*, 2007).

There is also the possibility that vasopressin and prolactin interact in the renal control of water reabsorption. Intravenous prolactin infusions into anaesthetized rats has a small diuretic effect which is in contrast with the pronounced dose-dependent antidiuresis seen in Brattleboro rats lacking vasopressin or in water-loaded normal control rats (Morrissey *et al.*, 2001). This effect does not appear to involve changes in glomerular filtration rate (Jones *et al.*, 2002).

3. Conclusion

It is clear that vasopressin, in addition to its direct effects, influences body function by means of interactions with other endocrine glands and control systems. These interactive effects are usually subtle but nevertheless enhance its overall regulatory influence on many physiological processes.

Bibliography

Andersson C., Lydrup M-L., Ferno M., Idvall I., Gustafsson J-A., Nilsson B-O. (2001). Immunocytochemical demonstration of oestrogen receptor b in blood vessels of the female rat. *J Endocrinol* 169: 241–247

Antunes-Rodriguez J., Ramalho M.J., Reis L.C., Menani J.V., Turrin M.Q.A., Gutkowska J., McCann S.M. (1991). Lesions of the hypothalamus and pituitary inhibit volume-expansion induced release of atrial natriuretic peptide. *Proc Natl Acad Sci* 88: 2956–2960

Antunes-Rodriguez J., De Castro M., Elias L.L.K., Valenca M.M., McCann S.M. (2004). Neuroendocrine control of body fluid metabolism. *Physiol Rev* 84: 169–208

Aoyagi T., Izumi Y., Hiroyama M., Matsuzaki T., Yasuoka Y., Sanbe A., Miyazaki H., Fujiwara Y., Nakayama Y., Kohda Y., Yamauchi J., Inoue T., Kawahara K., Saito H., Tomita K., Nonoguchi H., Tanoue A. (2008). Vasopressin regulates the renin-angiotensin-aldosterone system via V1a receptors in macula densa cells. *Am J Renal Physiol* 295: F100–F107

Auger C.J., De Vries G.J. (2002). Progestin receptor immunoreactivity within steroid-responsive vasopressin-immunoreactive cells in the male and female rat brain. *J Neuroendo* 14: 561–567

Axelson J.F., van Leeuwen F.W. (1990). Differential localization of estrogen receptors in various vasopressin synthesizing nuclei of the rat brain. *J Neuroendo* 2: 209–216

Bartelstone H.J., Nasmyth P.A. (1965). Vasopressin potentiation of catecholamine actions in dog, rat, cat, and rat aortic strip. *Am J Physiol* 208: 754–762

Baxter J.D., Young W.F. Jr., Webb P. (2003). Cardiovascular endocrinology: introduction. *Endo Rev* 24: 253–260

Boulkroun S., Le Moellic C., Blot-Chabaud M., Farman N., Courtois-Coutry N. (2005). Expression of androgen receptor and androgen regulation of NDRG2 in the rat renal collecting duct. *Pflugers Arch Eur J Physiol* 451: 388–394

Breyer M.D., Breyer R.M. (2000). Prostaglandin E receptors and the kidney. *Am J Physiol* 279: F12–F23

Charles C.J., Rademaker M.T., Richards A.M., Nicholls M.G. (2001). Adrenomedullin augments the neurohumoral response to haemorrhage in no-pregnant but not pregnant sheep. *J Endocrinol* 171: 363–371

Chou C-L., DiGiovanni S.R., Luther A., Lolait S.J., Knepper M.A. (1995). Oxytocin as an antidiuretic hormone II. Role of V2 vasopressin receptor. *Am J Physiol* 269: F78–F85

Couse J.F., Lindzey J., Grandien K., Gustafsson J.A., Korach K.S. (1997). Tissue distribution and quantitative analysis of estrogen receptor-a (Era) and estrogen receptor-b (ERb) messeneger ribonucleic acid in the wild-type and Era-knockout mouse. *Endocrinol* 138: 4613–4621

Cover P.O., Laycock J.F., Gartside I.B., Buckingham J.C. (1993). A role of vasopressin in the stress-induced inhibition of gonadotrophin secretion: studies in the Brattleboro rat. *J Neuroendocrinol* 3: 413–417

Crofton J.T., Ratcliff D.L., Brooks D.P., Share L. (1986). The metabolic clearance rate and pressor responses to vasopressin in male and female rats. *Endocrinol* 111: 1777–1781

Crofton J.T., Share L. (1990). Sexual dimorphism in vasopressin and cardiovascular response to haemorrhage in the rat. *Circ Res* 66: 1345–1353

Dawson C.A., Jhamandas J.H., Krukoff T.L. (1998). Activation by systemic angiotensin II of neurochemically identified neurons in rat hypothalamic paraventricular nucleus. *J Neuroendocrinol* 10: 453–459

Devost D., Zingg H.H. (2004). Homo- and hetero-dimeric complex formations of the human oxytocin receptor. *J Neuroendocrinol* 16: 372–377

Edwards R.M., Brooks D.P. (2001). Dopamine inhibits vasopressin action in the rat inner medullary collecting duct via a2-adrenoceptors. *J Pharm Exp Therap* 298: 1001–1006

Flores C.M., Muñoz D., Soto M., Kausel G., Romero A., Figueroa J. (2007). Copeptin, derived from isotocin precursor, is a probable prolactin releasing factor in carp. *Gen Comp Endocrinol*, 150: 343–54.

Garcia N.H., Pomposiello S.I., Garvin J.L. (1996). Nitric oxide inhibits ADH-stimulated osmotic water permeability in cortical collecting ducts. *Am J Physiol* 270: F206–F210

Gregory L.C., Quillen E.W., Keil L.C., Reid I.A. (1988). Effect of baroreceptor denervarion on the inhibition of renin release by vasopressin. *Endocrinol* 123: 319–327

Gudme C.N., Larsen A.L., Nielsen R. (2001). A2-adrenoceptors inhibit antidiuretic hormone-stimulated Na+ absorption across tight epithelia (*Rana esculenta*). *Pflugers Arch Eur J Physiol* 442: 346–352

Gutkowska J., Antunes-Rodrigues J., McCann S.M. (1997). Atrial natriuretic peptide in brain and pituitary gland. *Physiol Rev* 77: 466–515

Hartley D.E., Forsling M.L. (2002). Renal response to arginine vasopressin during the oestrous cycle in the rat: comparison of glucose and saline infusion using physiological doses of vasopressin. *Exp Physiol* 87: 9–15

Hashimoto H., Hyodo S., Kawasaki M., Mera T., Chen L., Soya A., Saito T., Fujihara H., Higuchi T., Takei Y., Ueta Y. (2005). Cenrally administered adrenomedullin 2 activates hypothalamic oxytocin-secreting neurons, causing elevated plasma oxytocin level in rats. *Am J Physiol* 289: E753–E761

Hebert R.L., Carmosino M., Saito O., Yang G., Jackson C.A., Qi Z., Bryer R.M., Natarajan C., Hata A.N., Zhang Y., Guan Y., Bryer M.D. (2005). Characterization of a rabbit prostaglandin F (2 alpha) receptor exhibiting G(i)-restricted signalling that inhibits water absorption in the collecting duct. *J Biol Chem* 280: 35028–35037

Henrich W.L., Walker B.R., Handelman W.A., Erickson A.L., Arnold P.E., Schrier R.W. (1986). Effects of angiotensin II on plasma antidiuretic hormone and renal water excretion. *Kidney Int* 30: 503–508

Hodaca T., Tsuneyoshi I., Boyle W.E. III, Onomoto M., Yonetani S., Hamasaki J., Katai R., Kunmura Y. (2005). Marked synergism between vasopressin and angiotensin II in a human isolated artery. *Crit Care Med* 33: 2613–2622

Hinson J.P., Kapas S., Smith D.M. (2000). Adrenomedullin, a multifunctional regulatory peptide. *Endo Rev* 21: 138–167

Hofbauer K.G., Zschiedrich H., Gros F. (1976). Regulation of renal release and intrarenal formationof angiotensin. Studies in the isolated perfused rat kidney. *Clin Exp Pharmacol Physiol* 3: 73–93

Holmqvist B., Olsson C.F., Svensson M.L., Svanborg C., Forsell J., Alm P. (2005). Expression of nitric oxide synthase isoforms in the mouse kidney: cellular localization and influence by lipopolysaccharide and Toll-like receptor 4. *J Mol Hist* 36: 499–516

Hrabovszky E., Kallo I., Hajszan T., Shughrue P.J., Merchenthaler I., Liposits Z. (1998). Expression of estrogen receptor-b messenger ribonucleic acid in oxytocin and vasopressin neurons of the rat supraoptic and paraventricular nuclei. *Endocrinol* 139: 2600–2604

Hughes A.K., Kohan D.E. (2006). Mechanism of vasopressin-induced contraction of renal medullary interstitial cells. *Nephron Physiol* 103: 119–124

Iyengar N., Laycock J.F. (1993). The cardiovascular response to haemorrhage in female rats is influenced by the estrous cycle. *Ann NY Acad Sci* 689: 603–605

Jochberger S., Wenzel V., Dunser M.W. (2005). Arginine vasopressin as a rescue vasopressor agent in the operating room. *Curr Opin Anaesthesiol* 18: 396–404

Jones G.G., Bagshaw L., Laycock J.F. (2002). Is the antidiuretic effect of recombinant prolactin mediated by changes in the glomerular filtration rate? *Endocrinol Abs* 3: P208

Kalamatianos T., Kallo I., Goubillon M.L., Coen C.W. (2004). Cellular expression of V1a vasopressin receptor mRNA in the female rat preoptic area: effect of oestrogen. *J Neuroendocrinol* 16: 525–533

Kalra P.R., Anker S.D., Coats A.J.S. (2001). Water and sodium regulation in chronic heart failure: the role of natriuretic peptides and vasopressin. *Cardiovasc Res* 51, 495-509

Konrads A., Hofbauer K.G., Werner U., Gross F. (1978). Effects of vasopressin and its deamino-D-arginine analogue on rennin release in the isolated perfused rat kidney. *Pflugers Arch* 377: 81–85

Laycock J.F., Lightman S. (1989). Cardiovascular interactions between vasopressin, angiotensin and noradrenaline in the Brattleboro rat. *Br J Pharmacol* 96: 347–355

Li M., Stallone J.N. (2005). Estrogen potentiates vasopressin-inducerd contraction of female rat aorta by enhancing cyclooxygenase-2 and thromboxane function. *Am J Physiol* 289: H1542–H1550

Loichot C., Krieger J.P., De Jong W., Nisato D., Imbs J.L., Barthelmebs M. (2001). High concentrations of oxytocin cause vasoconstriction by activating vasopressin V1a receptors in the isolated perfused rat kidney. *Naunyn Schmiedebergs Arch Pharmacol* 363: 369–375

Lon S, Szczepanska-Sadowska E & Szczypaczewska M (1996). Evidence that centrally released arginine vasopressin is involved in central pressor action of angiotensin II. *Am. J. Physiol.*, 270: H167–H173

Ludwig M., Leng G. (2006). Dendritic peptide release and peptide-dependent behaviours. *Nature Reviews* 7: 126–136

Mahon J.M., Allen M., Herbert J., Fitzsimmons J.T. (1995). The association of thirst, sodium appetite and vasopressin release with c-fos expression in the forebrain of the rat after intracerebroventricular injection of angiotensin II, angiotensin (1-7) or carbachol. *Neuroscience* 69: 199–208

Martin P.Y., Biancho M., Roger F., Niksic L., Feraille E. (2002). Arginine vasopressin modulates expression of neuronal NOS in rat renal medulla. *Am J Physiol* 283: F559–F568

McKinley M.J., Allen A.M., Clevers J., Denton D.A., Mendelsohn F.A. (1986). Autoradiographic localization of angiotensin receptors in sheep brain. *Brain Res* 375: 373–376

McKinley M.J., Allen A.M., Clevers J., Paxinos G., Mendelsohn F.A. (1987). Angiotensin receptor binding in human hypothalamus: autoradiographic localization. *Brain Res* 420: 375–379

McKinley M.J., McBurnie M.I., Mathai M.L. (2001). Neural mechanisms subserving central angiotensinergic influences on plasma rennin in sheep. *Hypertension* 37: 1375–1381

Medina P., Noguera I., Aldasoro M., Vila J.M., Flor B., Lluch S. (1997). Enhancement by vasopressin of adrenergic responses in human mesenteric arteries. *Am J Physiol* 272: H1087–H1093

Medina P., Acuna A., Martinez-Leon J.B., Otero E., Vila J.M., Aldasoro M., Lluch S. (1998). Arginine vasopressin enhances sympathetic constriction through the V1 vasopressin receptor in human saphenous vein. *Circulation* 97: 865–870

Meffre D., Delespierre B., Gouezou M., Leclerc P., Vinson G.P., Schmacher M., Stein D.G., Guennoun R. (2005). The membrane-associated progesterone-binding protein 25-Dx is expressed in brain regions involved in water homeostasis and is up-regulated after traumatic brain injury. *J Neurochem* 93: 1314–1326

Mendelsohn F.A., Allen A.M., Clevers J., Denton D.A, Tarjan E., McKinley M.J. (1988). Localization of angiotensin II receptor binding in rabbit brain by *in vitro* autoradiography. *J Comp Neurol* 270: 372–384

Mori T., Dickhout J.G., Cowley A.W. Jr. (2002). Vasopressin increases intracellular NO concentration via Ca(2+) signalling in inner medullary collecting duct. *Hypertension* 39: 465–469

Morrissey S.E., Baden-Fuller J., Murugananthan N., Whitehead S.A., Laycock J.F. (1996). Influence of oestrous cycle on the pressor recovery following haemorrhage in anaesthetized Brattleboro rats. *Eur J Endo* 134: 379–285

Murase T., Tian Y., Fang X.Y., Verbalis J.G. (2003). Synergistic effects of nitric oxide and prostaglandins on renal escape from vasopressin-induced antidiuresis. *Am J Physiol Regul Integr Comp Physiol* 284: R354–R362

Nielsen S., Terris J., Andersen D., Ecelberger C., Frokler J., Jonassen T., Marples D., Knepper M.A., Petersen J.S. (1997). Congestive heart failure in rats is associated with increased expression and targeting of aquaporin-2 water channel in collecting duct. *Proc Natl Acad Sci* 94: 5450–5455

Ortiz P.A., Garvin J.L. (2002). Role of nitric oxide in the regulation of nephron transport. *Am J Physiol* 282: F777–F784

Ortiz P.A., Garvin JL (2003). Cardiovascular and renal control in NOS-deficient mouse models. *Am J Physiol* 284: R628–R638

Ozaki Y., Soya A., Nakamura T., Matsumoto T., Ueta Y. (2004). Potentiation by angiotensin II of spontaneous excitatory postsynaptic currents in rat supraoptic magnocellular neurones. *J Neuroendocrinol* 16: 871–879

Palm I.F., van der Beek E.M., Wiegant V.M., Buijs R.M., Kalsbeek A. (1999). Vasopressin induces a luteinizing hormone surge in ovariectomised, estradiol-treated rats with lesions of the suprachiasmatic nucleus. *Neurosci* 93: 659–666

Palm I.F., Eline M., van der Beek E.M., Wiegant V.M., Buijs R.M., Kalsbeek A. (2001). The stimulatory effect of vasopressin on the luteinizing hormone surge in ovariectomized, estrasdiol-treated rats is time-dependent. *Brain Res* 901: 109–116

Palm I.F., Eline M., van der Beek E.M., Swarts J.M., van der Vliet J., Wiegant V.M., Buijs R.M., Kalsbeek A. (2002). Control of the estradiol-induced prolactin surge by the suprachiasmatic nucleus. *Endocrinol* 142: 2296–2302

Pavo I., Varga C., Szucs M., Laszlo F., Szecsi M., Gardi J., Laszlo F.A .(1995). Effects of testosterone on the rat renal medullary vasopressin receptor concentration and the antidiuretic response. *Life Sci* 56: 1215–1222

Pelosi G.G., Peres-Polon V.L., Correa F.M. (2006). Pressor effects of the injection of noradrenaline into different cerebroventricular spaces in anaesthetized rats. *Neurosci Lett* 397: 165–169

Petrie M.C., McDonald J.E., Hillier C., Morton J.J., McMurray J.J.V. (2001). Effects of adrenomedullin on angiotensin II stimulated atrial natriuretic peptide and arginine vasopressin secretion in healthy humans. *J Clin Pharmacol* 52 : 165–168

Pouzet B., Serradeil-Le-Gal C., Bouby N., Maffrand J.P., Le Fur G., Bankir L. (2001). Selective blockade of vasopressin V2 receptors reveals significant V2-mediated water reabsorption in Brattleboro rats with diabetes insipidus. *Nephrol Dial Transplant* 16: 725–734

Rubis B., Krozowski Z., Trzeciak W.H. (2006). Arginine vasopressin stimulates 11 beta-hydroxysteroid dehydrogenase type 2 expression in the mineralocorticoid target cells. *Mol Cell Endocrinol* 256: 17–22

Saad A.W., De Arruda Camargo A.L., Cerri S. P., Simoes S., Garcia G., Gutierrez I.L., Guarda I.,Guarda S.R. (2004). Influence of arginine vasopressin receptors and angiotensin receptor subtypes on the water intake and arterial blood pressure induced by vasopressin injected into the lateral septal area of the rat. *Autonom Neurosci* 111: 66–70

Schwartz J., Reid I.A. (1986). Role of the vasoconstrictor and antidiuretic activities of vasopressin in inhibition of renin secretion in conscious dogs. *Am J Physiol* 250: F92–F96

Segarra G., Medina P., Vila J.M., Chuan P., Domenech C., Lluch S. (2002). Increased contraction to noradrenaline by vasopressin in human renal arteries. *J Hypertension* 20: 1373–1379

Serradeil-Le-Gal C., Lacour C., Valette G., Garcia G., Foulon L., Galindo G., Bankir L., Ouzet B., Guillon G., Barberis C., Chicot D., Jard S., Vilain P., Garcia C., Marty E., Raufaste D., Brossard G., Nisato D., Maffrand J.P., Le Fur G. (1996). Characterization of SR 121463A, a highly potent and selective orally active vasopressin V2 receptor antagonist. *J Clin Invest* 98: 2729–2738

Shade R.E., Share L. (1975). Vasopressin release during nonhypotensive haemorrhage and angiotensin II infusion. *Am J Physiol* 228: 149–154

Spath M., Pavenstadt H., Petersen J., Schollmeyer P. (1996). Arginine vasopressin and oxytocin increase intracellular calcium and cAMP in human glomerular epithelial cells in culture. *Kid Blood Press Res* 19: 81–86

Stallone J.N. (1993). Role of endothelium in sexual dimorphism in vasopressin-induced contraction of rat aorta. *Am J Physiol* 265: H2073–H2080

Stallone J.N., Crofton J.T., Share L. (1991). Sexual dimorphism in vasopressin-induced contraction of rat aorta. *Am J Physiol* 260: H453–H458

Stallone J.N., Salisbury R.L., Fulton C.T. (2001). Androgen-receptor defect abolishes sex differences in nitric oxide and reactivity to vasopressin in rat aorta. *J Appl Physiol* 81: 2602–2610

Stocker S.D., Wilson M.E., Madden C.J., Lone U., Sved A.F. (2006). Intravenous 6-hydroxydopamine attenuates vasopressin and oxytocin secretion stimulated by haemorrhage and hypotension but not hyperosmolality in rats. *Am J Physiol* 291: R59–R67

Streefkerk J.O., Mathy M.J., Pfaffendorf M., van Zweiten P.A. (2002). Vasopressin-induced presynaptic facilitation of sympathetic neurotransmission in the pithed rat. *J Hypertens* 20: 1175–1180

Streefkerk J.O., Balt J.C., van Montfrans G.A., van Lieshout J.J., Pfaffendorf M., van Zweiten P.A. (2004). Vasopressin facilitates presynaptic sympathetic nerve activity in humans. *J Hypertens* 22: 551–555

Taylor A.H., Al-Azzawi F. (2000). Immunolocalization of oestrogen receptor beta in human tissues. *J Mol Endocrinol* 24: 145–155

Taylor M.M., Baker J.R., Samson W.K. (2005). Brain-derived adrenomedullin controls blood volume through the regulation of arginine vasopressin production and release. *Am J Physiol* 288: R1203–1210

Taylor M.M., Samson W.K. (2005). Stress hormone secretion is altered by central administration of intermedin/asdrenomedullin-2. *Brain Res* 1045: 199–205

Terrillon S., Durroux T., Mouillac B., Breit A., Ayoub M.A., Taulan M., Jockers R., Barberis C., Bouvier M. (2003). Oxytocin and vasopressin V1a and V2 receptors form constitutive homo- and hetero-dimers during biosynthesis. *Mol Endocrinol* 17: 677–691

Turgeon J.L., Carr M.C., Maki P.M., Mendelsohn M.E., Wise P.M. (2006). Complex actions of sex steroids in adipose tissue, the cardiovascular system, and brain: insights from basic science to clinical studies. *Endo Rev* 27: 575–605

Ueta Y., Serino R., Shibuya I., Kitamura K., Kangawa K., Russell J.A., Yamashita H. (2000). A physiological role for adrenomedullin in rats; a potent hypotensive peptide in the hypothalamo-neurohypophysial system. *Exp Physiol* 85: 163S–169S

Van Balkom B.W., Hoffert J.D., Chou C.L., Knepper M.A. (2004). Proteomic analysis of long-term vasopressin action in the inner medullary collecting duct of the Brattleboro rat. *Am J Physiol* 286: F216–F224

Voisin D.L., Simonian S.X., Herbison A.E. (1997). Identification of estrogen receptor-containing neurons projecting to the rat supraoptic nucleus. *Neurosci* 78: 215–228

Wang Y-X., Crofton J.T., Miller J., Sigman C.J., Liu H., Huber J.M., Brooks D.P., Share L. (1996). Sex difference in urinary concentrating ability of rats with water deprivation. *Am J Physiol* 270: R550–R555

Wang Y-X., Edwards R.M., Nambi P., Stack E.J., Pullen M., Share L., Crofton J.T., Brooks D.P. (2003). Sex difference in the antidiuretic activity of vasopressin in the rat. *Am J Physiol* 265: R1284–R1290

Wargent E.T., Burgess W.J., Laycock J.F., Balment R.J. (1999). Separate receptors mediate oxytocin and vasopressin stimulation of cAMP in rat inner medullary collecting duct cells. *Exp Physiol* 84: 17–25

Wegmann M., Nusing R.M. (2003). Prostaglandin E2 stimulates sodium reabsorption in MDCK C7 cells, a renal collecting duct principal cell model. *Prostaglandins Leukot Essent Fatty Acids* 69: 315–322

Wells C.C., Riazi S., Mankhey R.W., Bhatti F., Ecelberger C., Maric C. (2005). Diabetic nephropathy is associated with decreased circulating estradiol levels and imbalance in the expression of renal estrogen receptors. *Gender Med* 2: 227–237

Williams T.D.M., Laycock J.F., Lightman S.L., Guy R.L. (1988). Increased sensitivity to pressor hormones in central diabetes insipidus. *Eur J Clin Invest* 18: 375–379

Yamashita T., Liu X., Onaka T., Honda K., Saito T., Yagi K. (2001). Vasopressin differentially modulates noradrenaline release in the rat supraoptic nucleus. *Neuroreport* 12: 3509–3511

Yokoi H., Arima H., Murase T., Kondo K., Iwasaki Y., Uiso Y. (1996). Intracerebroventricular injection of adrenomedullin inhibits vasopressin release in conscious rats. *Neurosci Lett* 20: 65–67

Zelenina M., Christensen B.M., Palmer J., Nairn A.C., Nielsen S., Aperia A. (2000). Prostaglandin E(2) interaction with AVP: effects on AQP2 phosphorylation and distribution. *Am J Physiol* 278: F388–F394

Zhou L., Blaustein J.D., De Vries G.J. (1994). Distribution of androgen receptorimmunoreactivity in vasopressin- and oxytocin-immunoreactive neurons in the male rat brain. *Endocrinol* 134: 2622–2627

Zimmerman E.A., Nilaver G., Silverman A.J. (1984). Vasopressinergic and oxytocinergic pathways in the central nervous system. *Fed Proc* 43: 91–96

CHAPTER 9

UNDERSTANDING THE ROLE OF VASOPRESSIN IN THE HYPOTHALAMO-PITUITARY ADRENOCORTICAL AXIS

Julia Buckingham

Division of Neuroscience and Mental Health
Imperial College London, Hammersmith Campus
Du Cane Road, London W12 0NN
Email: j.buckingham@imperial.ac.uk

1. Introduction

Glucocorticoids exert wide-ranging effects in the body which, collectively, are essential for normal growth and development and for the maintenance of homeostasis. Severe, long-term disturbances in the circulating levels of glucocorticoids, which may be induced pathologically (e.g. Addison's disease or Cushing's syndrome), surgically (adrenal resection) or pharmacologically (e.g. administration of anti-inflammatory steroids), are well known to produce a plethora of unwanted effects. However, a growing body of data suggests that more subtle changes in the secretion and/or activity of glucocorticoids may also have serious deleterious effects if sustained for a long period. In particular, they may predispose the organism to a variety of diseases which are endemic in the western world and are also emerging in developing countries. These include type 2 diabetes, hypertension and depression.

Cortisol (the principal glucocorticoid in man) and its rodent counterpart, corticosterone, are synthesised from cholesterol in the adrenal cortex by zona fasciculata cells and released into the systemic circulation. The plasma profile of the steroids is rhythmic, reflecting the pulsatile pattern of release: pulse amplitude follows a distinct circadian pattern and, consequently, serum glucocorticoid concentrations are maximal just before waking and decline thereafter, reaching a nadir some 6–8 hours later. Glucocorticoids are also released in response to physical and/or emotional trauma. The 'stress response' is superimposed upon the existing circadian tone and varies in magnitude according to the nature, the intensity and the duration of the stimulus and the individual's previous experience (Buckingham, 2006).

The circadian and stress-induced secretion of the glucocorticoids is governed by the hypothalamo-pituitary axis (Fig. 1). The hypothalamus receives, monitors and integrates neural and humoral information from many sources. It thus acts as a sensor of changes in the external and internal environment and responds to adverse physical or emotional circumstances, and to circadian factors by activating the final common pathway which drives glucocorticoid synthesis. The first step in this pathway is the release of two hypothalamic neuropeptides, corticotrophin releasing hormone (CRH) and arginine vasopressin (AVP), into the hypothalamo-hypophysial portal vessels. These peptides act synergistically on specialised cells in the anterior pituitary gland, the corticotrophs, to cause release of the adrenocorticotrophic hormone (ACTH, or Corticotrophin) into the systemic circulation. Adrenocorticotrophin, in turn, targets zona fasciculata cells in the adrenal cortex and stimulates the synthesis and release of cortisol/corticosterone. The sensitivity of the hypothalamo-pituitary-adrenocortical (HPA) axis to incoming stimuli is modulated by a negative feedback system through which the sequential release of CRH/AVP and ACTH from the hypothalamus and anterior pituitary gland is inhibited by the glucocorticoids themselves. The magnitude of the HPA response to stress thus depends upon the pre-existing glucocorticoid tone (Buckingham, 2006). This review will focus specifically on the role of vasopressin within the HPA axis.

2. Historical Perspectives

The concept of neurohumoral control of the anterior pituitary gland emerged in the middle of the last century, due mainly to the elegant work of Harris and his colleagues (see Harris, 1952). Harris proposed that

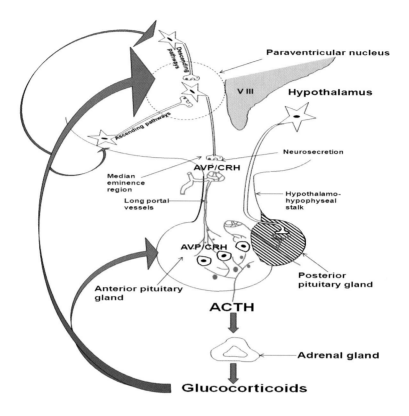

Figure 1. The hypothalamo-pituitary-adrenocortical axis and principal loci of glucocorticoid feedback control. ACTH, adrenocorticotrophic hormone; AVP, arginine vasopressin; CRH, corticotrophin releasing hormone. Note that the CRH/AVP secreting neurones are innervated by ascending nervous pathways from the brain-stem nuclei and by descending pathways from the limbic system and other centres (e.g. cortex). Circadian regulation is effected mainly via pathways from the suprachiasmatic nucleus (not shown). Local factors derived from glial cells (e.g. cytokines) and humoral factors (e.g. glucose) may also modulate the secretion of CRH/AVP. Similarly, locally produced substances also modulate the secretion of ACTH and glucocorticoids. Reprinted from Buckingham (2006), with permission.

ACTH secretion is driven by a single hypothalamic neurohormone, later termed the 'corticotrophin releasing factor' (CRF), and attempts to identify the active substance began in the mid-1950s. Early studies suggested that vasopressin may be the CRF (Martini and Monpurgo, 1955; McCann, 1957; McCann and Brobeck, 1954) and there was circumstantial evidence to support this view. For example, it was noted that stress often causes the release of both vasopressin and ACTH (Mirsky *et al.*, 1954) and that extracts of the posterior pituitary gland possess corticotrophin releasing activity (McCann, 1957). Furthermore, rats with lesions in the median eminence develop both diabetes insipidus and impaired ACTH secretion and also respond to exogenous vasopressin with increases in circulating ACTH (McCann and Brobeck, 1954; McCann and Fruit, 1957). Additionally, adrenalectomy induces a rise in hypothalamic vasopressin content which is normalised by corticosteroid replacement therapy (Sofroniew *et al.*, 1977). Other data, however, mitigated against a role for vasopressin. For example, Briggs and Munson (1955) found that vasopressin had no effect on ACTH release in rats sedated with pentobarbitone and morphine. Concern was expressed that the doses of vasopressin used by McCann's group to induce ACTH release in rats were supra-physiological and several hundred fold higher than those required to induce a maximal anti-diuretic effect (Saffran and Saffran, 1959). Evidence also emerged of a complete lack of correlation between plasma ACTH and vasopressin after nicotine treatment, water loading or water deprivation (McDonald *et al.*, 1957). Moreover, hypothalamic extracts from hypophysectomised rats were shown to contain a high degree of corticotrophin releasing activity but little pressor (de Wied, 1961).

Renewed interest in the potential role of vasopressin within the HPA axis emerged in the late 1970s. Studies performed *in vitro* on pituitary segments and isolated pituitary cells and also *in vivo* in rats in which the hypothalamus was lesioned surgically or pharmacologically, confirmed that vasopressin induces ACTH release. These studies also explored the nature of the dose-response curves to vasopressin and hypothalamic extracts (used as a source of the 'true' CRH) and revealed that the ACTH-releasing activity of vasopressin was very modest versus the tissue extract. Thus, in all the CRF assay systems tested, the efficacy (or maximal effect) of vasopressin was well below that of the 'CRF' contained within an hypothalamic extract (Buckingham and Hodges, 1977; Buckingham and van Wimersma Greidanus, 1977; Gillies *et al.*, 1978). Furthermore, vasopressin lacked potency and, therefore, concentrations well above those found in the systemic circulation were required to release ACTH. Together these findings indicated that vasopressin alone could not be the elusive CRF. Nonetheless, the possibility that vasopressin may have a role in the sequence of events leading to ACTH secretion retained some credence, largely on the basis that rats which congenitally lack vasopressin (Brattleboro strain) show impaired basal and stress-induced HPA activity, as evidenced by reductions in the resting ACTH and corticosterone levels and in the magnitude of the HPA response to stress (Buckingham and Leach, 1980; Krieger *et al.*, 1977).

To explore the potential role of vasopressin further, Gillies and Lowry focused on the use of extracts of the pituitary stalk-median eminence (SME) as a source of CRF (Gillies and Lowry, 1979). Using chromatography to separate the proteins within the SME prior to assay, they identified two peaks with CRF activity. The major peak eluted in the expected position of vasopressin and, when tested in the isolated pituitary cell assay, showed a concentration response curve which resembled that of synthetic vasopressin (i.e. low efficacy). However, when the two peak fractions were recombined, the full efficacy of the original extract was restored. In addition, the CRF activity of the SME extract was abolished by a specific anti-vasopressin antiserum. On the basis of these data, the authors proposed that vasopressin is indeed the CRH but that it requires a synergistic factor to exhibit its full biological activity (Gillies and Lowry, 1979).

Other findings however did not accord with this view. For example, hypothalamic extracts from Brattleboro rats were shown to possess significant corticotrophin releasing activity which, although reduced in terms of potency and efficacys versus extracts from control rats of the same parent strain, was more pronounced than that of vasopressin (Buckingham and Leach, 1980). Furthermore, in concentrations well below those required to stimulate ACTH release directly, vasopressin potentiated the activity of hypothalamic extracts from Brattleboro rats and restored its potency and efficacy to control levels (Buckingham, 1981). Additionally, in this study and in contrast to the findings of

Gillies and Lowry (1979), treatment of hypothalamic extracts from control rats with an anti-vasopressin antiserum reduced, but did not, abolish the corticotrophin releasing activity of the extracts. Taken together, these and other data led to the conclusion that vasopressin is not the major corticotrophin releasing hormone but that it fulfils an important role in the regulation of ACTH secretion by potentiating the biological activity of the principal corticotrophin releasing hormone which remained to be identified (Buckingham, 1981; Buckingham and Leach, 1980; Yates, *et al.*, 1971). Subsequently, a 41-amino acid residue peptide with strong CRF activity was isolated from ovine hypothalami (Vale, *et al.*, 1981) and heralded as the CRH. This peptide, and its rodent and human counterparts, proved to be a more powerful ACTH secretagogue than vasopressin, and it has since been shown to play a major role in the regulation of HPA function. However, CRH is not the sole hypothalamic regulator of ACTH secretion, but appears to act in concert with vasopressin, which readily potentiates its biological activity (Gillies *et al.*, 1982), and also possibly with other factors, such as oxytocin. Thus, some 25 years ago, a view emerged that vasopressin is one of two, or possibly more, physiologically significant corticotrophin releasing factors and that its principal role is to potentiate the biological activity of the other factors, notably CRH.

3. Localisation and Regulation of Vasopressin in the Hypothalamo-Pituitary-Adrenal Axis

Vasopressin is synthesised by three discrete populations of neurones in the hypothalamus. The first are magnocellular neurones which project from the paraventricular and supraoptic nuclei (PVN and SON) to the posterior pituitary gland (Fig. 2). These neurones are responsible for the secretion of vasopressin into the systemic circulation for delivery to its peripheral target tissues (e.g. kidney), but they may also have a role in stimulating ACTH secretion in conditions of acute stress (Holmes *et al.*, 1986). The second population comprises parvocellular neurones which originate in the PVN and project to the external zone of the median eminence (Figs. 2–4). These neurones secrete vasopressin into the

hypophysial portal vessels for direct transportation to the anterior
pituitary gland and are therefore principally concerned with the
regulation of ACTH secretion (Vandesande *et al.*, 1977; Wiegand and
Price, 1980; Zimmerman *et al.*, 1977). The third population arises in the
suprachiasmatic nucleus and projects to various hypothalamic loci,
including the PVN, and may thereby contribute to the circadian
regulation of CRH/vasopressin secretion.

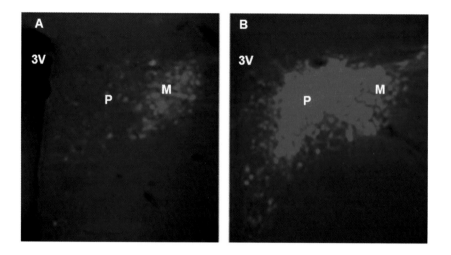

Figure 2. Micrographs of the mouse paraventricular nucleus (PVN) and median eminence
of transgenic mice expressing enhanced green fluorescent protein (eGFP) under the
control of the vasopressin promoter; eGFP thus serves as a surrogate marker of
vasopressin expression. The data compare the effects of sham-adrenalectomy (Panel A)
and adrenalectomy (Panel B). Note the strong expression of eGFP in the magnocellular
neurones of the PVN (M) in the sham-operated animals (Panel A) and the marked
increase in eGFP expression in the parvocellular neurones of the PVN (P) of the
adrenalectomised animals (Panel B). 3v = third ventricle. Reprinted from Shibata *et al.*
(2007), with permission.

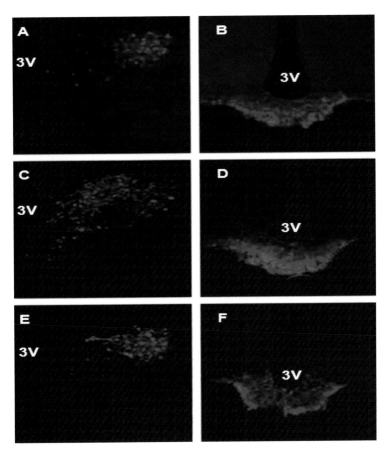

Figure 3. Micrographs of the mouse paraventricular nucleus (PVN) and median eminence of transgenic mice expressing enhanced green fluorescent protein (eGFP) under the control of the vasopressin promoter; eGFP thus serves as a surrogate marker of vasopressin expression. The data demonstrate the effects of sham-adrenalectomy (Panels A and B), adrenalectomy (Panels C and D) and adrenalectomy plus dexamethasone treatment (Panels E and F) on expression of eGFP and CRH in the PVN (Panels A, C and E) and the median eminence (Panels B, D and F). Note the increased expression of eGFP after adrenalectomy in the parvocellular region of the PVN (adjacent to the third ventricle, 3V, Panel C) and median eminence (Panel D) and its reversal by dexamethasone (Panels E and F). Reprinted from Shibata *et al.* (2007), with permission.

Studies involving *in situ* hybridisation and immunohistochemistry have shown a high degree of co-localisation of vasopressin and CRH within the parvocellular neurones of the PVN-median eminence tract. They have also provided evidence for differential control of vasopressin gene expression in the magnocellular and parvocellular neuronal populations. For example, in the magnocellular population, vasopressin expression is highly sensitive to osmotic stimuli, while in the parvocellular neurones it is enhanced by stress (e.g. restraint) and adrenalectomy and suppressed by exogenous glucocorticoids (Figs. 2–4, Shibata *et al.*, 2007).

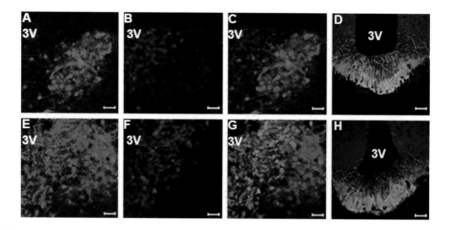

Figure 4. Micrographs of the mouse paraventricular nucleus (PVN) and median eminence of transgenic mice expressing enhanced green fluorescent protein (eGFP) under the control of the vasopressin promoter; eGFP thus serves as a surrogate marker of vasopressin expression. The data illustrate the effects of adrenalectomy (panels E–H) and sham-adrenalectomy (panels A–D) on the expression of eGFP and CRH in the parvocellular and magnocellular regions of PVN and the median eminence. Note that in the sham-operated controls, AVP (green) is localised mainly to the magnocellular region (panel A) while CRH (red) is found mainly in the parvocellular region (adjacent to the third ventricle, 3v panel B); there is little colocalisation of the two peptides in the PVN (panel C). Adrenalectomy causes a profound increase in AVP in the parvocellular region of the PVN (panel E) together with a more modest increase in parvocellular CRH (panel F); there is a significant degree of co-localisation of the peptides (panel G). Note also the abundance of eGFP in the median eminence of sham-operated and adrenalectomised rats and the co-localisation with CRH (Panels D and H). Reprinted from Shibata *et al.*, (2006) with permission.

Numerous workers have attempted to explore the relative importance of CRH and vasopressin in mediating the pituitary responses to different stressors. Several early studies made direct measurements of CRH and vasopressin in the portal blood of anaesthetised rats and sheep exposed to various stressors, using elegant surgical techniques to access the vessels, (Gibbs, 1985a, 1985b; Horn *et al.*, 1985; Plotsky, 1985; Plotsky *et al.*, 1985; Plotsky and Vale, 1984). These studies provided firm evidence that, as for other hypothalamic releasing hormones (e.g. CRH, Gonadotrophin releasing hormone GnRH), vasopressin is released in a pulsatile manner into the portal vessels, where it reaches concentrations well above those of peripheral blood, a finding that negated earlier concerns that vasopressin is not delivered to the pituitary gland in concentrations sufficient to elicit ACTH release. Haemorrhage (15%) causes marked increases in portal blood vasopressin and CRH and in plasma ACTH; the rise in ACTH is prevented by anti-CRH antisera, but vasopressin receptor antagonists are only partially effective in this regard (Plotsky *et al.*, 1985). By contrast, insulin-induced hypoglycaemia causes a marked increase in portal blood vasopressin without affecting CRH release (Plotsky, 1985; Plotsky *et al.*, 1985; Plotsky and Vale, 1984). Portal blood CRH is also unaffected by atrial pulsation and hypothermia but both stimuli reduce the plasma ACTH and portal blood AVP concentrations (Gibbs, 1985a, 1985b; Plotsky, 1985). Together, these findings led to suggestions that CRH and vasopressin show some degree of stimulus-selectivity and that in some instances (e.g. atrial pulsation, hypoglycaemia), AVP may fulfil a dynamic role in regulating ACTH release while the effects of CRH are permissive (Plotsky, 1985).

With the development of sophisticated semi-quantitative histological methods, notably *in situ* hybridisation (ISH), the majority of workers turned to measurements of CRH and vasopressin mRNA expression as indices of neuronal activity and peptide release. While this approach is undoubtedly more straightforward than portal blood sampling, it is limited by the fact that changes in mRNA expression can be brought about by many factors (e.g. altered degradation) and do not necessarily mirror the pattern of release of preformed peptide from stores in the axon terminals. Notwithstanding these criticisms, there is good evidence that acute stress (e.g. restraint, exposure to endotoxin) increases CRH and vasopressin mRNA expression in the parvocellular PVN (e.g. Harbuz *et al.*, 1994; Xia and Krukoff, 2003) and that these responses are sensitive to changes in the glucocorticoid *milieu* (Figs. 2–4, Shibata *et al.*, 2007). Analysis of the primary transcripts (i.e. heteronuclear RNA, hnRNA) has revealed a clear temporal dissociation in the expression pattern of the two genes in several stress paradigms (ether inhalation, hypertonic saline, forced swimming) and following micro-injection of noradrenaline into the PVN. In all cases, the release of ACTH is associated with a prompt but transient increase in CRH hnRNA. In contrast, the augmentation of vasopressin gene transcription is both delayed and prolonged (Helmreich *et al.*, 2001; Itoi *et al.*, 1999; Kovacs and Sawchenko, 1996; Ma and Lightman, 1998; Ma *et al.*, 1999; Rabadan-Diehl *et al.*, 1995). The mechanisms underpinning this differential response are not fully understood. There is evidence that the rapid increase in CRH gene transcription is due partly to protein kinase A (PKA)-induced phosphorylation of a transcription factor, 3'5'cyclic adenosine monophosphate (cAMP) response element binding protein (CREB), which targets specific cyclic AMP response elements (CREs) in the promoter (Itoi *et al.*, 2004; Kovacs and Sawchenko, 1996). The vasopressin promoter also includes several CREs and is sensitive to phospho-CREB (Emanuel *et al.*, 1998; Iwasaki *et al.*, 1997). However, induction of the vasopressin gene in the parvocellular PVN also appears to require newly synthesised factors, such as the products of the immediate early genes (e.g. c-fos), which may explain the delay in transcription (Kovacs *et al.*, 1998).

In the case of repeated stress, the induction of vasopressin gene transcription is generally preserved, even if the pituitary-adrenocortical response to the stimulus is blunted whereas the correlation between CRH gene expression and ACTH and corticosterone secretion is maintained. For example, rats adapt readily to restraint stress, and therefore the CRH hnRNA, and plasma ACTH and corticosterone responses, to successive episodes of restraint are all progressively attenuated. By contrast, the vasopressin mRNA response ensues (Volpi *et al.*, 2004). However rats do not adapt to chronic mild variable stress paradigms (CMVS, a model of repeated heterotypic stress in which rodents are exposed for several weeks to successive periods of mild but unpredictable stress with intervening periods of calm designed to mimic the everyday hassles of life); hence CRH and vasopressin gene expression, plasma ACTH and corticosterone levels are all raised at the end of the test period (Herman *et al.*, 1995).

Marked dissociations between CRH and vasopressin gene transcription have been widely reported in prolonged (chronic) stress, for example in models in which an inflammatory response develops and then resolves over a period of days (e.g. experimentally induced arthritis or allergic encephalomyelitis). However, in these models, it is vasopressin gene expression that correlates with ACTH release and a view has emerged that vasopressin is the dominant factor driving ACTH secretion in chronic stress. For example, in adjuvant-induced arthritis, increases in plasma ACTH and corticosterone emerge just before or at the time of onset of the clinical symptoms of disease. They continue to rise, correlating with disease progression and severity, and then decline as the disease regresses to return to normal on recovery. Increases in CRH mRNA expression in the parvocellular PVN occur early in the disease and precede the appearance of disease symptoms. However, in contrast to the secretion of ACTH and corticosterone, CRH mRNA expression declines as the inflammation progresses, as does the release of CRH into the hypophophysial portal blood (Aguilera, 1994; Harbuz *et al.*, 1992). By contrast, vasopressin gene transcription and portal blood vasopressin both increase markedly as inflammation progresses, suggesting a critical role for AVP in effecting the pituitary adrenocortical response to the disease (Chowdrey *et al.*, 1995).

Pharmacological and genetic studies have provided further evidence that AVP plays an important part in the regulation of HPA function. Significantly, studies in mice null for CRH or the pituitary CRH receptor (CRH-R1) indicate that vasopressin is able to maintain adequate HPA activity for survival in the absence of CRH (Muglia *et al.*, 1995; Timpl *et al.*, 1998). Simultaneous blockade of the pituitary CRH-R1 and the pituitary vasopressin receptor (V1bR) with selective antagonists (CP154,526 and SSR149415 respectively) abolishes the ACTH response to ether, forced swimming and restraint. However, V1b blockade alone does not affect the response to forced swimming although it attenuates the responses to ether and restraint, thus confirming earlier evidence that the release of vasopressin shows a degree of stress selectivity (Ramos, Troncone and Tufik, 2006). Similar, although not entirely complementary, data have emerged from studies using V1bR-null mice. Tanoue *et al.* (2004) reported that the circulating concentrations of ACTH and corticosterone are reduced in V1bR-null mice versus wild-type controls, as also is the ACTH response to a forced swim test. By contrast, others claimed that the basal ACTH and corticosterone levels are unaffected by V1bR gene deletion but that marked disturbances in stress-induced ACTH secretion are apparent (Stewart *et al.*, 2008b). In particular, this group reported marked reductions in the ACTH and corticosterone responses to hypoglycaemia (Lolait *et al.*, 2007a), novel environment (Stewart *et al.*, 2008b), acute (30 minutes) endotoxin exposure and alcohol (Lolait *et al.*, 2007b). They also noted a blunting of the ACTH, but not the corticosterone, responses to acute and repeated restraint (15 or 30 minutes) or forced swimming (Stewart *et al.*, 2008a), although paradoxically their earlier data indicated that the response to acute (30 min) restraint was unaffected by V1bR gene deletion (Lolait *et al.*, 2007a). Despite these discrepant findings, these studies emphasise the importance of vasopressin in regulating ACTH secretion.

The neural and humoral substrates that underpin the differential activation of the CRH and vasopressin genes are also poorly understood although the sensitivity of the vasopressin gene to the glucocorticoid *milieu* is well documented (Ma *et al.*, 1997; Shibata *et al.*, 2007, Figs. 2 and 3). Furthermore, there is evidence that, in the rat, the vasopressin gene is preferentially suppressed in pregnancy (*vs.* the CRH gene) when the HPA axis is refractory to stress (Ma *et al.*, 2005) whereas in the neonatal stress hyporesponsive phase the CRH gene expression is suppressed and vasopressin appears to be responsible for driving the attenuated pituitary response (Zelena *et al.*, 2008). Other data suggest that AVP may contribute to the emergence of the sexual dimorphisms in HPA activity (Ferrini *et al.*, 1997) and, while the CRH gene is positively regulated by oestrogens (Buckingham, 2006), vasopressin expression in the parvocellular PVN is sensitive to androgen status and is thus increased by orchidectomy (Seale *et al.*, 2004). Further studies are now required to understand the hierarchal pathways which determine the differential responses of the CRH and vasopressin genes to stressors of differing intensity and nature.

4. Mechanism of Vasopressin Action in the Pituitary Gland

Binding and functional studies using selective vasopressin agonists and antagonists provided early evidence that the pituitary vasopressin receptor is similar to the type 1 vasopressin receptor located in blood vessels (Antoni, 1984; Buckingham, 1987). These studies also revealed that, while all corticotrophs bind CRH, only approximately 50–80% bind AVP and these belong mainly to the large corticotroph subpopulation (Childs and Unabia, 1990). Molecular studies subsequently identified two distinct type 1 vasopressin receptor species, termed V1aR and V1bR (sometimes also called V3). The V1a receptor is expressed mainly in blood vessels and also in the brain whereas the V1b receptor is found in the anterior pituitary gland (Antoni, 1993) and also in a number of regions of the brain, in particular the hypothalamus, amygdala, cerebellum, the circumventricular organs and the median eminence (Hernando *et al.*, 2001). Both receptors belong to the seven transmembrane domain, G-protein coupled superfamily of receptors, and both are positively coupled to phospholipase C. Activation of the receptors thus leads to the generation of inositol trisphosphate and activation of protein kinase C (PKC) within the target cell. Confirmation of the importance of the V1bR within the pituitary has been provided by evidence that vasopressin alone or in combination with CRH fails to influence ACTH release from pituitary cells from V1bR-null mice (Lolait *et al.*, 2007a). Pharmacological studies have been more limited due to the lack of selective ligands. However, recent structure-activity relationship studies have pinpointed the importance of amino acid residue 4 in determining specificity for the V1bR and to the development selective agonists (e.g. 1, deamino-[Leu4, Lys8] vasopressin, Pena *et al.*, 2007) and antagonists (e.g. SR149415), which will provide useful tools for further research.

The actions of vasopressin in the pituitary gland differ from those of CRH in several respects. Both peptides readily stimulate the release of preformed ACTH into the circulation. However, the effects of vasopressin, unlike those of CRH, are refractory to the regulatory effects of glucocorticoids (Rabadan-Diehl and Aguilera, 1998). Furthermore, unlike CRH, vasopressin does not induce pro-opiomelanocortin (POMC, the ACTH precursor) synthesis or corticotroph mitogenesis, although a recent paper has argued a role for vasopressin and the V1bR in mediating the mitogenic response of the corticotrophs to adrenalectomy (Subburaju and Aguilera, 2007).

The mechanism by which AVP potentiates the ACTH releasing activity of CRH is surprisingly poorly understood. The pituitary CRH receptor (CRH-R1) is positively coupled to adenyl cyclase; thus, CRH-driven ACTH release is affected by increased intracellular cAMP and activation of PKA. Vasopressin signals via phospholipase C but also potentiates the increase in intracellular cAMP induced by CRH (Giguere and Labrie, 1982; Labrie et al., 1987). This phenomenon has been attributed to PKC-dependent cross-talk between the two signalling pathways which may augment receptor-adenyl cyclase signalling and/or suppress the activity of phosphodiesterase (the enzyme that degrades cAMP). However, more recent studies in birds have raised the possibility that heterodimerisation of the receptors may underpin the enhanced cAMP accumulation (Mikhailova et al., 2007). In addition, there is evidence that vasopressin increases CRH binding to corticotrophs (Childs and Unabia, 1990), although it is doubtful whether this alone could account for the increase in efficacy associated with the two peptides in combination.

A considerable amount of attention has focused on the mechanisms that regulate the expression of the V1bR in the anterior pituitary gland. In many cases, there is a good correlation between V1bR number and the pituitary response to stress (Aguilera, 1994), and V1bR expression is increased in conditions of chronic stress (Volpi et al., 2004), emphasising the importance of vasopressin in this state. Thus, in repeated homotypic stress paradigms, the enhanced response to the introduction of a novel stress is associated with upregulation of the receptors (Aguilera, 1994), although paradoxically pituitary cells exposed to vasopressin *in vitro* rapidly undergo desensitisation due to receptor internalisation and subsequent sensitisation due to receptor dephosphorylation (Hassan and Mason, 2005). Interestingly, V1bR mRNA expression does not always correlate with V1bR binding, suggesting that there may be differential control of transcription and post-transcriptional events (Aguilera *et al.*, 2003; Rabadan-Diehl *et al.*, 1995) as well as receptor recycling and degradation. For further details, see Volpi *et al.* (2004).

5. Clinical Implications

From a clinical perspective, the advances in our understanding of the vasopressinergic control of ACTH secretion have opened two main areas of study. The first has explored the potential value of vasopressin analogues in the differential diagnosis of Cushing's disease and the second the role of vasopressin and the V1b-R in the aetiology of depression.

Desmopressin (deamino-8D-arginine vasopressin, DDAVP) is a long-acting vasopressin analogue which shows a high degree of selectivity for the V2 (renal) receptor and negligible V1aR-mediated pressor activity. Hence, it is used clinically to treat hypothalamic diabetes insipidus and nocturnal enuresis. Its activity at the pituitary V1bR is uncertain. Desmopressin has little effect on ACTH secretion when given as an infusion in man (Gaillard *et al.*, 1988) or applied to rat pituitary tissue *in vitro* (Buckingham, 1987). However, it has been reported to show weak agonist activity at the V1bR (Dinan *et al.*, 1999) and, in accord with this, it has been shown to potentiate the ACTH releasing activity of CRF in an *in vitro* system (Buckingham, 1987) and to stimulate ACTH release in patients with Cushing's disease (Nieman *et al.*, 1986). The latter finding raised the question that desmopressin may be a useful aid to the differential diagnosis of pituitary versus ectopic ACTH-dependent Cushing's disease, in those cases where the tumour defied detection by MRI. Data based on venous sampling suggested that desmopressin was inferior to CRH in this regard, perhaps because the V1bR is commonly expressed in ectopic tumours (Newell-Price *et al.*, 1999; Tsagarakis *et al.*, 2002).

However, a more recent study in which blood was taken from the antecubital vein and the right and left petrosal sinuses 5 and 10 minutes after desmopressin injection, demonstrated a clear difference in the ratio of venous:sinus blood ACTH in patients with pituitary-dependent Cushing's disease and ectopic ACTH secreting tumours. Therefore, the authors concluded that the combination of desmopressin and petrosal sinus sampling provides a safe and effective diagnostic procedure and a potential alternative to CRH (Castinetti *et al.*, 2007). In addition, desmopressin combined with low dose dexamethasone may provide a useful adjunct in the differential diagnosis of Cushing's disease and the pseudo-Cushingoid states that emerge in depression, alcoholism and visceral obesity, for example (Pecori Giraldi *et al.*, 2007). Other workers have noted abnormal vasopressin receptor expression in adrenal tissue in ACTH-independent macronodular adrenal hyperplasia and suggested that ectopic expression of V1bR and V2R may contribute to the aetiology of the disease (Lee *et al.*, 2005) and that hyper-responsiveness of the adrenal gland to vasopressin is a frequent characteristic of patients with adrenal nodules (Suzuki *et al.*, 2008).

Hyperactivity of the HPA axis is frequently observed in subjects with major depression. In particular, subjects show raised morning cortisol levels and a loss of sensitivity to the feedback actions of the glucocorticoids, and failure to suppress cortisol in the combined dexamethasone-CRH test (Deuschle *et al.*, 1997; Holsboer *et al.*, 1984; Zobel *et al.*, 1999). Divergent views have been expressed as to whether the disturbances in HPA functions are causal or consequential of the disease process. Nevertheless, a growing body of evidence now supports the premise that overexpression of CRH and impaired actions of cortisol in the brain, in particular in the limbic system, are causal in the pathogenesis (Modell *et al.*, 1997; Nemeroff *et al.*, 1984). Therefore, both CRH-R1 and the glucocorticoid receptor (GR) are important targets for novel antidepressant therapies (reviewed in Thomson and Craighead, 2008).

In recent years, increasing attention has focused on the potential role of vasopressin in this regard. As discussed earlier, chronic stress increases the expression of vasopressin in the parvocellular PVN and the secretion of the peptide into the hypophysial portal vessels. It also upregulates the expression of V1bR and thereby augments the pituitary response to vasopressin. Vasopressin is released into the limbic system where it is strongly implicated in triggering the behavioural responses to psychological stress, including the processes of learning, memory and anxiety-related behaviours (reviewed in Frank and Landgraf, 2008). Depressed patients show increases in circulating vasopressin (van Londen *et al.*, 1998), in pituitary vasopressin sensitivity (Dinan *et al.*, 1999) and in the number of vasopressin-positive cells in the PVN (Merali *et al.*, 2006).

There is also limited evidence to link increases in vasopressin with anxiety states in man (e.g. post-traumatic stress disorder, de Kloet *et al.*, 2008). Studies in experimental animals based upon pharmacological approaches, natural mutants (e.g. Brattleboro rat), selective gene targeting (e.g. V1b-null mice) and RNA silencing (e.g. downregulation of V1aR expression) have provided evidence of a role for vasopressin and its receptors in various behavioural states (reviewed in Surget and Belzung, 2008). While the data are not entirely consistent, a substantial body of evidence supports the premise that V1aR is concerned with anxiety-type responses whereas the V1bR is implicated in 'depressive-like' behaviours. Thus, the V1aR antagonist, d(CH$_2$)5Tyr(Me)-AVP, shows anxiolytic activity in some, but not all, test paradigms (Everts and Koolhaas, 1999; Liebsch *et al.*, 1996), and may induce coping strategies in conditions of stress (Ebner *et al.*, 2002).

On the other hand, the V1bR antagonist (SR149415) shows 'anti-depressant activity' in several models of depression, e.g. forced swim test (Griebel *et al.*, 2002) and chronic mild variable (unpredictable) stress (Alonso *et al.*, 2004), while also exhibiting anxiolytic properties in social interaction tests for example (Shimazaki *et al.*, 2006). This compound also attenuates the HPA response to forced swim as does V1bR gene deletion (Stewart *et al.*, 2008a). Furthermore, the initial increase in HPA activity induced by tricylic antidepressants and selective 5-hydroxytryptamine (5-HT) uptake inhibitors is attenuated in V1bR null mice (Stewart *et al.*, 2008a). Taken together, these and other preclinical data raise the possibility that V1bR antagonists have potential for further development as therapeutic agents for the treatment of depression and other stress-related mental health disorders. If progressed to the clinic, there are arguments for focusing trials on those specific cohorts of patients that show dysregulation of the HPA axis. Such trials may not only provide insight to the therapeutic potential of these compounds, but also to the role of vasopressin, the V1bR and the HPA axis in the aetiology of the disease.

6. Conclusion

Our understanding of the role of vasopressin in the regulation of HPA function has emerged slowly over a period of 50 years. After the controversies of the early years, there can now be little doubt that vasopressin has a fundamental role in driving ACTH secretion in health and disease and that it acts, at least in part, by synergising with CRH. It is evident that vasopressin contributes to the regulation of basal ACTH release and to the response to acute stress. However, increasing evidence suggests that it is particularly important in maintaining HPA activity in conditions of chronic stress and that modulation of the vasopressinergic drive to the corticotrophs may also underpin the adaptive responses of the axis to certain physiological factors, in particular during the neonatal phase and in pregnancy. The possibility that dysfunction of the vasopressinergic system within the HPA axis may contribute to disease pathology is receiving increasing attention with emerging data pointing to a potential place for vasopressin receptor antagonists in the treatment of depression and certain anxiety states.

Bibliography

Aguilera G. (1994). Regulation of pituitary ACTH secretion during chronic stress. *Front Neuroendocrinol* 15: 321–350

Aguilera G., Volpi S., Rabadan-Diehl C. (2003). Transcriptional and post-transcriptional mechanisms regulating the rat pituitary vasopressin V1b receptor gene. *J Mol Endocrinol* 30: 99–108

Alonso R., Griebel G., Pavone G., Stemmelin J., Le Fur G., Soubrie P. (2004). Blockade of CRF(1) or V(1b) receptors reverses stress-induced suppression of neurogenesis in a mouse model of depression. *Mol Psychiatry* 9: 278–286

Antoni F.A. (1984). Novel ligand specificity of pituitary vasopressin receptors in the rat. *Neuroendocrinology* 39: 186–188

Antoni F.A. (1993). Vasopressinergic control of pituitary adrenocorticotropin secretion comes of age. *Front Neuroendocrinol* 14: 76–122

Briggs F.N., Munson P.L. (1955). Studies on the mechanism of stimulation of ACTH secretion with the aid of morphine as a blocking agent. *Endocrinology* 57: 205–219

Buckingham J.C. (1981). The influence of vasopressin on hypothalamic corticotrophin releasing activity in rats with inherited diabetes insipidus. *J Physiol* 312: 9–16

Buckingham J.C. (1987). Vasopressin receptors influencing the secretion of ACTH by the rat adenohypophysis. *J Endocrinol* 113: 389–396

Buckingham J.C. (2006). Glucocorticoids: exemplars of multi-tasking. *Br J Pharmacol* 147 Suppl 1: S258–268

Buckingham J.C., Hodges J.R. (1977). The use of corticotrophin production by adenohypophysial tissue *in vitro* for the detection and estimation of potential corticotrophin releasing factors. *J Endocrinol* 72: 187–193

Buckingham J.C., Leach J.H. (1980). Hypothalamo-pituitary-adrenocortical function in rats with inherited diabetes insipidus. *J Physiol* 305: 397–404

Buckingham J.C., van Wimersma Greidanus T.B. (1977). The effects of neurohypophyseal hormones and their analogues on corticotrophin release. *J. Endocrinol* 72: 9P

Castinetti F., Morange I., Dufour H., Jaquet P., Conte-Devolx B., Girard N., Brue T. (2007). Desmopressin test during petrosal sinus sampling: a valuable tool to discriminate pituitary or ectopic ACTH-dependent Cushing's syndrome. *Eur J Endocrinol* 157: 271–277

Childs G.V., Unabia G. (1990). Rapid corticosterone inhibition of corticotropin-releasing hormone binding and adrenocorticotropin release by enriched populations of corticotropes: counteractions by arginine vasopressin and its second messengers. *Endocrinology* 126: 1967–1975

Chowdrey H.S., Larsen P.J., Harbuz M.S., Jessop D.S., Aguilera G., Eckland D.J., Lightman S.L. (1995). Evidence for arginine vasopressin as the primary activator of the HPA axis during adjuvant-induced arthritis. *Br J Pharmacol* 116: 2417–2424

de Kloet C.S., Vermetten E., Geuze E., Wiegant V.M., Westenberg H.G. (2008). Elevated plasma arginine vasopressin levels in veterans with posttraumatic stress disorder. *J Psychiatr Res* 42: 192–198

de Wied D. (1961). An assay of corticotrophin-releasing principles in hypothalamic lesioned rats. *Acta Endocrinol (Copenh)* 37: 288–297

Deuschle M., Schweiger U., Weber B., Gotthardt U., Korner A., Schmider J., Standhardt H., Lammers C.H., Heuser I. (1997). Diurnal activity and pulsatility of the hypothalamus-pituitary-adrenal system in male depressed patients and healthy controls. *J Clin Endocrinol Metab* 82: 234–238

Dinan T.G., Lavelle E., Scott L.V., Newell-Price J., Medbak S., Grossman A.B. (1999). Desmopressin normalizes the blunted adrenocorticotropin response to corticotropin-releasing hormone in melancholic depression: evidence of enhanced vasopressinergic responsivity. *J Clin Endocrinol Metab* 84: 2238–2240

Ebner K., Wotjak C.T., Landgraf R., Engelmann M. (2002). Forced swimming triggers vasopressin release within the amygdala to modulate stress-coping strategies in rats. *Eur J Neurosci* 15: 384–388

Emanuel R.L., Iwasaki Y., Arbiser Z.K., Velez E.M., Emerson C.H., Majzoub J.A. (1998). Vasopressin messenger ribonucleic acid regulation via the protein kinase A pathway. *Endocrinology* 139: 2831–2837

Everts H.G., Koolhaas J.M. (1999). Differential modulation of lateral septal vasopressin receptor blockade in spatial learning, social recognition, and anxiety-related behaviors in rats. *Behav Brain Res* 99: 7–16

Ferrini M.G., Grillo C.A., Piroli G., de Kloet E.R., De Nicola A.F. (1997). Sex difference in glucocorticoid regulation of vasopressin mRNA in the paraventricular hypothalamic nucleus. *Cell Mol Neurobiol* 17: 671–686

Frank E., Landgraf R. (2008). The vasopressin system — from antidiuresis to psychopathology. *Eur J Pharmacol* 583: 226–242

Gaillard R.C., Riondel A.M., Ling N., Mulle, A.F. (1988). Corticotropin releasing factor activity of CRF 41 in normal man is potentiated by angiotensin II and vasopressin but not by desmopressin. *Life Sci* 43: 1935–1944

Gibbs D.M. (1985a). Inhibition of corticotropin release during hypothermia: the role of corticotropin-releasing factor, vasopressin, and oxytocin. *Endocrinology* 116: 723–727

Gibbs D.M. (1985b). Measurement of hypothalamic corticotropin-releasing factors in hypophyseal portal blood. *Fed Proc* 44: 203–206

Giguere V., Labrie F. (1982). Vasopressin potentiates cyclic AMP accumulation and ACTH release induced by corticotropin-releasing factor (CRF) in rat anterior pituitary cells in culture. *Endocrinology* 111: 1752–1754

Gillies G., Lowry P. (1979). Corticotrophin releasing factor may be modulated vasopressin. *Nature* 278: 463–464

Gillies G., Van Wimersma Greidanus T.B., Lowry P.J. (1978). Characterization of rat stalk median eminence vasopressin and its involvement in adrenocorticotropin release. *Endocrinology* 103: 528–534

Gillies G.E., Linton E.A., Lowry P.J. (1982). Corticotropin releasing activity of the new CRF is potentiated several times by vasopressin. *Nature* 299: 355–357

Griebel G., Simiand J., Serradeil-Le Gal C., Wagnon J., Pascal M., Scatton B., Maffrand J.P., Soubrie P. (2002). Anxiolytic- and antidepressant-like effects of the non-peptide vasopressin V1b receptor antagonist, SSR149415, suggest an innovative approach for the treatment of stress-related disorders. *Proc Natl Acad Sci USA* 99: 6370–6375

Harbuz M.S., Jessop D.S., Lightman S.L., Chowdrey H.S. (1994). The effects of restraint or hypertonic saline stress on corticotrophin-releasing factor, arginine vasopressin, and proenkephalin A mRNAs in the CFY, Sprague-Dawley and Wistar strains of rat. *Brain Res* 667: 6–12

Harbuz M.S., Rees R.G., Eckland D., Jessop D.S., Brewerton D., Lightman S.L. (1992). Paradoxical responses of hypothalamic corticotropin-releasing factor (CRF) messenger ribonucleic acid (mRNA) and CRF-41 peptide and adenohypophysial proopiomelanocortin mRNA during chronic inflammatory stress. *Endocrinology* 130: 1394–1400

Harris G.W. (1952). The neural control of the pituitary gland. London; Arnold.

Hassan A., Mason D. (2005). Mechanisms of desensitization of the adrenocorticotropin response to arginine vasopressin in ovine anterior pituitary cells. *J Endocrinol* 184: 29–40

Helmreich D.L., Itoi K., Lopez-Figueroa M.O., Akil H., Watson S.J. (2001). Norepinephrine-induced CRH and AVP gene transcription within the hypothalamus: differential regulation by corticosterone. *Brain Res Mol Brain Res* 88: 62–73

Herman J.P., Adams D., Prewitt C. (1995). Regulatory changes in neuroendocrine stress-integrative circuitry produced by a variable stress paradigm. *Neuroendocrinology* 61: 180–190

Hernando F., Schoots O., Lolait S.J., Burbach J.P. (2001). Immunohistochemical localization of the vasopressin V1b receptor in the rat brain and pituitary gland: anatomical support for its involvement in the central effects of vasopressin. *Endocrinology* 142: 1659–1668

Holmes M.C., Antoni F.A., Aguilera G., Catt K.J. (1986). Magnocellular axons in passage through the median eminence release vasopressin. *Nature* 319: 326–329

Holsboer F., Von Bardeleben U., Gerken A., Stalla G.K., Muller O.A. (1984). Blunted corticotropin and normal cortisol response to human corticotropin-releasing factor in depression. *N Engl J Med* 311: 11–27

Horn A.M., Robinson I.C., Fink G. (1985). Oxytocin and vasopressin in rat hypophysial portal blood: experimental studies in normal and Brattleboro rats. *J Endocrinol* 104: 211–224

Itoi K., Helmreich D.L., Lopez-Figueroa M.O., Watson S.J. (1999). Differential regulation of corticotropin-releasing hormone and vasopressin gene transcription in the hypothalamus by norepinephrine. *J Neurosci* 19: 5464–5472

Itoi K., Jiang Y.Q., Iwasaki Y., Watson S.J. (2004). Regulatory mechanisms of corticotropin-releasing hormone and vasopressin gene expression in the hypothalamus. *J Neuroendocrinol* 16: 348–355

Iwasaki Y., Oiso Y., Saito H., Majzoub J.A. (1997). Positive and negative regulation of the rat vasopressin gene promoter. *Endocrinology* 138: 5266–5274

Kovacs K.J., Arias C., Sawchenko P.E. (1998). Protein synthesis blockade differentially affects the stress-induced transcriptional activation of neuropeptide genes in parvocellular neurosecretory neurons. *Brain Res Mol Brain Res* 54: 85–91

Kovacs K.J., Sawchenko P.E. (1996). Regulation of stress-induced transcriptional changes in the hypothalamic neurosecretory neurons. *J Mol Neurosci* 7: 125–133

Krieger D.T., Liotta A., Brownstein M.J. (1977). Corticotropin releasing factor distribution in normal and Brattleboro rat brain, and effect of deafferentation, hypophysectomy and steroid treatment in normal animals. *Endocrinology* 100: 227–237

Labrie F., Giguere V., Meunier H., Simard J., Gossard F., Raymond V. (1987). Multiple factors controlling ACTH secretion at the anterior pituitary level. *Ann NY Acad Sci* 512: 97–114

Lee S., Hwang R., Lee J., Rhee Y., Kim D.J., Chung U.I., Lim S.K. (2005). Ectopic expression of vasopressin V1b and V2 receptors in the adrenal glands of familial ACTH-independent macronodular adrenal hyperplasia. *Clin Endocrinol (Oxf)* 63: 625–630

Liebsch G., Wotjak C.T., Landgraf R., Engelmann M. (1996). Septal vasopressin modulates anxiety-related behaviour in rats. *Neurosci Lett* 217: 101–104

Lolait S.J., Stewart L.Q., Jessop D.S., Young W.S. 3rd, O'Carroll A.M. (2007a). The hypothalamic-pituitary-adrenal axis response to stress in mice lacking functional vasopressin V1b receptors. *Endocrinology* 148: 849–856

Lolait S.J., Stewart L.Q., Roper J.A., Harrison G., Jessop D.S., Young W.S. 3rd, O'Carroll A.M. (2007b). Attenuated stress response to acute lipopolysaccharide challenge and ethanol administration in vasopressin V1b receptor knockout mice. *J Neuroendocrinol* 19: 543–551

Ma S., Shipston M.J., Morilak D., Russell J.A. (2005). Reduced hypothalamic vasopressin secretion underlies attenuated adrenocorticotropin stress responses in pregnant rats. *Endocrinology* 146: 1626–1637

Ma X.M., Levy A., Lightman S.L. (1997). Rapid changes of heteronuclear RNA for arginine vasopressin but not for corticotropin releasing hormone in response to acute corticosterone administration. *J Neuroendocrinol* 9: 723–728

Ma X.M., Lightman S.L. (1998). The arginine vasopressin and corticotrophin-releasing hormone gene transcription responses to varied frequencies of repeated stress in rats. *J Physiol* 510: 605–614

Ma X.M., Lightman S.L., Aguilera G. (1999). Vasopressin and corticotropin-releasing hormone gene responses to novel stress in rats adapted to repeated restraint. *Endocrinology* 140: 3623–3632

Martini L., Monpurgo C. (1955). Neurohumoral control of the release of adrenocorticotrophic hormone. *Nature* 175: 1127–1128

McCann S.M. (1957). The ACTH-releasing activity of extracts of the posterior lobe of the pituitary *in vivo*. *Endocrinology* 60: 664–676

McCann S.M., Brobeck J.R. (1954). Evidence for a role of the supraopticohypophyseal system in regulation of adrenocorticotrophin secretion. *Proc Soc Exp Biol Med* 87: 318–324

McCann S.M., Fruit A. (1957). Effect of synthetic vasopressin on release of adrenocorticotrophin in rats with hypothalamic lesions. *Proc Soc Exp Biol Med* 96: 566–567

McDonald R.K., Wagner H.N.J., Weise V.K. (1957). Relationship between endogenous antidiuretic hormone activity and ACTH release in man. *Proc Soc Exp Biol Med* 96: 652–655

Merali Z., Kent P., Du L., Hrdina P., Palkovits M., Faludi G., Poulter M.O., Bedard T., Anisman H. (2006). Corticotropin-releasing hormone, arginine vasopressin, gastrin-releasing peptide, and neuromedin B alterations in stress-relevant brain regions of suicides and control subjects. *Biol Psychiatry* 59: 594–602

Mikhailova M.V., Mayeux P.R., Jurkevich A., Kuenzel W.J., Madison F., Periasamy A., Chen Y., Cornett L.E. (2007). Heterooligomerization between vasotocin and corticotropin-releasing hormone (CRH) receptors augments CRH-stimulated 3',5'-cyclic adenosine monophosphate production. *Mol Endocrinol* 21: 2178–2188

Mirsky I.A., Stein M., Paulisch G. (1954). The secretion of an antidiuretic substance into the circulation of adrenalectomized and hypophysectomized rats exposed to noxious stimuli. *Endocrinology* 55: 28–39

Modell S., Yassouridis A., Huber J., Holsboer F. (1997). Corticosteroid receptor function is decreased in depressed patients. *Neuroendocrinology* 65: 216–222

Muglia L., Jacobson L., Dikkes P., Majzoub J.A. (1995). Corticotropin-releasing hormone deficiency reveals major fetal but not adult glucocorticoid need. *Nature* 373: 427–432

Nemeroff C.B., Widerlov E., Bissette G., Walleus H., Karlsson I., Eklund K., Kilts C.D., Loosen P.T., Vale W (1984). Elevated concentrations of CSF corticotropin-releasing factor-like immunoreactivity in depressed patients. *Science* 226: 1342–1344

Newell-Price J., Jorgensen J.O., Grossman A. (1999). The diagnosis and differential diagnosis of Cushing's syndrome. *Horm Res* 51(Suppl 3): 81–94

Nieman L.K., Chrousos G.P., Oldfield E.H., Avgerinos P.C., Cutler G.B. Jr., Loriaux D.L. (1986). The ovine corticotropin-releasing hormone stimulation test and the dexamethasone suppression test in the differential diagnosis of Cushing's syndrome. *Ann Intern Med* 105: 862–867

Pecori Giraldi F., Pivonello R., Ambrogio A.G., De Martino M.C., De Martin M., Scacchi M., Colao A., Toja P.M., Lombardi G., Cavagnini F. (2007). The dexamethasone-suppressed corticotropin-releasing hormone stimulation test and the desmopressin test to distinguish Cushing's syndrome from pseudo-Cushing's states. *Clin Endocrinol (Oxf)* 66: 251–257

Pena A., Murat B., Trueba M., Ventura M.A., Bertrand G., Cheng L.L., Stoev S., Szeto H.H., Wo N., Brossard G., Serradeil-Le Gal C., Manning M., Guillon G. (2007). Pharmacological and physiological characterization of d[Leu4, Lys8]vasopressin, the first V1b-selective agonist for rat vasopressin/oxytocin receptors. *Endocrinology* 148: 4136–4146

Plotsky P.M. (1985). Hypophyseotropic regulation of adenohypophyseal adrenocorticotropin secretion. *Fed Proc* 44: 207–213

Plotsky P.M., Bruhn T.O., Vale W. (1985). Evidence for multifactor regulation of the adrenocorticotropin secretory response to hemodynamic stimuli. *Endocrinology* 116: 633–639

Plotsky P.M., Vale W. (1984). Hemorrhage-induced secretion of corticotropin-releasing factor-like immunoreactivity into the rat hypophysial portal circulation and its inhibition by glucocorticoids. *Endocrinology* 114: 164–169

Rabadan-Diehl C., Aguilera G. (1998). Glucocorticoids increase vasopressin V1b receptor coupling to phospholipase C. *Endocrinology* 139: 3220–3226

Rabadan-Diehl C., Lolait S.J., Aguilera G. (1995). Regulation of pituitary vasopressin V1b receptor mRNA during stress in the rat. *J Neuroendocrinol* 7: 903–910

Ramos A.T., Troncone L.R., Tufik S. (2006). Suppression of adrenocorticotrophic hormone secretion by simultaneous antagonism of vasopressin 1b and CRH-1 receptors on three different stress models. *Neuroendocrinology* 84: 309–316

Saffran M., Saffran J. (1959). Adenohypophysis and adrenal cortex. *Ann Rev Physiol* 21: 403–444

Seale J.V., Wood S.A., Atkinson H.C., Harbuz M.S., Lightman S.L. (2004). Gonadal steroid replacement reverses gonadectomy-induced changes in the corticosterone pulse profile and stress-induced hypothalamic-pituitary-adrenal axis activity of male and female rats. *J Neuroendocrinol* 16: 989–998

Shibata M., Fujihara H., Suzuki H., Ozawa H., Kawata M., Dayanithi G., Murphy D., Ueta Y. (2007). Physiological studies of stress responses in the hypothalamus of vasopressin-enhanced green fluorescent protein transgenic rat. *J Neuroendocrinol* 19: 285–292

Shimazaki T., Iijima M., Chaki S. (2006). The pituitary mediates the anxiolytic-like effects of the vasopressin V1B receptor antagonist, SSR149415, in a social interaction test in rats. *Eur J Pharmacol* 543: 63–67

Sofroniew M.V., Weindl A., Wetzstein R. (1977). Immunoperoxidase staining of vasopressin in the rat median eminence following adrenalectomy and steroid substitution. *Acta Endocrinol* 85: 94

Stewart L.Q., Roper J.A., Scott Young W. 3rd, O'Carroll A.M., Lolait S.J. (2008a). The role of the arginine vasopressin Avp1b receptor in the acute neuroendocrine action of antidepressants. *Psychoneuroendocrinology* 33: 405–415

Stewart L.Q., Roper J.A., Young W.S. 3rd, O'Carroll A.M., Lolait S.J. (2008b). Pituitary-adrenal response to acute and repeated mild restraint, forced swim and change in environment stress in arginine vasopressin receptor 1b knockout mice. *J Neuroendocrinol* 20: 597–605

Subburaju S., Aguilera G. (2007). Vasopressin mediates mitogenic responses to adrenalectomy in the rat anterior pituitary. *Endocrinology* 148: 3102–3110

Surget A., Belzung C. (2008). Involvement of vasopressin in affective disorders. *Eur J Pharmacol* 583: 340–349

Suzuki S., Uchida D., Koide H., Tanaka T., Noguchi Y., Saito Y., Tatsuno I. (2008). Hyper-responsiveness of adrenal gland to vasopressin resulting in enhanced plasma cortisol in patients with adrenal nodule(s). *Peptides* 29: 1767–1772

Tanoue A., Ito S., Honda K., Oshikawa S., Kitagawa Y., Koshimizu T.A., Mori T., Tsujimoto G. (2004). The vasopressin V1b receptor critically regulates hypothalamic-pituitary-adrenal axis activity under both stress and resting conditions. *J Clin Invest* 113: 302–309

Thomson F., Craighead M. (2008). Innovative approaches for the treatment of depression: targeting the HPA axis. *Neurochem Res* 33: 691–707

Timpl P., Spanagel R., Sillaber I., Kresse A., Reul J.M., Stalla G.K., Blanquet V., Steckler T., Holsboer F., Wurst W. (1998). Impaired stress response and reduced anxiety in mice lacking a functional corticotropin-releasing hormone receptor 1. *Nat Genet* 19: 162–166

Tsagarakis S., Tsigos C., Vasiliou V., Tsiotra P., Kaskarelis J., Sotiropoulou C., Raptis S.A., Thalassinos N. (2002). The desmopressin and combined CRH-desmopressin tests in the differential diagnosis of ACTH-dependent Cushing's syndrome: constraints imposed by the expression of V2 vasopressin receptors in tumors with ectopic ACTH secretion. *J Clin Endocrinol Metab* 87: 1646–1653

Vale W., Spiess J., Rivier C., Rivier J. (1981). Characterization of a 41-residue ovine hypothalamic peptide that stimulates secretion of corticotropin and beta-endorphin. *Science* 213: 1394–1397

van Londen L., Kerkhof G.A., van den Berg F., Goekoop J.G., Zwinderman K.H., Frankhuijzen-Sierevogel A.C., Wiegant V.M., de Wied D. (1998). Plasma arginine vasopressin and motor activity in major depression. *Biol Psychiatry* 43: 196–204

Vandesande F., Dierickx K., De Mey J. (1977). The origin of the vasopressinergic and oxytocinergic fibres of the external region of the median eminence of the rat hypophysis. *Cell Tissue Res* 180: 443–452

Volpi S., Rabadan-Diehl C., Aguilera G. (2004). Vasopressinergic regulation of the hypothalamic pituitary adrenal axis and stress adaptation. *Stress* 7: 75–83

Wiegand S.J., Price J.L. (1980). Cells of origin of the afferent fibers to the median eminence in the rat. *J Comp Neurol* 192: 1–19

Xia Y., Krukoff T.L (2003). Differential neuronal activation in the hypothalamic paraventricular nucleus and autonomic/neuroendocrine responses to I.C.V. endotoxin. *Neuroscience* 121: 219–231

Yates F.E., Russell S.M., Dallman M.F., Hodge G.A., McCann S.M., Dhariwal A.P. (1971). Potentiation by vasopressin of corticotropin release induced by corticotropin-releasing factor. *Endocrinology* 88: 3–15

Zelena D., Domokos A., Barna I., Mergl Z., Haller J., Makara G.B. (2008). Control of the hypothalamo-pituitary-adrenal axis in the neonatal period: adrenocorticotropin and corticosterone stress responses dissociate in vasopressin-deficient Brattleboro rats. *Endocrinology* 149: 2576–2583

Zimmerman E.A., Stillman M.A., Recht L.D., Antunes J.L., Carmel P.W., Goldsmith P.C. (1977). Vasopressin and corticotropin-releasing factor: an axonal pathway to portal capillaries in the zona externa of the median eminence containing vasopressin and its interaction with adrenal corticoids. *Ann NY Acad Sci* 297: 405–419

Zobel A.W., Yassouridis A., Frieboes R.M., Holsboer F. (1999). Prediction of medium-term outcome by cortisol response to the combined dexamethasone-CRH test in patients with remitted depression. *Am J Psychiatry* 156: 949–951

CHAPTER 10

VASOPRESSIN: THE CENTRAL SYSTEMS

Gareth Leng and Simone Meddle

Centre for Integrative Physiology
College of Medicine and Veterinary Medicine
George Square, University of Edinburgh, Edinburgh EX8 9XD
Email: gareth.leng@ed.ac.uk, simone.meddle@ed.ac.uk

1. Introduction

Physiology textbooks often consider vasopressin by its other name, antidiuretic hormone (ADH), a name which implies that its most important role is to regulate water balance by exerting effects upon the kidney and peripheral vasculature. But from an evolutionary perspective, the hormonal role of vasopressin was a relatively late development, and one that accompanied rather than replaced older behavioural functions. We have only recently come to appreciate that these behavioural roles persist in mammals, and it now seems that vasopressin plays an important role in behaviour including social behaviours, emotionality and learning and memory.

2. Peptide Signalling in the Brain

Cells in the mammalian brain communicate using a wide variety of chemical signals. Most (if not all) neurones have at least one neurotransmitter, usually the excitatory neurotransmitter glutamate or the inhibitory neurotransmitter gamma aminobutyric acid (GABA), but sometimes acetylcholine, dopamine, serotonin, adrenaline or noradrenaline. In addition, most neurones also use other messenger molecules, including nitric oxide, adenosine, adenosine triphosphate (ATP) and cannabinoids. Some of these messengers act on other neurones, but some act back on the cell of origin (autoregulatory signals). Others act on the afferent nerve endings that impinge on a neurone (retrograde signals) on glial cells, and some on local blood vessels. These messengers can act locally over a very short time scale or act for prolonged periods and over considerable distances.

The largest family of signalling molecules is the neuropeptides. At least a hundred different peptides are released by neurones, including endorphins, hypocretins, neuromedins, releasing hormones, tachykinins, oxytocin and vasopressin. These act at specific, high affinity, G-protein coupled receptors, expressed on particular subsets of neurones, and often there is more than one receptor subtype, coupled to different intracellular pathways. Peptides can act at diverse targets, and have wide-ranging influences on those targets, not only through acting at different receptors, but also because many of the receptors are coupled to various signalling pathways in different cell types. Many peptides have a direct influence on membrane excitability, but they can also affect gene transcription, and thereby affect the phenotype of the target cell. They can also influence synaptogenesis, and affect the 'hard wiring' of neuronal circuits. In addition, they can act on glial cells, influencing the local morphology and regulating the secretory activity of neurones, and on blood vessels, influencing local blood flow. Many peptides, when injected centrally, have remarkably coherent effects on behaviour; angiotensin II, for instance, induces thirst, and neuropeptide Y induces voracious eating. Vasopressin is one of the most interesting — it induces aggression.

3. Evolution of Vasopressin Systems

Vasopressin is one of the most abundant peptides in the mammalian brain; its receptors are widely distributed, and we probably know more about its actions in the brain than any other peptide. Vasopressin is one of two peptide hormones of the posterior pituitary gland, the other, oxytocin, differing from vasopressin by just one amino acid. They seem to have been derived by gene duplication from a common ancestral peptide. As far as we know, every vertebrate has at least one vasopressin-like peptide and at least one oxytocin-like peptide, so this gene duplication must have taken place early in evolutionary history. Earthworms, leeches, octopuses, snails and other multicellular invertebrates generally lack a pituitary gland, but all have at least one 'neurohypophysial' peptide. In these invertebrates, a peptide closely related to vasopressin is produced by specialized nerve cells and is important for governing behaviours, including feeding and reproductive. So vasopressin, or something very similar, has been with us for much of our evolutionary history, and for most of that time it was exclusively a neuropeptide — a messenger between nerve cells, important in regulating instinctive or programmed behaviours. See also Chapter 2.

4. Behavioural Effects in Mammals

In mammals, vasopressin and oxytocin have a wide range of behavioural effects (Fig. 1). Oxytocin is important for maternal behaviour in several species, and in the female prairie vole, it is instrumental in forging monogamous partner bonds. These roles seem to tally with behavioural observations that indicate more general effects of oxytocin on 'social behaviours' (Neumann, 2008). Oxytocin has been described as anti-anxiolytic for its ability to increase exploratory activity, and especially for olfactory investigations by mice of other mice. In humans intranasal application of oxytocin has been reported to enhance 'trust' (Baumgartner *et al.*, 2008). In addition, oxytocin facilitates sexual responsiveness in female rats and sexual behaviour in male rats, and there have been reports of similar effects in humans. Vasopressin has effects on behaviour that appear intriguingly different, yet complementary to the effects of oxytocin: in male prairie voles, vasopressin enhances the expression of aggression directed towards other males, behaviour that seems territorial, designed to protect a mate from other males or to defend a nest.

The behavioural effects of oxytocin and vasopressin do not consistently accompany peripheral secretion of these hormones, and concentrations measured in the cerebrospinal fluid (CSF) do not change in parallel with

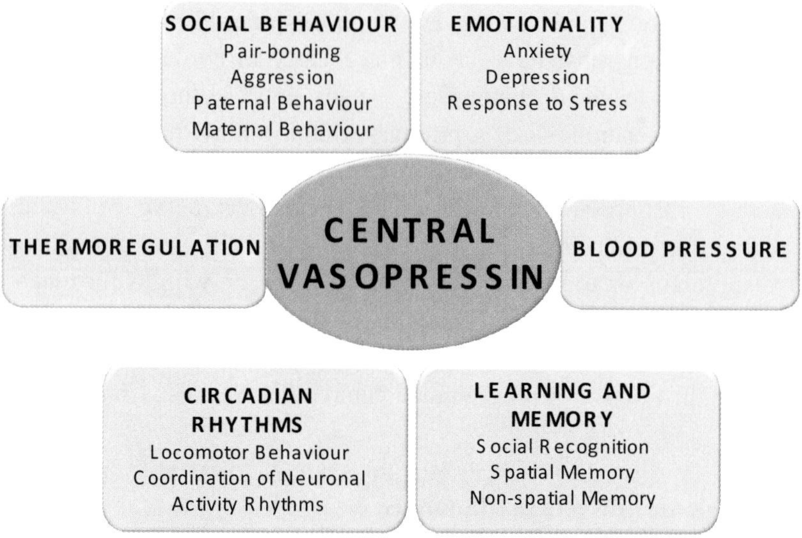

Figure 1. Behavioural effects of vasopressin. Vasopressin has a wide range of behavioural effects. The action of vasopressin on behaviour is through its central release and action via V1a and V1b receptors. There is a very effective blood-brain barrier for vasopressin so what is released from the pituitary does not re-enter the brain in significant amounts.

blood concentrations. The natural conclusion has been that the oxytocin and vasopressin measured in CSF or extracellular fluid in different brain areas, and which presumably mediate behavioural actions do not derive from magnocellular neurones. However, this conclusion has been thrown into doubt by the discovery that magnocellular neurones can regulate central release of their peptide independently of peripheral secretion (Ludwig and Leng, 2006; Leng and Ludwig, 2006).

Most peptidergic neurones also synthesize a conventional neurotransmitter; for instance, the neuropeptide Y/agouti related protein (NPY/AGRP) neurones of the arcuate nucleus synthesize the inhibitory neurotransmitter GABA. Conventional transmitters are packaged in small clear vesicles, and are found mainly at synapses. Peptides are packed into larger vesicles that have an electron-dense core; few of these vesicles are found at synapses, and they do not seem to need specialized sites for their release. For magnocellular neurones, vesicles that contain vasopressin or oxytocin can be released from the nerve terminals but also from axon swellings, undilated axons, soma and dendrites. In the brain, most of the vesicles that contain vasopressin are in the dendrites of magnocellular neurones, and these are likely to be the main source of central release. This is probably true of many, if not all, other peptides as well; large dense-cored vesicles are usually distributed throughout the neuronal cytoplasm and, as more than 80% of the cell volume of a typical neurone is in its dendrites, this is where most large vesicles are found. Whereas electron microscopic profiles of synapses in the central nervous system might typically show one or two large dense-core vesicles present (sometimes as many as six or seven), the abundance of such vesicles in dendrites of vasopressin neurones is similar to that typically found in endocrine cells, such as somototrophs or gonadotrophs. Importantly, secretion is regulated differentially from specific compartments. In axons and nerve terminals, secretion is determined by calcium entry through voltage-dependent calcium channels that open as a result of spike activity, but in the soma and dendrites, calcium release from the intracellular stores of the endoplasmic reticulum also plays a major role, and can trigger release independently of spike activity. See also Chapter 11.

5. Chemical Coding in Neural Networks: Early Evidence of Complexity

Until the 1980s, the brain seemed to be a grey sort of place; there were unimaginably many neurones (10 billion or more in the human brain) and many more connections between them (typically 10,000 for each neurone). We did not understand much about how the brain processed information, but there seemed to be more than enough computational power in the sheer volume of connections in the brain for it to do whatever it liked, however it liked. Distinctions between different types of neurones seemed to be almost beside the point. Several neurotransmitters were known of, but it was far from clear why there was really any need for more than two. One neurotransmitter to excite and one to inhibit seemed ample for the type of 'Boolean algebra' that was how the brain was thought to do its computations.

However, in the 1970s, Fuxe and his co-workers in Sweden took neuroanatomy to a new level of detail by refining the art of visualising catecholaminergic neurones (see Fuxe and Jonsson, 1973), and then by assembling an armamentarium of techniques for studying them. The map of the brain that they unveiled was remarkable. Only three sites contained noradrenergic neurones: the A1 cell group in the nucleus of the solitary tract, the A2 group in the ventrolateral medulla, and the A6 group in locus coeruleus. At each site, there were just a few hundred noradrenergic neurones, but fibres from these neurones permeated virtually the whole brain; whatever these few neurones were doing, it seemed that the whole brain had to know about it. What these noradrenergic neurones actually did though, was not clear; they seemed to be important for virtually everything: for appetite, noradrenaline was then the most potent known orexigenic factor; for reproduction, pulses of luteinizing hormone, secreted from the anterior pituitary, were triggered by pulses of noradrenaline; also for blood pressure regulation, thermoregulation, thirst, stress responses, moods, and much more.

Fuxe saw that it was hard to reconcile the diffusely distributed nature of the noradrenergic fibres with the idea that they carried precise information, and he also recognised that noradrenaline release from these fibres was not confined to synapses, but spilled over into the extracellular fluid, meaning that this information could not be specifically targeted. Noradrenaline seemed to be released and perhaps acted in a way that was somehow half hormone, half neurotransmitter. Fuxe named this new mode of communication 'volume transmission', and speculated that diffusion of noradrenaline through the brain was not uniform, but would occur preferentially along particular channels, bounded by glial cells, carried by 'canals' in the brain (see Fuxe *et al.*, 2007). The idea that the noradrenergic systems were part of a non-specific 'activating' system also arose partly to make sense of why such an apparently crude messenger system was needed at all, and partly to account for why this system appeared to be important for so many things.

But any idea that the noradrenergic systems were an exception to the ordered layout of logically structured processing elements elsewhere in the brain was short lived. By the end of the 20th century, the grey and ordered map of the brain had been replaced by a 'Jackson Pollack' extravagance of disordered colour. The first colour to be added was for vasopressin, as immunocytochemical techniques mapped out a rich and diverse network of vasopressin cells. This was a foretaste of things to come: now we know of more than 100 different peptides that are expressed in particular small populations of neurones, all of which signal to other neurones via specific receptors.

Vasopressin is packaged within neurones at a high density, in large vesicles. When released, it has a long half-life in the brain (typically minutes) and it acts at receptors that are sensitive to nanomolar concentrations. By contrast, conventional neurotransmitters are released from abundant small vesicles, but have a biological half-life of just a few milliseconds. They act at low affinity ionotropic receptors, so have an immediate, direct effect on neuronal excitability, but one that is very short lasting.

Exactly why the brain needs this exuberant diversity of signalling systems is a topic of huge interest and considerable importance, and studies of the vasopressin system have been very influential in our present understanding of brain function. However, it is difficult to even begin talking about the central vasopressin systems without acknowledging that our understanding of them has been in almost constant flux for thirty years, and this should warn us that today's 'knowledge' may be as ephemeral as yesterday's was. These unsettled notions do not seem to be the product of reckless speculation, arising, as it were, from a swamp of ignorance; the vasopressin systems have been the subject of close attention from electrophysiologists, molecular biologists, anatomists, chemists and behavioural neuroendocrinologists.

More is known about magnocellular vasopressin neurones than about almost any other type of neurone, and what we have learned from them has progressively changed our understanding of the brain.

6. Behavioural Effects of Vasopressin: History of the Idea

The possibility that the brain might be amongst the targets for the actions of vasopressin was first seriously explored by David de Wied and his co-workers in the 1960s. Like Karl Lashley (1938) before him, de Wied believed that strong motivational drives must have a deep rooted instinctive basis, and that threats to an organism's homeostasis should powerfully activate such drives. He suspected that a shortage of water should initiate goal-seeking cognitive behaviour in animals; he thought that this might be the product of a hormonal feedback action on the brain, and he set about testing this by behavioural experiments (see de Wied, 1997).

The model that he chose for his experiments was the Brattleboro rat (see Bohus and de Wied, 1998). This rat strain has hereditary hypothalamic diabetes insipidus; there is a single base deletion in the coding region for the vasopressin precursor, and the aberrant peptide that is produced cannot be properly packaged into neurosecretory vesicles, so no detectable vasopressin is secreted. De Wied noted that this rat had several behavioural abnormalities, some of which seemed to reflect deficits in memory processing, and some of which could be corrected by replacing the absent vasopressin by giving a vasopressin agonist systemically. This bold hypothesis ran into problems in the following years, and it is worth recalling now, not because its truth has endured, but because it provided the incentive for research that ultimately led to a radically new vision of how the brain processes information.

When de Wied first published his accounts of the Brattleboro rat, it was assumed that vasopressin could reach the brain readily from the pituitary gland. However, this is not so: there is a very effective blood-brain barrier for vasopressin, and what is released from the pituitary does not re-enter the brain in significant amounts. The experiments of de Wied thus needed a new interpretation to understand how the cognitive deficits of Brattleboro rats could be rescued by systemically administered vasopressin. Part of the answer turned out to be almost embarrassingly mundane. The Brattleboro rat maintains approximate fluid and electrolyte balance by drinking copious amounts of water while excreting equally copious amounts of dilute urine. Perhaps unsurprisingly, its sleep rhythms are disrupted by these necessities. When some antidiuretic function is restored by an exogenous vasopressin agonist, the rat seems to sleep better and generally perform better in a range of cognitive tasks. However, even as this was becoming clear, it was also emerging that vasopressin clearly did act in the brain, at least when it was injected directly into it. Doses that were far too low to be systemically effective were found to have a wide variety of effects, including on blood pressure and body temperature, as well as effects on an intriguing but confusing set of behaviours.

7. Vasopressin's Diverse Central Actions

With the advent of high affinity radio-labelled agonists for vasopressin, it became clear that the brain was indeed rich in vasopressin receptors, and that certain limbic regions, including predictably the hippocampus, but also the amygdala, the septum, bed nucleus of the stria terminalis, olfactory bulb, many parts of the hypothalamus, and regions of the caudal brainstem and spinal cord, all expressed high affinity vasopressin binding sites in abundance. Further studies using *in situ* hybridisation histochemistry (to identify cells that transcribe the receptor gene) have clarified that vasopressin V1a and V1b receptors are both expressed in many different brain regions, while V2 receptors seem to be absent. In addition to widespread distribution in the brain, the V1b receptor is prominent in the anterior pituitary gland, particularly within corticotrophs.

The vasopressin that acts at these receptors in the brain does not come from the pituitary gland either directly, by some kind of retrograde flow, or via the blood. The concentrations of vasopressin and oxytocin in CSF or brain extracellular fluid are consistently higher than in blood, and they do not change in parallel. This must mean that large amounts of vasopressin and oxytocin are released within the brain, and this release is at least semi-independent of secretion from the pituitary. The key question is then if vasopressin cannot get into the brain from the blood, then are these receptors an irrelevant curiosity? Perhaps they are the product of some incidental gene mutation that has little cost and no maladaptive consequences? Vasopressin is released within the brain, although where from, and how it is released, is still the subject of controversy.

What we know of the physiological actions of central vasopressin release comes from experiments, mainly in rodents, that involve giving a vasopressin agonist or an antagonist, either into the CSF, usually via a lateral cerebral ventricle, or into a discrete brain region by micro-injection. Development of specific agonists and antagonists for vasopressin receptors has been a popular area of research, and one breakthrough was using desmopressin in the treatment of excess urine production in patients with central diabetes insipidus. Desmopressin acts on the V2 receptors in the renal collecting ducts, and V2 anatgonists are effective in treatment of hypernatraemia. Other selective antagonists such as the V1b antagonist (SSR149415) can be given orally and are effective in rodents for reducing aggression and anxiety behaviour (Blanchard *et al.*, 2005). See also Chapter 5.

8. Sources of Vasopressin in the Brain

The vasopressin cells of the brain were mapped in detail by immunocytochemical studies in the 1980s (Fig. 2). There is so much vasopressin in the magnocellular neurones that to stain them by immunocytochemistry requires no special techniques. Indeed, the density of staining in these cells exceeded that in any other cells to such a great extent that at first it was suspected that the staining seen in some other cells was a weak cross-reaction of the antiserum with some other substance. However, with careful controls, it became clear that the staining seen in some locations did indeed reflect synthesis of vasopressin, and this was confirmed when *in situ* hybridisation histochemistry localised vasopressin mRNA to these same places. These studies showed that, as well as the magnocellular vasopressin neurones, there are several populations of parvocellular vasopressin cells in the paraventricular nucleus. Some of them project to the median eminence to

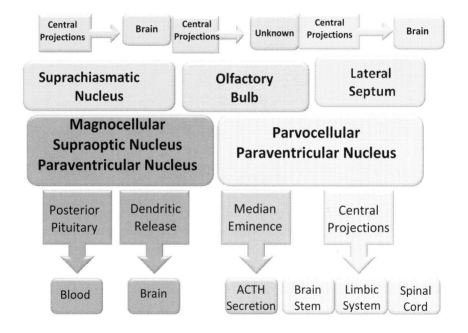

Figure 2. The sources of vasopressin. As well as the magnocellular vasopressin neurones, there are several populations of parvocellular vasopressin cells in the paraventricular nucleus. Other parvocellular vasopressin neurones are found in the lateral septum, suprachiasmatic nucleus and olfactory bulb.

secrete vasopressin into the hypothalamo-hypophysial portal circulation, to regulate the secretion of adrenocorticotrophic hormone (ACTH) (see Chapter 9). Other parvocellular populations project centrally, innervating many other brain regions.

In addition, there is a large population of vasopressin cells in the suprachiasmatic nucleus of the hypothalamus, and also populations in the lateral septum and olfactory bulb.

It is possible to measure vasopressin release at particular brain sites, either by push-pull perfusion or by microdialysis, although both techniques have problems. Push-pull perfusion tends to cause considerable local damage; microdialysis causes less damage, but as the recovery of peptides using current probes is only a few percent of the extracellular concentrations, the time resolution of microdialysis studies is poor. Typically, basal concentrations of vasopressin are measurable only in microdialysis samples collected over about 30 minutes.

9. Sex Dfferences in the Vasopressin System

We have known that there are sex differences in the vasopressin system since the early 1980s when it was shown by De Vries and colleagues that vasopressin fibre density is higher in the lateral septum of males than in females. They were able to increase vasopressin fibre density in this region in female and castrated male rats by giving testosterone (De Vries *et al.*, 1983). More evidence for actions of gonadal steroids on the vasopressin system was published a decade later, when androgen receptors were located in non-magnocellular vasopressin neurones. Oestrogens may also have a direct effect on the vasopressin system, as oestrogen receptor beta is expressed by magnocellular neurones (Sladek and Somponpun, 1994). Gonadal steroids also appear to affect the expression of vasopressin receptors, as gonadectomy decreases V1a mRNA expression and receptor binding in the hypothalamus of hamsters (Young *et al.*, 2000).

10. Central Actions of Vasopressin

a) *Vasopressin in cardiovascular regulation*

Vasopressin injected peripherally evokes a potent increase in blood pressure as a result of its pressor activity at many peripheral vascular beds, but vasopressin can also transiently raise blood pressure when injected into the brain at very low doses, and this is independent of any effect on vasculature, as the arterioles of the brain do not express vasopressin receptors. The response to centrally injected vasopressin is thus a neurogenic pressor response.

The physiology underlying these pharmacological observations is unclear, but there is now an accepted role for spinally-projecting vasopressin in sympathetic regulation of the cardiovascular system. An expansion of blood volume triggers a reflex increase in heart rate that is mediated via sympathetic nerves, mainly as a result of activation of volume receptors at the venous-atrial junctions of the heart. Stimulation of these volume receptors also leads to an inhibition of renal sympathetic nerve activity. This reflex depends on the paraventricular nucleus: cardiac atrial afferents, acting via GABA interneurones in the paraventricular nucleus, inhibit spinally projecting vasopressin neurones that project to renal sympathetic neurones, and lesions of these spinally projecting neurones abolish the reflex (Coote, 2005). See also Chapter 7.

b) *Vasopressin in thermoregulation*

When we think of the body's defences against infection, we usually think of the immune system, but the brain also has an important part to play in both defending against infection and in facilitating healing. The full range of mechanisms by which the brain directs these processes is far from clear, but many of the inflammatory cytokines that are released in response to injury or infection signal to the hypothalamus, and especially to the paraventricular nucleus. One way in which the brain mounts a defence against infection is by generating a high body temperature; fever is not a consequence of a viral infection *per se*, but is a centrally evoked response that can weaken or kill the invading virus.

The paraventricular nucleus has an important role in generating fever in response to viral infection, and it seems that centrally released vasopressin is involved in modulating this. Central injections of vasopressin will reduce body temperature, and particularly the elevated body temperature of a fever (Rothwell, 1994).

c) *Vasopressin in stress responses, anxiety and depression*

It is often assumed that vasopressin is likely to be involved in behaviours that are adaptive responses to stressors, given that it is made by the paraventricular neurones that regulate secretion of the stress hormone ACTH. Some studies of vasopressin release in different brain areas have indeed indicated that vasopressin is released centrally in a variety of stressful conditions, and in response to fear, but what vasopressin does that might be useful in these circumstances is unclear. Vasopressin may act to enhance both the expression and learning of fear by modulating the integration of information in the amygdala (Debiec, 2005). Existing evidence suggests that excessive fear may lead to anxiety disorders.

In addition to anxiety, vasopressin impacts on depression-related behaviour. Chronic forced swim stress is used in rodents as a model for depression and to investigate coping behaviour. Such tests are associated with increases in vasopressin release particularly in the paraventricular nucleus and the amygdala. Interestingly, Brattleboro rats show better coping behaviour than wild-types. Much evidence indicates a role for vasopressin in regulating the hypothalamo-pituitary axis (HPA) in both humans and rodents, and rats bred for abnormal HPA axis activity have provided a useful model to study relationships between the neuroendocrine system and behavioural disorders. Rats bred to display greater anxiety and depressive type behaviour have enhanced activity of the HPA axis including the vasopressin system (Landgraf, 2006). Single nucleotide polymorphisms (SNPs) may explain the increased transcription of vasopressin the paraventricular nucleus in this phenotype. A family history of depression also increases the likelihood of developing the condition, and this is highly correlated with above normal plasma vasopressin. This elevation and increased vasopressin in the paraventricular nucleus in depressed patients is thought to reflect disregulation of the HPA axis (Landgraf, 2006).

The V1a receptor is clearly important for controlling depression and anxiety, as V1a knockout mice display low anxiety (Egashira *et al.*, 2007) and anxiety, as measured on the elevated plus maze (EPM), is reduced following targeted V1a mRNA antisense oligodeoxynucleotide delivery to the septum (Landgraf *et al.*, 1995). Central actions of V1a antagonists produce antidepressant-like effects in rats but V1b also modulates depression like behaviour. The nonpeptide V1b receptor antagonists attenuate stress-related behaviour in rodents and increase coping behaviour (Griebel *at al.*, 2005). The development of such orally active selective V1b antagonists, with their anxiolytic effect, may provide future treatment for excessive anxiety and stress in humans.

d) *Vasopressin in social behaviours*

Perhaps the best evidence of the hormone-like nature of the behavioural effects of vasopressin comes from studies of pair bonding (Insel and Young, 2001; Ferguson *et al.*, 2002; Bielsky *et al.*, 2005). In prairie voles, the male forms a monogamous bond with a female after mating; this is quite rare in mammals, even for other species of vole. After mating, the male becomes aggressive towards other males, a kind of "jealousy" that is the mark, in prairie voles, of the pair bond. This aggression is facilitated by vasopressin within the brain, and can be attenuated by blocking vasopressin actions. In prairie voles, the vasopressin V1a receptor has a distribution in the brain quite unlike that of promiscuous montane voles. Indeed, the distribution is quite variable, even between different voles, because of a high variability in the V1a receptor gene (Donaldson and Young, 2008). This, and individual variations are predictive of differences in both receptor distribution and social behaviour (Hammock and Young, 2005). Moreover, experimental manipulation of this gene, either through transgenic mutations or adenoviral gene transfer, show that behavioural changes accompany alterations in the distribution of V1a receptors (Landgraf *et al.*, 2003).

Thus, it is not the distribution of vasopressin fibres in the brain that determines the behaviour, but the distribution of vasopressin receptors.

To date, the effects of vasopressin in social behaviour have been mostly described in males and in particular in relation to aggressive behaviour in a resident intruder paradigm (Ferris *et al.*, 2006). It is clear that components of vasopressin-facilitated aggression depend upon prior learning and experience. The plasticity in aggression may be linked to social status but also early life experience. For instance, unpaired male prairie voles do not usually demonstrate territorial aggression unless they are exposed post-natally to vasopressin (Stribley and Carter, 1999). The environment also plays a direct programming role as adult male rats separated from their mothers as pups exhibit higher levels of aggression and vasopressin mRNA expression in the paraventricular nucleus than males that have not experienced early life stress (Veenema *et al.*, 2006).

For most aggression studies, the male Syrian hamster has been the animal model of choice as they are a highly aggressive solitary species. Flank marking is a stereotypic form of scent marking displayed by socially dominant males, and this behaviour is increased in a dose-dependant manner following vasopressin microinjections into the hypothalamus (Ferris *et al.*, 1984). Aggression in this species appears to be regulated by both types of vasopressin receptors, since V1a antagonists block vasopressin facilitated flank marking (Ferris *et al.*, 1993, 2006) and aggression is attenuated in hamsters given oral V1b antagonists (Blanchard *et al.*, 2005).

Aggression and V1a binding in the anterior hypothalamus and paraventricular nucleus is correlated with social isolation in hamsters, and subordinate Syrian hamsters have fewer vasopressin immunoreactive labelled neurones and display increased flank marking when treated with vasopressin, compared to dominants (Ferris *et al.*, 1989). For vasopressin to be effective in facilitating aggression in hamsters, social isolation for weeks is required (Caldwell and Albers, 2004), highlighting the importance of social experience and status. Central vasopressin projections from the medial amygdala and bed nucleus of the stria terminalis to the lateral septum are important for aggression and appear to be sex-steroid dependent. In male mice bred for short attack latency there are fewer vasopressin neurones in the bed nucleus of the stria terminalis and less vasopressin innervation in the lateral septum than in long attack latency mice. Transgenic male mice bred with V1b receptor inactivation are less aggressive (Wersinger *et al.*, 2007) and studies on this mouse line indicate that V1b receptors are important for coupling social context to the display of appropriate behaviour. However, V1a-receptor deficient mice do not display reduced aggression, and it has been hypothesised that there is developmental compensation in these animals. Even in humans, there is evidence that vasopressin is associated with aggression; healthy men with a life history of general and directed aggression have elevated CSF concentrations of vasopressin (Coccaro *et al.*, 1998). Future studies will be important in elucidating the neuroanatomical regions involved and the role vasopressin plays in the regulation of male aggression.

There is evidence that vasopressin promotes and regulates parental care. For instance, male California mice provide more parental care than white-footed male mice. They are also more aggressive to intruders in the presence of pups, and have higher levels of vasopressin and V1a expression in the bed nucleus of the stria terminalis and hypothalamus (Bester-Meredith *et al.*, 1999). Recent studies in the California mouse have shown that experimental reduction in paternal care influences the development of aggression and is also associated with increased vasopressin in the paraventricular nucleus in the male offspring. There are differences in V1a receptor distribution between monogamous, parental and non-monogamous, non-parental vole species, hinting that these receptors may regulate parental behaviour. But its not just rodents that exhibit changes in their vasopressin system with fatherhood. Experienced marmoset fathers have higher levels of V1a labelled dendritic spines in the prefrontal cortex than non-parental males (Kozorovitskiy *et al.*, 2006). This raises the question as to what is the neural mechanism underlying these reorganisational changes in vasopressin signalling in these fathers. If such changes occur in non-human primates, do we expect similar changes in human fathers too?

Maternal behaviour is complex, but it is also promoted and regulated by vasopressin. A study in rats (Bosch and Neumann, 2008) has elegantly shown that maternal care is impaired by locally blocking vasopressin receptors in the brain using vasopressin antagonists or by antisense oligodeoxynucleotides. The vasopressin system is activated around the time of birth, so it is not surprising to find that central vasopressin facilitates maternal care, including defence of the pups from intruders. This defence, termed 'maternal aggression', is impaired in V1b-receptor deficient mice (Wersinger *et al.*, 2007).

The most social of all mammals is the human — we form elaborate complex networks of social bonds, and it has been suggested that pair-bonding is a critical factor in the evolutionary development of the 'social brain'. It is not yet known whether similar central vasopressin mechanisms are also important for human pair-bonding, but there is a reported association between one of the human vasopressin V1a polymorphisms and traits reflecting pairbonding behaviour in men, including partner bonding, perceived marital problems, and marital status (Walum *et al.*, 2008). Further studies are also required to reveal whether disturbances in the vasopressin system in the perinatal period are related to postnatal depression or psychosis in women. If vasopressin is crucial for the display of parental behaviour, therapeutic intervention using drugs to manipulate the vasopressin system provides a potentially exciting possibility to develop treatments for behavioural disorders.

e) *Vasopressin in learning and memory*

Social memory is important for all social interactions as it allows animals to recognise individuals so that they can display the appropriate behaviour towards that individual. In rodents, most social cues are olfactory, whereas in primates these cues are mainly visual or auditory. Social recognition tests are employed to examine social memory and the processing of olfactory cues and memories in rodents is vasopressin-dependent. For instance, individual recognition in rats relies on vasopressin projections from the medial amygdala and bed nucleus of the stria terminalis to the lateral septum (Dantzer and Bluthé, 1993), and manipulation of the vasopressin system within the lateral septum influences social memory and discrimination (Landgraf *et al.*, 1995, 2003). Such contradictory results may be explained by the fact that endogenous vasopressin released within the lateral septum can act to favour simple stimulus processing like olfactory recognition over complex stimulus processing, in which the dorsal hippocampus is required (Englemann, 2008). Studies using vasopressin-receptor deficient mice have built on these findings and suggest that V1a receptors may be involved with the integration of olfactory cues while V1b receptors are more associated with the motivation of behavioural responses via the formation and retrieval of memories associated with chemosensory cues from social encounters (Wersinger *et al.*, 2004, 2008).

Vasopressin also has effects on non-social memory. In both spatial and non-spatial tasks, vasopressin enhances not only memory consolidation but also memory retrieval (Gulpinar and Yegen, 2004). During non-spatial passive avoidance trials, in which animals receive a foot shock after entering the dark compartment of a light dark box, vasopressin administration improves passive avoidance learning (Kovacs *et al.*, 1986). Rodent spatial learning and working memory is normally quantified by performance on a radial arm maze or Morris water maze.

In the mid eighties, Packard and Ettenberg (1985) showed that working memory is improved by peripherally administered vasopressin. Other studies designed to study reference memory, such as the hole board search task, showed improvement in both long- and short-term memory with vasopressin (Vawter *et al.*, 1997) and as discussed earlier, Brattleboro heterozygotes demonstrated poorer working memory performance than wild-type controls (Aarde and Jentsch, 2006).

The V1a appears also to be critical for spatial task performance in the eight-arm radial maze as transgenic V1a knockout mice or wild-type mice, given a selective V1aR antagonist, have impaired short term memory. Interestingly, V1b knockout mice have no such impairment

(Egashira *et al.*, 2004). Effects on memory of peripheral administration of vasopressin may just reflect changes in the arousal state. Studies in men have shown that a vasopressin analogue enhances reaction times and arousal but not memory itself (Beckwith *et al.*, 1983; Gais *et al.*, 2002), although other human memory studies have reported that vasopressin treatment is more effective in enhancing memory in men compared to women (Pietrowsky *et al.*, 1988).

11. Parvocellular Vasopressin Cells of the Paraventricular Nucleus

In the rat brain, and probably in the brains of all mammals, there are at least four functionally distinct vasopressin systems, and three of these are present in the paraventricular nucleus. Apart from the magnocellular neurosecretory neurones, the paraventricular nucleus contains at least two populations of parvocellular vasopressin neurones. One population comprises neurosecretory neurones that project to the median eminence, releasing their contents into the hypothalamo-pituitary portal circulation. These hypophysiotropic neurones regulate the secretion of ACTH, and are part of the hypothalamo-pituitary adrenal stress axis. They are interesting for many reasons, not least because their biochemical phenotype appears quite 'plastic'. At pituitary corticotrophs, both vasopressin and corticotrophin releasing factor (CRF) can trigger ACTH secretion; they act at separate receptors, but their combined effect is synergistic. CRF and vasopressin are made in the same parvocellular neuroendocrine neurones, but in amounts that vary according to physiological circumstances. It seems that the expression of CRF, but not that of vasopressin, is subject to negative feedback by glucocorticoids. Accordingly, in chronically stressed animals, vasopressin expression is high, apparently continually activated by the continuing stressful challenge, but CRF expression is diminished because of the prolonged secretion of glucocorticoids. Therefore, in response to chronic stress, the neurones progressively change their biochemical phenotype, from being mainly 'CRF cells' to being mainly 'vasopressin cells' (Ma *et al.*, 1999). See also Chapter 9.

Whether these parvocellular neurones also project within the brain is not clear, but they probably do. The paraventricular nucleus contains other vasopressin cells that only project centrally; many of these project down the spinal cord, and others innervate many regions of the brainstem and limbic system. Indeed, it is far from clear exactly how many functionally distinct vasopressin populations there are in the paraventricular nucleus. These centrally projecting neurones have usually been thought to be the substrate for most vasopressin-dependent behaviours.

12. The Suprachiasmatic Nucleus

There is a large vasopressin cell population in the suprachiasmatic nucleus (SCN), and vasopressin was the first neuropeptide to be described in the area of the hypothalamus now known as the 'biological clock'. The SCN is the major circadian rhythm generator in mammals, and the ~10,000 neurones of the SCN express a family of so-called 'clock genes'. The protein products of these genes regulate the expression of other clock genes to produce a slow, cyclically repeating cascade of gene expression, with a period of around 24 hours. This rhythm is entrained every day by light signals from photoreceptors in the retina which, through their input via the retinohypothalamic tract, produce a circadian rhythm in the animal's motor activity that is locked to the light-dark cycle.

Interactions amongst the clock genes have been studied extensively, but it is not clear how the gene rhythms affect SCN neurones in ways that enable the rhythms to be communicated to other neurones. For example, the clock gene Period 1 is expressed rhythmically in SCN neurones, and its expression is correlated with neuronal electrical activity, but if there is a causal link between clock gene expression and neuronal excitability, we do not know what it is. The functional significance of the changes in activity is also not clear; there is no consistent correlation between Period 1 expression and circadian rhythms of locomotor activity. While it is often thought that the subpopulations of SCN neurones oscillate in synchrony to produce a single, coherent output, some suspect that there are several, independently regulated oscillator populations within the SCN, producing a family of rhythms with varied phase relationships.

Vasopressin is released as part of these rhythms, and its release may be measured *in vivo*, with vasopressin peaking in the CSF during the day. For neurones in the SCN to generate these strong rhythms that influence so many essential physiological functions, coordination of neuronal activity is likely to be very important. The circadian rhythmicity of rodent locomotor behaviour implicates vasopressin. For example, SCN cultures taken from common voles lacking rhythmic wheel running activity do not produce a circadian rhythm in vasopressin release (Jansen *et al.*, 1999). The vasopressin cells in the SCN express vasopressin receptors, and rhythms in V1a mRNA expression have been observed in the SCN of rats (Kalamatianos *et al.*, 2004), so it is possible that vasopressin released within the SCN helps to 'bind' the activity of a subset of these neurones together. Ageing causes a decrease in circadian activity and vasopressin is likely to play a role in this as the number of vasopressin cells in the SCN decreases in older animals (Van der Zee *et al.*, 1999).

Thus the peptides released by SCN neurones are internal mechanisms of neuronal coordination, but are also important signals for the brain beyond. Transplant experiments in hamsters have shown that ablation of the SCN destroys circadian activity rhythms, but these rhythms could be restored by SCN transplants into the third ventricle, even if the transplants were enclosed by a semi-permeable polymeric capsule (Silver *et al.*, 1996). The capsule prevented axonal outgrowth, but signals could still exchange by diffusion between transplant and host, and thus the SCN (like neural pacemakers in the invertebrates Drosophila and silkmoths) can sustain circadian rhythms by a diffusible signal.

13. The Magnocellular Vasopressin System

The magnocellular vasopressin system (see Armstrong, 1995; Leng *et al.*, 1998) consists of about 9000 large magnocellular neurones, each typically with a soma about 20 μm in diameter. These cells comprise a 'cloud' of neurones in the anterior hypothalamus, within which are several foci of aggregation. Each of the two supraoptic nuclei contains about 2,000 vasopressin cells (and about 1,000 oxytocin cells); the paraventricular nuclei have fewer vasopressin cells and more oxytocin cells. There are also several small 'accessory' nuclei between these most prominent aggregations, the largest of which is the nucleus circularis.

Each magnocellular neurone has a single long axon that projects to the posterior pituitary gland via the internal zone of the median eminence and the neural stalk. These axons have very few collateral branches that end within the hypothalamus, but in the posterior pituitary, about 2000 nerve endings arise like "buds" from each axon. The cells have between one and three large dendrites, up to several hundred microns long. In the supraoptic nucleus these dendrites project to the ventral surface of the brain, where they form a dense plexus. These dendrites are characterized by very large swellings, of up to 15 μm in diameter, which show dense peptide immunostaining. See also Chapter 11.

Vasopressin is abundant in all compartments of the magnocellular neurones, packaged in large dense-core vesicles. The two supraoptic nuclei of a rat contain about 27 ng of vasopressin, each dendrite containing tens of thousands of these vesicles, each of which contains about 85,000 molecules of vasopressin (see Leng and Ludwig, 2008). The magnocellular neurones also make several other neuroactive peptides which are co-packaged and co-secreted with vasopressin (though in much smaller amounts). These co-existing peptides include dynorphin, galanin and apelin.

The afferent pathways to the supraoptic nucleus have been well studied. There are inputs from many brain areas, but the most substantial inputs arise from structures adjacent to the anterior wall of the third ventricle, including from two circumventricular organs: the subfornical organ and the organum vasculosum of the lamina terminalis. These are the source of excitatory projections that use glutamate as a neurotransmitter and inhibitory projections that use GABA, and they also signal via several peptides, including angiotensin II, which is excitatory to vasopressin cells. There is also a major direct innervation from the ventrolateral medulla, including from noradrenergic neurones of the A1 cell group; these A1 neurones produce several peptides, including neuropeptide Y. However, much of the afferent input to the vasopressin cells is relayed via the so-called perinuclear zone dorsal and lateral to the nucleus, which includes both GABA and glutamate neurones, and also cholinergic neurones.

14. Dendritic Localization of Peptides

Studies on dendritic vasopressin release have been assisted by the fact that magnocellular neurones aggregate into compact and homogenous nuclei and, because the axons have few if any collaterals, studies of dendritic release can be accomplished without contamination by synaptic release. In these dendrites, vesicle exocytosis can be regulated by Ca^{2+} entry but also by intracellular Ca^{2+} release. Large amounts of Ca^{2+} are sequestered in the endoplasmic reticulum, and release from these stores is regulated by second-messenger pathways. Thus the dendrites contain two mechanisms for regulated secretion of vesicles: activity-dependent release, whereby spikes regulate release from a readily-releasable pool of vesicles via Ca^{2+} entry, and store-regulated release, triggered by agonists that induce intracellular Ca^{2+} release. These pathways can be activated independently of each other. For example, after systemic osmotic stimulation, vasopressin is released both into the blood and from the dendrites, but the temporal profiles of release are dissociated. Osmotic stimulation promptly activates secretion into the blood, but dendritic release is apparently delayed by more than one hour compared to axonal secretion, and it persists for much longer. Such dissociation between dendritic and axonal release was the first clear indication that the presumption that all central actions of vasopressin reflect the activity of centrally-projecting parvocellular neurones needed reconsideration.

15. Vasopressin as an Autoregulator of Vasopressin Cell Activity

In the supraoptic nucleus, both the electrical activity of vasopressin cells and the dendritic release of vasopressin are orchestrated by the local actions of vasopressin. Both V1a and the V1b receptors are expressed by vasopressin cells, and a complex cascade of second messenger interactions results from the binding of vasopressin to these receptors (Sabatier *et al.*, 2004), and one consequence is to trigger vasopressin release from the dendrites. The dendrites lie close to each other, and the local concentrations of vasopressin are extremely high, as every vesicle that is released there introduces about 85,000 molecules of vasopressin into the narrow clefts of the extracellular space. The concentrations from even a single vesicle are so high that vasopressin released from one dendrite is not only a signal that feeds back on its cell of origin, but also a signal that affects at least those cells with neighbouring dendrites. The effects of vasopressin on the electrical activity of vasopressin cells are mainly inhibitory. However, the effects on dendritic release have a positive feedback effect — once vasopressin release is triggered, it will become self-sustaining and long-lasting.

Elevation of intracellular $[Ca^{2+}]$ has another important consequence: it primes dendritic stores of peptides to make them available for subsequent activity-dependent release (Ludwig *et al.*, 2002, 2005). Spike activity in vasopressin neurones *in vivo* does not always result in significant dendritic oxytocin release, but after exposure to agents that mobilise Ca^{2+} from intracellular stores, dendritic peptide release in response to depolarising stimuli is dramatically potentiated. Priming is a long-lasting phenomenon; its effects persist for at least 90 minutes. The cellular mechanisms of priming may involve actions on translation/protein processing such as local synthesis of proteins that support exocytosis. Furthermore, it may entail changes in vesicle tethering, maturation of docked vesicles and/or active vesicle transport. Studies using electron microscopy indicate that priming involves a relocation of vesicles closer to sites of secretion (Tobin *et al.*, 2004), resulting in augmentation of the readily-releasable pool of vesicles that are then available for conventional activity-dependent release.

16. Conclusion

Neuropeptides are not like neurotransmitters. Neurotransmitters, acting at synapses, have a spatial specificity conferred by the anatomy of neuronal projection sites, and a temporal specificity conferred by tight coupling of transmitter release to electrical activity and rapid breakdown or re-uptake at the site of release. Neuropeptides appear to be more like classical hormones: their long half-lives mean that they can survive for long enough to diffuse to sites that may be distant from where they are released. Even in the CSF, vasopressin is present at concentrations high enough to activate the high-affinity peptide receptors that are present in many brain regions. Peripheral hormonal signals are interpreted by receptors distant from the sites of secretion, and thus the information carried by these signals is encoded in the temporal, not the spatial, pattern of secretion, and the same may be true in the brain — it may be the rhythms of vasopressin release that matter, as much or more than where it is released. Indeed, mismatches between receptor distribution and peptidergic innervation are far from unusual: Herkenham (1987) suggested that they may be more the norm than the exception.

There is a reticence to use the term 'hormone' for peptides released into the brain, as hormones are often thought of as substances released into the blood. But the important feature of hormones is not the route by which they travel, but that they are messengers between one group of cells and another, distant group. Communication over a distance implies coordination among the cells of origin, so the message they generate is coherent, and it implies that the targets are specialized to receive that message. In suggesting that vasopressin's actions in the brain are analogous to peripheral endocrine signals, we are emphasising that the actions of vasopressin in the brain may depend more on the distribution of its receptors than on the specific sites of release.

Bibliography

Aarde S.M., Jentsch J.D. (2006). Haploinsufficiency of the arginine-vasopressin gene is associated with poor spatial working memory performance in rats. *Horm Behav* 49: 501–508

Armstrong W.E. (1995). Morphological and electrophysiological classification of hypothalamic supraoptic neurons. *Prog Neurobiol* 47: 291–339

Baumgartner T., Heinrichs M., Vonlanthen A., Fischbacher U., Fehr E. (2008). Oxytocin shapes the neural circuitry of trust and trust adaptation in humans. *Neuron* 58: 639–650

Beckwith B.E., Couk D.I., Till T.S. (1983). Vasopressin analog influences the performance of males on a reaction time task. *Peptides* 4: 707–709

Bester-Meredith J.K., Young L.J., Marler C.A. (1999). Species differences in paternal behavior and aggression in peromyscus and their associations with vasopressin immunoreactivity and receptors. *Horm Behav* 36: 25–38

Bielsky I.F., Hu S.B., Ren X., Terwilliger E.F., Young L.J. (2005). The V1a vasopressin receptor is necessary and sufficient for normal social recognition: a gene replacement study. *Neuron* 47: 503–513

Blanchard R.J., Griebel G., Farrokhi C., Markham C., Yang M., Blanchard D.C. (2005). AVP V1b selective antagonist SSR149415 blocks aggressive behaviors in hamsters. *Pharmacol Biochem Behav* 80: 189–194

Bohus B., de Wied D. (1998). The vasopressin deficient Brattleboro rats: a natural knockout model used in the search for CNS effects of vasopressin. *Prog Brain Res* 119: 555–573

Bosch O.J., Neumann I.D. (2008). Brain vasopressin is an important regulator of maternal behavior independent of dams' trait anxiety. *Proc Natl Acad Sci USA* 105: 17139–17144

Caldwell H.K., Albers H.E. (2004). Effect of photoperiod on vasopressin-induced aggression in Syrian hamsters. *Horm Behav* 46: 444–449

Coccaro E.F., Kavoussi R.J., Hauger R.L., Cooper T.B., Ferris C.F. (1998). Cerebrospinal fluid vasopressin levels: correlates with aggression and serotonin function in personality-disordered subjects. *Arch Gen Psychiatry* 55: 708–714

Coote J.H. (2005). A role for the paraventricular nucleus of the hypothalamus in the autonomic control of heart and kidney. *Exp Physiol* 90: 169–173

Dantzer R., Bluthé R.M. (1993). Vasopressin and behavior: from memory to olfaction. *Regul Pept* 45: 121–125

Debiec J. (2005). Peptides of love and fear: vasopressin and oxytocin modulate the integration of information in the amygdala. *Bioessays* 27: 869–873

De Vries G.J., Best W., Sluiter A.A. (1983). The influence of androgens on the development of a sex difference in the vasopressinergic innervation of the rat lateral septum. *Brain Res* 284: 377–380

De Wied D. (1997). The neuropeptide story. Geoffrey Harris Lecture. *Front Neuroendocrinol* 18: 101–113.

Donaldson Z.R., Young L.J. (2008). Oxytocin, vasopressin, and the neurogenetics of sociality. *Science* 322: 900–904

Egashira N., Tanoue A., Higashihara F., Mishima K., Fukue Y., Takano Y., Tsujimoto G., Iwasaki K., Fujiwara M. (2004). V1a receptor knockout mice exhibit impairment of spatial memory in an eight-arm radial maze. *Neurosci Lett* 356: 195–198

Engelmann M. (2008). Vasopressin in the septum: not important versus causally involved in learning and memory — two faces of the same coin? *Prog Brain Res* 170: 389–395

Ferguson J.N., Young L.J., Insel T.R. (2002). The neuroendocrine basis of social recognition. *Front Neuroendocrinol* 23: 200–224

Ferris C.F. (2005). Vasopressin/oxytocin and aggression. *Novartis Found Symp* 268: 190–198

Ferris C.F., Albers H.E., Wesolowski S.M., Goldman B.D., Luman S.E. (1984). Vasopressin injected into the hypothalamus triggers a stereotypic behavior in golden hamsters. *Science* 224: 521–523

Ferris C.F., Axelson J.F., Martin A.M., Roberge L.F. (1989). Vasopressin immunoreactivity in the anterior hypothalamus is altered during the establishment of dominant/subordinate relationships between hamsters. *Neuroscience* 29: 675–83

Ferris C.F., Delville Y., Grzonka Z., Luber-Narod J., Insel T.R. (1993). An iodinated vasopressin (V1) antagonist blocks flank marking and selectively labels neural binding sites in golden hamsters. *Physiol Behav* 54: 737–747

Ferris C.F., Lu S.F., Messenger T., Guillon C.D., Heindel N., Miller M., Koppel G., Robert Bruns F., Simon N.G. (2006). Orally active vasopressin V1a receptor antagonist, SRX251, selectively blocks aggressive behavior. *Pharmacol Biochem Behav* 83: 169–174

Frazier C.R., Trainor B.C., Cravens C.J., Whitney T.K., Marler C.A. (2006). Paternal behavior influences development of aggression and vasopressin expression in male California mouse offspring. *Horm Behav* 50: 699–707

Fuxe K., Jonsson G. (1973). The histochemical fluorescence method for the demonstration of catecholamines. Theory, practice and application. *J Histochem Cytochem* 21: 293–311

Fuxe K., Dahlström A., Höistad M., Marcellino D., Jansson A., Rivera A., Diaz-Cabiale Z., Jacobsen K., Tinner-Staines B., Hagman B., Leo G., Staines W., Guidolin D.,

Kehr J., Genedani S., Belluardo N., Agnati L.F. (2007). From the Golgi-Cajal mapping to the transmitter-based characterization of the neuronal networks leading to two modes of brain communication: wiring and volume transmission. *Brain Res Rev* 55: 17–54

Gais S., Sommer M., Fischer S., Perras B., Born J. (2002). Post-trial administration of vasopressin in humans does not enhance memory formation (vasopressin and memory consolidation). *Peptides* 23: 581–583

Griebel G., Stemmelin J., Gal C.S., Soubrié P. (2005). Non-peptide vasopressin V1b receptor antagonists as potential drugs for the treatment of stress-related disorders. *Curr Pharm Des* 11: 1549–1559

Gülpinar M.A., Yegen B.C. (2004). The physiology of learning and memory: role of peptides and stress. *Curr Protein Pept Sci* 5: 457–473

Hammock E.A., Young L.J. (2005). Microsatellite instability generates diversity in brain and sociobehavioral traits. *Science* 308: 1630–1634

Herkenham M. (1987). Mismatches between neurotransmitter and receptor localizations in brain: observations and implications. *Neuroscience* 23: 1–38

Insel T.R., Young L.J. (2001). The neurobiology of attachment. *Nat Rev Neurosci* 2: 129–136

Kalamatianos T., Kalló I., Coen C.W. (2004). Ageing and the diurnal expression of the mRNAs for vasopressin and for the V1a and V1b vasopressin receptors in the suprachiasmatic nucleus of male rats. *J Neuroendocrinol* 16: 493–501

Kovács G.L., Veldhuis H.D., Versteeg D.H., De Wied D. (1986). Facilitation of avoidance behavior by vasopressin fragments microinjected into limbic-midbrain structures. *Brain Res* 371: 17–24

Kozorovitskiy Y., Hughes M., Lee K., Gould E. (2006). Fatherhood affects dendritic spines and vasopressin V1a receptors in the primate prefrontal cortex. *Nat Neurosci* 9: 1094–1095

Landgraf R. (2006). The involvement of the vasopressin system in stress-related disorders. *CNS Neurol Disord Drug Targets* 5: 167–179

Landgraf R., Gerstberger R., Montkowski A., Probst J.C., Wotjak C.T., Holsboer F., Engelmann M. (1995). V1 vasopressin receptor antisense oligodeoxynucleotide into septum reduces vasopressin binding, social discrimination abilities, and anxiety-related behavior in rats. *J Neurosci* 15: 4250–4258

Landgraf R., Frank E., Aldag J.M., Neumann I.D., Sharer C.A., Ren X., Terwilliger E.F., Niwa M., Wigger A., Young L.J. (2003). Viral vector-mediated gene transfer of the vole V1a vasopressin receptor in the rat septum: improved social discrimination and active social behaviour. *Eur J Neurosci* 18: 403–411

Lashley K.S. (1938). Experimental analysis of instinctive behavior, *Psychol Rev* 45: 445–471

Leng G., Brown C.H., Russell J.A. (1998). Physiological pathways regulating the activity of magnocellular neurosecretory cells. *Prog Neurobiol* 56: 1–31

Leng G., Ludwig M. (2006). Information processing in the hypothalamus: peptides and analogue computation. *J Neuroendocrinol* 18: 379–392

Ludwig M., Leng G. (2006). Dendritic peptide release and peptide-dependent behaviours. *Nat Rev Neurosci* 7: 126–136

Ludwig M., Sabatier N., Bull P.M., Landgraf R., Dayanithi G., Leng G. (2002). Intracellular calcium stores regulate activity-dependent neuropeptide release from dendrites. *Nature* 418: 85–89

Ludwig M., Bull P.M., Tobin V.A., Sabatier N., Landgraf R., Dayanithi G., Leng G. (2005). Regulation of activity-dependent dendritic vasopressin release from rat supraoptic neurones. *J Physiol* 564: 515–522

Ma X.M., Lightman S.L., Aguilera G. (1999). Vasopressin and corticotropin-releasing hormone gene responses to novel stress in rats adapted to repeated restraint. *Endocrinology* 140: 3623–3632

Neumann I.D. (2008). Brain oxytocin: a key regulator of emotional and social behaviours in both females and males. *J Neuroendocrinol* 20: 858–65

Packard M.G., Ettenberg A. (1985). Effects of peripherally injected vasopressin and des-glycinamide vasopressin on the extinction of a spatial learning task in rats. *Regul Pept* 11: 51–63

Pietrowsky R., Fehm-Wolfsdorf G., Born J., Fehm H.L. (1988). Effects of DGAVP on verbal memory. *Peptides* 9: 1361–1366

Rothwell N.J. (1994). CNS regulation of thermogenesis. *Crit Rev Neurobiol* 8: 1–10

Sabatier N., Shibuya I., Dayanithi G. (2004). Intracellular calcium increase and somatodendritic vasopressin release by vasopressin receptor agonists in the rat supraoptic nucleus: involvement of multiple intracellular transduction signals. *J Neuroendocrinol* 16: 221–236

Silver R., LeSauter J., Tresco P.A., Lehman M.N. (1996). A diffusible coupling signal from the transplanted suprachiasmatic nucleus controlling circadian locomotor rhythms. *Nature* 382: 810–813

Sladek C.D., Somponpun S.J. (2004). Oestrogen receptor beta: role in neurohypophyseal neurones. *J Neuroendocrinol* 16: 365–371

Stribley J.M., Carter C.S. (1999). Developmental exposure to vasopressin increases aggression in adult prairie voles. *Proc Natl Acad Sci USA* 96: 12601–1264

Tobin V.A., Hurst G., Norrie L., Dal Rio F.P., Bull P.M., Ludwig M. (2004). Thapsigargin-induced mobilization of dendritic dense-cored vesicles in rat supraoptic neurons. *Eur J Neurosci* 19: 2909–2912

Van der Zee E.A., Jansen K., Gerkema M.P. (1999). Severe loss of vasopressin-immunoreactive cells in the suprachiasmatic nucleus of aging voles coincides with reduced circadian organization of running wheel activity. *Brain Res* 816: 572–579

Vawter M.P., De Wied D., Van Ree J.M. (1997). Vasopressin fragment, AVP-(4-8), improves long-term and short-term memory in the whole board search task. *Neuropeptides* 31: 489–494

Veenema A.H., Blume A., Niederle D., Buwalda B., Neumann I.D. (2006). Effects of early life stress on adult male aggression and hypothalamic vasopressin and serotonin. *Eur J Neurosci* 24: 1711–1720

Walum H., Westberg L., Henningsson S., Neiderhiser J.M., Reiss D., Igl W., Ganiban J.M., Spotts E.L., Pedersen N.L. Eriksson E., Lichtenstein P. (2008). Genetic variation in the vasopressin receptor 1a gene (AVPR1A) associates with pair-bonding behavior in humans. *Proc Natl Acad Sci USA* 105: 14153–14156

Wersinger S.R., Kelliher K.R., Zufall F., Lolait S.J., O'Carroll A.M., Young W.S. 3rd. (2004). Social motivation is reduced in vasopressin 1b receptor null mice despite normal performance in an olfactory discrimination task. *Horm Behav* 46: 638–645

Wersinger S.R., Caldwell H.K., Martinez L., Gold P., Hu S.B., Young W.S. 3rd. (2007). Vasopressin 1a receptor knockout mice have a subtle olfactory deficit but normal aggression. *Genes Brain Behav* 6: 540–551

Wersinger S.R., Temple J.L., Caldwell H.K., Young W.S. 3rd. (2008). Inactivation of the oxytocin and the vasopressin (Avp) 1b receptor genes, but not the Avp 1a receptor gene, differentially impairs the Bruce effect in laboratory mice (*Mus musculus*). *Endocrinology* 149: 116–121

Young L.J., Wang Z., Cooper T.T., Albers H.E. (2000). Vasopressin (V1a) receptor binding, mRNA expression and transcriptional regulation by androgen in the Syrian hamster brain. *J Neuroendocrinol* 12: 1179–1185

CHAPTER 11

VASOPRESSIN SECRETION: MECHANISMS OF CONTROL OF SECRETION FROM THE POSTERIOR PITUITARY GLAND

Gareth Leng

Centre for Integrative Physiology
College of Medicine and Veterinary Medicine, University of Edinburgh
George Square, Edinburgh EH8 9XD
Email: gareth.leng@ed.ac.uk

1. Introduction

The hormones of the anterior pituitary gland are peptides made by the endocrine cells, packaged in large stores of secretory vesicles awaiting a signal to be secreted. That signal is likely to be a blood-borne releasing factor (usually another peptide), which generally acts by stimulating the release of calcium from intracellular stores which in turn triggers the calcium-dependent exocytosis of some of the vesicles' contents. The two hormones of the posterior pituitary gland, vasopressin and its close relative oxytocin, are also peptides made, not by pituitary cells, but by magnocellular neuroendocrine neurones of the hypothalamus. In the cell bodies of these neurones, vasopressin and oxytocin are packaged into large membrane-bound neurosecretory vesicles, much like the vesicles that contain anterior pituitary hormones. These large dense-core vesicles (LDCVs, see later) are then transported along the axons of these neurones to be stored in axonal swellings and nerve endings, awaiting signals to trigger their release into the blood. Like the hormones of the anterior pituitary gland, secretion of these vesicles is by calcium-dependent exocytosis, but for the magnocellular neurones, the calcium trigger comes as calcium entry into the nerve terminals through channels that open in response to action potentials, the electrical signals that pass down the axons from the hypothalamus (Seward *et al.*, 1995).

2. Synthesis and Storage of Vasopressin

The posterior pituitary gland contains a very large store of vasopressin. Normal basal levels of vasopressin could be maintained for approximately one month, but if the demand is high, the store is rapidly depleted. After two or three days without water, the pituitary content will be only about 10% of its usual level. The vasopressin that is secreted is replaced by newly made vasopressin, but this replenishment takes time. In a steady state, newly made LDCVs arrive at the terminals at a rate that closely matches the rate of secretion or degradation of old vesicles, and so the pituitary content stays roughly constant. However, when the rate of vasopressin secretion increases, although there is a correspondingly increase in the rate of synthesis, there is an inevitable delay between activating synthesis and replenishing the stores.

We do not know exactly what causes vasopressin synthesis to increase in response to dehydration, but it seems likely that the increase in synthesis is a response to the same cellular stimuli that result in an increase in secretion. The signal to increase synthesis results first in increased mRNA expression, and only later in increased protein production after a delay of about two hours. Then, the newly made protein must be packaged and shipped down to the pituitary gland, a journey of several hours more, by which time the pituitary stores will already have fallen. This deficit will only be made up after the demand for extra secretion has subsided, when the same lag in signalling means that augmented supplies of vasopressin will still be transported to the pituitary gland for several hours after the rate of synthesis has been turned down to normal again.

Because of this delay in making extra vasopressin to meet an upsurge in demand, it is only prudent to maintain a substantial reserve of vasopressin at the pituitary gland. However, to sustain this reserve, it is important that only a small part of these stores is available for release at any given time, i.e. a store that is not too easily squandered. Exactly how secretion is rationed is not fully understood. It is not the case that there are only a limited number of sites at which vasopressin can be secreted; rather, it seems that LDCVs can be exocytosed from any part of the vasopressin cell membrane, from the nerve endings and from the many very large axonal swellings that contain most of the vesicles in the pituitary gland, but also even from the undilated sections of the axons and from the soma and dendrites in the hypothalamus, as we shall see later. For magnocellular vasopressin and oxytocin neurones, there are many more LDCVs in the axon swellings than in nerve endings, but in the nerve endings, more of the LDCVs are close to the plasma membrane, and this seems to be what is important for determining release probability. The number of exocytotic events seems to be proportional to the number of LDCVs close to the plasma membrane, and this is equally true for all parts of the cell: nerve terminals, axon swellings, undilated axons, soma and dendrites. The axon swellings contain many more LDCVs that the axon terminals, but more vasopressin is secreted from the nerve endings because they are smaller, and so more of the LDCVs are close to the cell membrane than in a swelling. Perhaps the very largest of the swellings close to the nerve terminals (Herring bodies) contain LDCVs that cannot be released. They can contain up to 15% of the total vesicle content of the pituitary gland and here the vesicles appear to be in the process of enzymatic degradation (Kruslovic *et al.*, 2005). However, during prolonged stimulation, the nerve terminals become progressively depleted and secretion from the swellings assumes increasingly greater importance.

To maintain stable, physiologically effective concentrations of vasopressin in the systemic circulation, despite relatively rapid degradation, the vasopressin system maintains a rate of synthesis and secretion that is massive by the standards of most neurones. Yet, for any one vasopressin neurone, even during a period of very high demand, secretion from its terminal fields seems to be a very disorderly process. At any one terminal the average secretion rate must be very low, and apparently governed by random, stochastic processes. We can reconstruct what might be happening as follows. Phasic bursts of action potentials are generated in the cell bodies in the hypothalamus, and are propagated down the axons to the nerve terminals in the neural lobe. When a burst of spikes arrives at a nerve terminal, the terminal is depolarised and voltage-gated calcium channels open. The entry of calcium through these channels triggers the exocytosis of vasopressin-containing vesicles. It seems that these calcium channels occur in clusters, and so a vesicle that is close to a channel cluster will see a larger calcium signal than a vesicle that is further away. We do not really know however what controls the movement of vesicles inside the axon. Is there a 'conveyer belt' system ferrying vesicles from deep stores to the membrane, perhaps at a rate related to the calcium signal, or are the vesicles bumping about randomly, with the statistics of random processes doing the job of rationing supply according to the reserve level in a perfectly adequate way? For the moment, we need note only that at any one terminal, a burst of spikes that lasts 10 or 20 seconds probably releases at most just one vesicle of vasopressin. That is enough vasopressin, given the large number of nerve terminals from each of several thousand neurones, to raise the physiological concentration of vasopressin in the systemic circulation to the level required to activate the high affinity receptors in the kidney to evoke a strong antidiuresis. This is a message we must remember for later, when we consider the central release of vasopressin.

3. The Magnocellular Vasopressin Neurones

There are about 9,000 magnocellular vasopressin neurones in the rat brain, all of which send an axon, their one and only axon, to the posterior pituitary gland. There, each axon gives rise to about 2,000 nerve endings and swellings, each of which is filled with neurosecretory vesicles: membrane-bound packets of vasopressin ready to be released into the systemic circulation (Morris, 1976a, 1976b; Nordmann, 1977). The posterior pituitary gland, sometimes called the neural lobe or neurohypophysis, lacks a blood-brain barrier. The blood vessels have fenestrations that allow vasopressin secreted from these nerve endings to enter the bloodstream without impediment.

Magnocellular neurones make their secretory products, package them in vesicles, transport them to their release sites, and regulate their release in many respects like any other neurone regulates the release of a conventional transmitter. The nerve endings in the pituitary have thus often been likened to synaptic endings of any neurone, perhaps misleadingly because there are important differences. The neurosecretory vesicles that contain vasopressin are larger than the small synaptic vesicles that neurones use to package conventional neurotransmitters (about 200 nm in diameter compared to the 40–50 nm of typical small synaptic vesicles). When seen under an electron microscope, neurosecretory vesicles have an opaque electron-dense core so they are often described as large dense-core vesicles (LDCVs). The core consists of tightly folded aggregations of the prohormone product of the vasopressin gene, including vasopressin and its associated neurophysin. As discussed later, each vesicle contains up to 85,000 molecules of the peptide hormone (Nordmann and Morris, 1984), a much larger 'payload' than is carried by the conventional small synaptic vesicles which usually contain about 5,000 molecules of neurotransmitter. Probably more importantly, the molecular machinery that guides exocytosis of these LDCVs is not the same as for the release of conventional synaptic vesicles.

More helpfully, there is the non-trivial difference of scale. Most neurones make just enough of their secretory products to survive passing across the tiny synaptic clefts that separate one neurone's nerve endings from another neurone's dendrite. Magnocellular vasopressin cells must make enough vasopressin to reach the kidneys from the pituitary gland, and this is one of the things that makes these cells a wonderful 'model system' in neuroscience. They make so much peptide that it is relatively easy to study the molecular biology, the biochemistry and the cell biology that is involved in peptide production, packaging and secretion. Another powerful reason is that the output of these neurones can be measured relatively easily — for example by radioimmunoassay of blood samples — and this output can be related both to *function*, the clearly adaptive physiological functions of vasopressin being antidiuresis and vasoconstriction, and to *mechanisms*, the electrical and biochemical activities of the vasopressin neurones.

Furthermore, many of these neurosecretory neurones are aggregated into relatively discrete hypothalamic nuclei. The rat brain contains about 9,000 of these neurones, of which about 30% are in the supraoptic nucleus and about 20% of which are in the paraventricular nucleus. The remainder are scattered quite widely throughout the anterior hypothalamus, with a few smaller aggregations — the so-called accessory magnocellular nuclei — the largest of which is the nucleus circularis which lie midway between the supraoptic and paraventricular nuclei. The paraventricular nucleus is a complex mosaic of many different neuronal types. As well as the magnocellular neuroendocrine neurones that project to the posterior pituitary gland, some of which make vasopressin and some oxytocin, there are smaller parvocellular neuroendocrine neurones that project to the primary capillaries of the hypothalamo-adenohypophysial portal system in the median eminence. Their release into this portal system is associated with their control of hormone secretion from the anterior pituitary gland. Some of these neurones synthesise vasopressin, and vasopressin secreted at the median eminence reaches the anterior pituitary corticotroph cells in high enough concentrations to influence corticotrophin (also known as adrenocorticotrophic hormone, ACTH) secretion. Other parvocellular neurones synthesise corticotrophin releasing hormone (CRH), which also regulates ACTH secretion, while yet others synthesise both vasopressin and CRH. Vasopressin and CRH are synergistic co-factors that regulate ACTH secretion. Other parvocellular neurons make thyrotrophin releasing hormone, which regulates secretion of thyrotrophin (thyroid stimulating hormone) from the thyrotrophes of the anterior pituitary. Many other neurones in the paraventricular nucleus, including other populations that make vasopressin, oxytocin and CRH, are not neuroendocrine neurones, but project centrally to many different parts of the brain.

In the rat, the supraoptic nucleus contains just two types of neurones, and about 70% of these produce vasopressin, the remainder producing oxytocin. For the experimental neuroscientist, the supraoptic nucleus is located very conveniently on the ventral surface of the brain, abutting the optic chiasma, so it is possible to dissect it relatively easily and cleanly for biochemical studies. Indeed, it is equally easy to keep the cells alive in slices or chunks of hypothalamus, and study them *in vitro*. Importantly, the supraoptic nucleus contains essentially just the cell bodies and dendrites of magnocellular neurones, for the axons of the magnocellular neurones leave the nucleus without giving rise to any collateral branches within its boundaries. At least, these are the only neurones in the nucleus, although there are other cell types present. The supraoptic nucleus also contains a large population of glial cells, these being specialised astrocytes with long processes which enshroud all the magnocellular neurones (Armstrong, 1995). These glial cells are important for many reasons. To some extent they can act as insulating sheaves, limiting (controlling) cross-talk between neurones. They also, like glial cells throughout the brain, regulate the environment of the magnocellular neurones, by mopping up excess neurotransmitter resulting from spillover of synaptic release for instance, and buffering the changes in extracellular electrolyte concentrations that accompany electrical activity (Oliet and Piet, 2004). These cells are dynamic components of the supraoptic nucleus: their morphology changes in different physiological circumstances, and they can release products (in particular taurine) that can directly affect neuronal excitability. The significance of these changes remains controversial in that it is not clear to what extent they are adaptations to changing metabolic demands, and to what extent they might actively promote adaptations in neuronal behaviour.

Finally, the supraoptic and paraventricular nuclei are amongst the most densely vascularised parts of the brain. Since the cells are so metabolically active, it is possible that this dense vascularity simply reflects their high demand for metabolic sustenance. Although these nuclei are within the blood-brain barrier and the blood vessels are unfenestrated, it is also possible that some blood-borne factors may have privileged access to the magnocellular neurones through specific transport mechanisms.

4. Regulation of Vasopressin Secretion

When we think of vasopressin cells, we tend to think first of their response to changes in osmotic pressure mediated by osmoreceptors, as this is a consequence of dehydration, and the antidiuretic actions of vasopressin at the kidney have obvious adaptive benefits in these circumstances. There are several physiological circumstances in which vasopressin secretion is adaptive, and these are associated with different afferent neural pathways.

Dehydration, as caused by the unavailability of drinking water, is a complex stimulus as it threatens both electrolyte and plasma volume homeostasis. A fall in plasma volume also activates vasopressin cells, following stimulation of low pressure atrial receptors (volume receptors) that relay in the brainstem. Vasopressin helps to defend plasma volume by limiting fluid loss in the urine, and also helps to maintain blood pressure by its vasopressor actions on peripheral vascular beds. Low peripheral blood pressure detected by baroreceptors in the carotid sinus and aortic arch also sends signals to the brain as well as via activation of the renal renin-angiotensin system. Circulating angiotensin II, released in response to the fall in arterial blood pressure, exerts central effects via the subfornical organ (SFO), a specialised sensory site in the forebrain just anterior and dorsal to the hypothalamus. It acts here to stimulate thirst (the thirst that is needed to stimulate drinking in order to replenish plasma volume), and also to stimulate vasopressin secretion by a direct projection from the subfornical organ to the magnocellular vasopressin neurones. Interestingly, this projection from the subfornical organ also uses angiotensin II as one of its messenger molecules.

There are many different circumstances in which plasma volume falls or electrolyte imbalance is threatened. Evaporative water loss in hot weather can cause the unusual combination of a loss of body water that is exceeded by the loss of sodium, because of the salt lost in sweating. This presents a difficult homeostatic challenge, because any increase in water intake alone would exacerbate the hyponatraemia. However, vasopressin secretion is absolutely indicated, because the threat to homeostasis presented by a fall in plasma volume is the more acute one. In these circumstances, many animals also develop a marked craving for salt — a specific 'sodium appetite' in conjunction with the increased vasopressin secretion. Another condition associated with acute fluid loss is in response to the ingestion of a perceived toxin which induces diarrhoea and/or vomiting. Not all animals vomit, but some do, including of course humans, and powerful nauseogenic stimuli trigger massive vasopressin secretion in man, possibly to counter the fluid loss during vomiting. Finally, vasopressin secretion in a conscious animal is regulated not only in response to actual perturbations of electrolyte and volume balance, but also in anticipation of such changes. Thus vasopressin secretion falls when water is drunk, and increases during the intake of food (and salt), *before* these have had time to be absorbed. These stimuli reach the magnocellular neurones by a variety of routes (see Leng *et al.*, 1998). Visceral information arrives via projections from the brainstem, notably by a noradrenergic projection from the A1cell group of the ventrolateral medulla which probably carries cardiovascular-related information and possibly also mediates vagal information.

From the forebrain, there are substantial projections to the vasopressin neurones from the SFO as already mentioned, and from the organum vasculosum of the lamina terminalis (OVLT). These two structures, believed to contain the osmoreceptors, are unusual in that they are very densely vascularised regions of the brain, lacking an effective blood-brain barrier, and thus are sites where neurones can respond to blood-borne factors that do not enter the brain. These regions contain cells that respond to angiotensin II as mentioned earlier, but also to other peptide hormones of peripheral origin, including relaxin, atrial natriuretic peptide, endothelin, leptin and many others. The SFO and the OVLT project directly to the magnocellular neurones but also project indirectly, via a midline structure known as the nucleus medianus. These three interconnected regions are collectively known as the region anterior and ventral to the third ventricle (AV3V). This region is critical for the regulation not only of vasopressin secretion but also for the regulation of thirst and natriuresis, and lesions in this area result in a syndrome of chronic hypernatraemia associated with a relative absence of thirst. These anterior projections to the vasopressin neurones are functionally mixed however, and they include inhibitory effects mediated by gamma-aminobutyric acid (GABA), excitatory effects mediated by glutamate as well as complex peptide-mediated effects.

Some of the input arising from the SFO and OVLT are activated by changes in systemic osmotic pressure. Some of the afferent neurones are directly osmosensitive (the osmoreceptors), as are the magnocellular neurones themselves. Thus the interacting osmoresponsive regions are sometimes called the "osmoreceptor complex" of the forebrain (Leng *et al.*, 1982; Bourque *et al.*, 2002, 2007).

Whether the magnocellular vasopressinergic cells are activated by direct or indirect influences upon them, for instance by afferent input from other brain regions, the actual determinant of vasopressin secretion from the neural lobe is the electrical activity of the vasopressin neurones. Action potentials (spikes) are generated in the cell bodies in the hypothalamus in response to stimuli detected directly by the vasopressin cells and to afferent stimuli from other brain regions, and these action potentials are propagated down the axons. For example, with prolonged dehydration, magnocellular vasopressin cells are progressively depolarised. This is partly because of their intrinsic osmosensitivity: they express a specialised stretch-sensitive type of membrane ion channel. When a rise in the extracellular osmotic pressure causes a vasopressin cell to shrink because of the osmotic withdrawal of intracellular water, these channels open, depolarising the vasopressin cell. This depolarisation is linearly proportional to the osmotic pressure change. In addition, there are similar specialised osmoreceptor cells in those areas of the brain that project to the vasopressin cells, notably in the SFO and the OVLT. Thus, with progressive dehydration, vasopressin cells are directly depolarised and also receive a large increase in synaptic input — in fact a large increase in both excitatory and inhibitory postsynaptic potentials, as both GABA and glutamate are released in the supraoptic nucleus in response to a rise in osmotic pressure. Consequently, vasopressin cells increase their discharge rate from a basal level of about one action potential (spike)/second on average to a maximum sustained rate of about ten spikes/second, and this increase is approximately linear with the increase in plasma osmotic pressure.

The vasopressin neurones are not spontaneously active; in the absence of any synaptic input, their resting potential lies about 10 mV below the threshold for initiation of sodium spikes. The direct depolarising effect of increases in osmotic pressure is not large, and at the extreme end of the physiological range only amounts to a few millivolts — not enough to reach spike threshold, and so if the neurones are completely deafferented, vasopressin secretion stops. However, even in normonatraemic conditions when there is little vasopressin secretion, the neurones are continually bombarded by a huge amount of synaptic input. There seems to be an almost equal input of inhibitory and excitatory postsynaptic potentials — ipsps and epsps — mostly mediated by GABA and glutamate, respectively, although the cells also receive a noradrenergic input, especially from the A1 cell group of the ventrolateral medulla, and are influenced by many different peptidergic signals. The input, being balanced, has little overall effect on the mean resting potential of vasopressin cells, but it means that the membrane potential is rapidly and continually being perturbed. Spikes arise when a depolarising perturbation is large enough to reach the spike threshold, so the significance of the directly induced osmotic depolarisation is that it makes this more likely to happen.

5. Stimulus-Secretion Coupling in the Neural Lobe

Each magnocellular vasopressin neurone has just one axon, which runs directly from the hypothalamus into the posterior pituitary gland. As mentioned earlier, in the pituitary gland that axon gives rise to many large swellings and neurosecretory endings that are full of neurosecretory LDCVs containing vasopressin. These LDCVs are much bigger that the small synaptic vesicles that contain conventional neurotransmitters, and very like the vesicles contained in cells of the anterior pituitary gland that contain other peptide hormones.

Bandaranaake (1971) estimated that, in the rat, about 18,000 nerve cells project to the neural lobe; about half of these are vasopressin neurones and half are oxytocin neurones. Nordmann (1977) used ultrastructural morphometry studies to estimate that each of these neurones gives rise to 436 swellings and 1,840 nerve endings in the neural lobe. He also estimated that each swelling contains 2,240 LDCVs, and each ending 258 LDCVs, on average; each axon also contains some LDCVs in its undilated parts — about 12% of all vesicles are in these. Thus each neurone has about 1.5 million LDCVs in its whole axonal arborisation in the neural lobe, giving approximately 2.6×10^{10} LDCVs for the whole gland. In the rat, the neural lobe contains about 1 μg of vasopressin and a similar amount of oxytocin; exactly how much depends on the age and physiological status of the rat. From this, it can be calculated that each LDCV contains about 40,000 molecules of vasopressin (vasopressin has a molecular weight of about 1,000). In an independent study, Morris (1976b) calculated a lower figure for the total number of LDCVs: he concluded that the rat neural lobe contains 1.44×10^{10} LDCVs in total, giving an estimated 0.72×10^{10} that contain vasopressin; he calculated that each contains about 85,000 molecules of peptide.

Magnocellular neurones synthesise vasopressin on an almost industrial scale — enough to maintain sufficiently high concentrations in the systemic circulation to ensure an appropriate level of antidiuresis. In a normal hydrated conscious rat, the physiological concentration of vasopressin in the circulation is typically about 1 pg/ml. The plasma volume for such a rat is approximately 20 ml but the total distribution volume is larger than this since vasopressin is not confined to the plasma compartment. As the total extracellular volume would be about 50 ml in a 300 g rat, the peripheral content of vasopressin is about 50 pg. The fast phase of vasopressin clearance from the rat circulation is related to its half-life of approximately 2–5 minutes, so to maintain this concentration requires a secretion rate of approximately 0.3 pg/s, i.e. 28 ng/24 hours. This is equivalent to secretion of about 2,300 LDCV/s, so under basal conditions one vesicle is secreted from each vasopressin cell about every 3 seconds, and 2–3 vesicles/s at times of higher demand when plasma levels reach the upper end of the physiological range at about 10–12 pg/ml (Leng and Ludwig, 2008).

However, under many experimental (and physiological) circumstances, plasma vasopressin concentrations are much higher than this. The most commonly used anaesthetic for the study of vasopressin secretion in the rat is urethane (ethyl carbamate), which is used because it gives a very stable, deep anaesthesia without the loss of normal physiological neuroendocrine reflexes. However, urethane itself is a strong osmotic stimulus, and this together with the trauma of acute surgery means that the basal plasma vasopressin concentration in a urethane-anaesthetised rat is typically 50–100 pg/ml.

In these circumstances the mean basal discharge rate of vasopressin cells is about 3–4 spikes/s, as estimated independently by many workers in various conditions (Bicknell *et al.*, 1984). If the plasma vasopressin concentration is 85 pg/ml say, then this means that there is 4,250 pg of vasopressin in the peripheral extracellular volume. Given the half-life of vasopressin, about 20 pg/s must be secreted from the neural lobe to maintain this concentration. This is about 15 LDCV/s for every vasopressin neurone, giving a calculated secretion rate of 4 LDCV/neurone/spike. Of course, more vasopressin is released at higher cell firing rates. Leng *et al.* (1994) stimulated the neural lobes of anaesthetised rats at an average frequency of 10 Hz for 90 minutes, achieving a plasma vasopressin concentration of 220 pg/ml after 15 minutes; this requires a secretion rate of say 28.3 pg/s, achieved by secretion of 49 LDCVs/s from each neurone — this, over 90 minutes, would result in the secretion of 2.3×10^9 LDCVs in all, about 250,000 from each neurone. In these conditions, we can calculate that about 488 spikes are required on average to release one LDCV from a nerve ending — very close to the estimate of the number required under basal conditions of urethane anaesthesia.

Thus to achieve a relatively high sustainable rate of secretion each vasopressin neuron must secrete, on average, less than one LDCV per minute from each of its nerve terminals. In fact, this is an overestimate, as many vesicles are released not from nerve terminals but from axonal swellings. To release each LDCV requires, on average, about 500 action potentials to invade a terminal. At first, this seems to be an extraordinarily profligate arrangement, with a considerable amount of activity for such a small effect. However, we must consider what the vasopressin system must achieve in order to be effective.

6. Vasopressin as an Autoregulator of Vasopressin Cell Activity

There are three known vasopressin receptor subtypes, known as V1a, V1b and V2. The V2 subtype has so far not been shown to be expressed in the brain, but mRNA expression for both the V1a and V1b receptor has been reported at many different sites, including the supraoptic nucleus (Hurbin *et al.*, 1998) where both are specifically expressed by vasopressin neurones (and not by oxytocinergic neurones).

A complex cascade of second messenger interactions results from the binding of vasopressin to these receptors (Sabatier *et al.*, 2004b). There is an increase in intracellular calcium ion concentration, partly as a consequence of calcium mobilisation from thapsigargin-sensitive stores in the endoplasmic reticulum, and partly as a result of calcium ion entry through voltage-gated membrane channels, and this can trigger extensive release of vasopressin from the dendrites of the magnocellular neurones. When active vasopressin cells are exposed to vasopressin they are inhibited (Ludwig and Leng, 1997), but inactive cells are excited (Gouzenes *et al.*, 1998). The mechanisms underlying these dual effects are unclear. Any increase in intracellular calcium ion concentration will have consequences for calcium-activated K^+ channels, and this will tend to hyperpolarise vasopressin cells and inhibit their electrical activity. Thus one possibility is that when vasopressin cells are active, the depolarising effect of potentiating voltage-sensitive Ca^{2+} channels is minimal, but the enhancement of the intracellular Ca^{2+} concentration will lead to hyperpolarisation through Ca^{2+}-activated K^+ conductance. In other words, the dual action may arise through non-linearities in the relationships between membrane potential and Ca^{2+} entry, and between the intracellular Ca^{2+} concentration and K^+ conductance.

Thus the mechanisms of action of vasopressin on vasopressin cells are many and messy, but the net result of vasopressin release in the supraoptic nucleus will be that the most active cells become less active and the least active cells become more active, with the population of cells tending to become more homogeneous. Whatever the cellular mechanisms, the effects of vasopressin on vasopressin cells appear to represent *population signalling*, not intrinsic autoregulation. The dendrites of vasopressin cells lie close to each other, and measurements of vasopressin in dialysates of the supraoptic nucleus imply very high local concentrations, so we may assume that vasopressin released from one dendrite is not only a signal that feeds back on the cell of origin but also affects at least those cells with adjacent dendrites. Active vasopressin cells will tend to activate neighbours that are quiescent and inhibit neighbours that are active. Thus when there is a physiological demand for a high level of vasopressin secretion, this ensures that the "load" is shared fairly throughout the vasopressin cell population.

7. Phasic Firing

The above description, although accurate, is a little misleading because vasopressin cells do not fire at a consistent steady rate but in a highly patterned manner, with bursts of action potentials separated by periods of silence. This phasic firing of vasopressin cells in the rat is now well described and relatively well understood. Typically, phasic firing consists of bursts that last for between 20 and 60 seconds, separated by silent periods of 20 to 30 seconds. Within each burst, the firing rate is usually between 4 and 10 spikes/s; this is relatively constant within a burst, and is consistent from one burst to the next in any one cell (Fig. 1). With slowly progressing dehydration, these bursts gradually become more frequent and more intense in each cell. When osmotic pressure rises more acutely, phasic cells tend to fire continuously at a progressively increasing frequency as the osmotic pressure is rising, settling down again into a phasic firing pattern only once the osmotic pressure is again stable (Fig. 2).

Phasic firing is the consequence of a sequence of activity-dependent changes in vasopressin cell excitability. When a flurry of excitatory post-synaptic potentials (EPSPs) depolarises the vasopressin cell enough to exceed the spike threshold, the membrane potential of the soma rapidly rises in a classical action potential. At first, voltage-dependent sodium channels open, depolarising the membrane, followed by voltage-sensitive rectifying potassium channels which repolarise it again. In addition, voltage-sensitive calcium channels open, resulting in a large

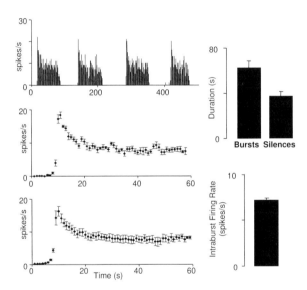

Figure 1. Vasopressin cells discharge spikes in a characteristic 'phasic' firing pattern. At the top left is an extract from a record of the firing rate of a single vasopressin neurone in the supraoptic nucleus of a urethane-anaesthetized rat. In this cell, spikes occur in bursts that last about 60 seconds separated by long silent periods. The firing rate is highest at the start of the bursts and settles into a 'plateau' level. The middle trace shows the mean (with standard error) of the firing rate of this cell within bursts, showing the average burst shape more clearly. Below this is the average burst profile of several vasopressin cells, showing how consistent this profile is. On the right, the bars show average burst and silence durations and average intraburst firing rates from a sample of vasopressin cells recorded in this way. Adapted from Sabatier *et al.* (2004).

calcium influx into the cell. This influx in turn opens another class of slowly inactivating calcium-dependent potassium channels which hyperpolarise the cell after the action potential for up to 40 ms causing what is known as a *hyperpolarising afterpotential*. However, other still slower depolarising channels open and so, after the post-spike hyperpolarisation, there is a late rebound depolarisation called a *depolarising afterpotential*. These late, slow depolarising events can summate to form what is called a 'plateau potential' that acts like a pedal to support further spike activity — a burst of spikes that often lasts for 40 seconds and sometimes for much longer (Fig. 3).

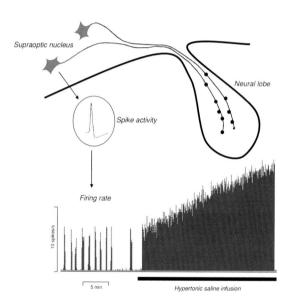

Figure 2. The magnocellular neurones that secrete vasopressin project from the hypothalamus to the pituitary neural lobe, and it is possible to record the electrical (spike) activity of these cells by placing a recording microelectrode into the supraoptic nucleus of a urethane-anaesthetized rat. Many of these cells fire phasically, and if the plasma osmotic pressure is raised progressively, as here by a slow i.v. infusion of hypertonic saline, the cells increase their spike activity. Typically, vasopressin cells fire continuously while the osmotic pressure is rising fast, and their firing rate increases linearly with the change in osmotic pressure. Adapted from Leng *et al.* (2001).

A burst thus reflects a plateau potential that is established as a regenerative response to spike activity, i.e. spike activity results in the opening of slowly inactivating depolarising membrane conductances. This plateau potential brings the resting potential of the vasopressin cell to within just a few millivolts of the spike threshold and sustains it there,

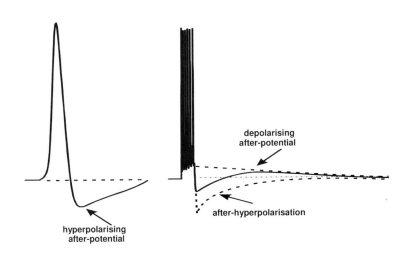

Figure 3. Some of the intrinsic mechanisms that are important in shaping the burst profiles. Every spike in a vasopressin cell is followed by a hyperpolarising after-potential; this causes the cell to be relatively refractory for 40 ms or so after a spike, so there will be no further spikes within this time. Because of this, the maximum instantaneous firing rates seen in these cells under physiological conditions are no more than about 25 spikes/s, and these are usually only seen at the start of bursts. When the effects of this have died away, there is a relative depolarisation because the spike has resulted in the opening of slowly inactivating depolarising conductances causing a long-lasting *depolarisation after-potential (DAP)*. The DAP makes the cell relatively excitable for another 100ms or more, and if it does fire again in this time, there will be a further DAP. These successive DAPs can summate to form a plateau potential which will sustain repetitive firing — the phasic burst.

so that spikes are triggered by EPSPs relatively often, and these spikes maintain the plateau potential. Eventually, the plateau mechanism is inactivated as a result of the prolonged spike activity. This is due in part to dynorphin, an opioid peptide released by the vasopressin cells, which acts back on the cell of origin to block the depolarising mechanism that sustains the plateau (Brown *et al.*, 1999). It is also partly because of yet another class of slowly inactivating calcium-activated potassium channels mediating a gradually accumulating hyperpolarisation called an *afterhyperpolarisation* which differs from the hyperpolarising afterpotential by its very slow prolonged time-course. Furthermore, it is in part because of other signals generated by the cell that act back upon the afferent nerve endings. For instance, vasopressin cells produce the gaseous transmitter nitric oxide in response to raised intracellular calcium, and this triggers GABA release from afferent nerve endings. Vasopressin cells also produce adenosine and endocannabinoids that suppress excitatory synaptic input. Collectively, these mechanisms ensure that bursts of spikes will come to an end and be followed by a period of relative inexcitability. Thus each vasopressin cell has complex intrinsic properties that ensure that it alternates between periods of activity and periods of silence (see Brown and Bourque, 2006).

Although individual vasopressin cells fire in intermittent bursts in response to dehydration, this does not mean that vasopressin secretion into the blood is intermittent. The vasopressin cells are not wholly independent of each other, but still their discharge activity is asynchronous, so the activity of the population as a whole increases relatively linearly and smoothly as osmotic pressure rises. Although the cells are asynchronous, they do communicate with each other via vasopressin itself, released in large amounts from the magnocellular dendrites.

8. Physiological Significance of Phasic Firing

If vasopressin cells do not fire phasically in order to produce a pulsatile pattern of vasopressin secretion, then it is natural to wonder why they fire phasically at all. This question was answered by studies of stimulus secretion coupling that took advantage of the anatomical fact that the neural lobe essentially contains just the axons and terminals of the neurosecretory neurones. The neural lobe of a rat or mouse, if kept in warm, oxygenated medium with an ionic composition similar to that of extracellular fluid, will retain for many hours the ability to secrete vasopressin in response to stimuli that depolarise the neurosecretory nerve endings, particularly in response to action potentials triggered in the axons by electrical stimuli. This simple *in vitro* preparation became an extremely important experimental model for understanding exactly how electrical activity propagated down the axons is coupled to secretion.

Some of the first experiments with this preparation addressed the question of why vasopressin neurones fire in their characteristic phasic pattern (see Leng and Brown, 1997). An answer soon appeared: they do so apparently because, for any one nerve terminal, this pattern is the most efficient stimulus for secreting vasopressin (Dutton and Dyball, 1979; Cazalis *et al.*, 1985). It seems that the secretion of vasopressin is facilitated, up to a point, by an increasing spike frequency, mainly because this produces a facilitation of calcium entry into the terminal that is a much more potent stimulus for exocytosis. However, this facilitation of secretion is not sustained; it is subject to a process called 'fatigue'. Exactly what underlies fatigue is unclear, and to some extent it probably merely reflects the temporary exhaustion of a readily releasable pool of LDCVs, but it might also reflect a hyperpolarisation of the terminal by activation of calcium-activated potassium channels. Whatever the explanation, the most efficient spike frequency for triggering vasopressin secretion is about 13 Hz — close to the maximum firing rate that vasopressin cells can sustain. A high rate of secretory efficiency cannot be maintained for more than a few tens of seconds; and a few tens of seconds of silence is needed for full recovery from fatigue.

As a consequence, the phasic discharge pattern of vasopressin cells appears to be about optimally efficient for secretion, in the sense of achieving a given secretion with the fewest action potentials (see Fig. 4).

Why it might be important that the vasopressin cells are efficient in this sense is less clear, as many other neurones in the brain are active at very much higher frequencies of spike activity than the vasopressin neurones are even capable of. One possibility, that must be substantially speculative, is that spike activity in vasopressin cells presents a real hazard. Their spikes have a very large calcium component, and this influx is important to regulate secretion from the soma and dendrites, as we shall see later, but probably also to regulate gene expression. However, excessive calcium entry is certainly potentially damaging to neurones in general. The demands on vasopressin neurones are also peculiarly unremitting. A lack of available drinking water will mean a progressively increasing demand for vasopressin secretion that may persist for days. Most neurones, when presented with a constant stimulus will adapt; this is not an option that is open to the vasopressin system. Accordingly, it seems possible that the vasopressin cells have evolved to be quite parsimonious in how they generate spikes in order to ensure that sustained intense activation is not unduly damaging.

If electrical hyperactivity indeed predisposes vasopressin cells to damage, we might consider the consequences of hyperactivation for a population of vasopressin cells whose responses to osmotic stimulation are very heterogeneous. The cells most sensitive to osmotic stimuli will be most strongly excited, and most likely to die. Their death would result in less vasopressin secretion, leading to raised osmotic pressure, and an enhanced excitatory drive to the surviving vasopressin cells, with risk of further damage to the most sensitive of the remainder, and so on. The vasopressin system would drift to a higher set point for osmoregulation, with progressively fewer cells surviving to share the demands of response to acute osmotic challenge. Interestingly, there may be pathological examples of exactly such a vicious circle in the vasopressin system.

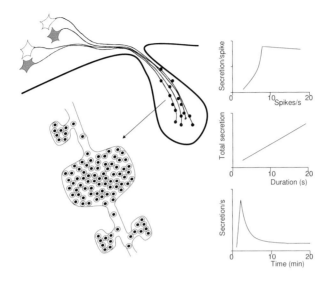

Figure 4. Phasic firing is efficient for releasing vasopressin from the neural lobe. The evidence for this has come mainly from experiments measuring secretion from the isolated neural lobe *in vitro*. The neural lobe contains no neuronal cell bodies, just the terminal regions of the magnocellular neurone axons. Each of these axons contains a very large number of nerve terminals and a smaller number of much larger axonal "swellings". Both of these compartments are densely filled with the large dense core vesicles that contain vasopressin, and vesicles can be released by both compartments. When the neural lobe is stimulated electrically *in vitro*, as Dutton and Dyball (1979) showed, the phasic pattern of stimulation was more effective than continuous stimulation, and this was partly because higher frequencies are disproportionately more effective at stimulating secretion than lower frequencies. Subsequently, Shaw *et al.* (1984) showed that the total secretion increases with the duration of stimulation up to about 20 seconds, and Bicknell *et al.* (1984) showed that when stimulation is continued beyond this, the efficiency of release declines again, a process called 'fatigue'.

9. Diabetes Insipidus: The Consequences of Failure of Vasopressin Release

Hypothalamic diabetes insipidus is rare in humans, but the most common heritable manifestation of this disease has some features that may cast light on how the vasopressin system compensates for degradation with age. Typically, familial hypothalamic diabetes insipidus is expressed not from birth, as would be expected from a failure to produce vasopressin, but appears suddenly in adulthood, as an abrupt loss of detectable vasopressin. In every case of late onset disease, the mutation affects a single allele of the vasopressin gene. Carriers of this gene are initially asymptomatic because the normal allele can produce enough vasopressin to sustain apparently normal water and electrolyte balance. So what goes wrong later?

Vasopressin is synthesised from its larger prohormone, enzymatic cleavage of which yields vasopressin, the larger neurophysin protein, a signal peptide and a glycopeptide. The seventy characterised kindreds with familial hypothalamic diabetes insipidus exhibit many different mutations, but in every case the mutation does not affect that part of the gene which codes for vasopressin, but results in the production of a mutated neurophysin. Although neurophysin is a large polypeptide that is packaged with vasopressin and secreted in equimolar amounts, we now believe that neurophysin has no biological role other than as an intracellular carrier of vasopressin. Yet mutations in the coding region for neurophysin have severe consequences, and this seems to be because the correct folding of the neurophysin-containing prohormone molecule is essential for aggregation and packaging into the neurosecretory vesicles. Aberrant forms of neurophysin do not enter the secretory pathway, but remain in the cell body where they are normally disposed of by autophagocytosis. However, the aberrant proteins can also accumulate in the cell body, with ultimately toxic effects on the cell.

It seems most likely that when the synthesis of vasopressin is increased, synthesis of the aberrant peptide may exceed the cell's capacity to dispose of it, resulting in accumulations of aberrant peptide which lead to cell death. Alternatively, it may simply represent functional inactivation of the vasopressin cell. The disease, when it manifests itself, does so abruptly rather than progressively. One likely explanation is that mutant peptide accumulates mostly in the relatively active cells, causing these to be the most likely to fail. As the most active cells die, the pressure on the remainder to sustain effective antidiuresis increases, causing others to fail. The more cells die, the greater the secretory stress on the remainder, resulting in a progressively escalating rate of cell death and the appearance of a sudden onset of symptoms.

Bibliography

Armstrong W.E. (1995). Morphological and electrophysiological classification of hypothalamic supraoptic neurons. *Prog Neurobiol* 47: 291–339

Bicknell R.J., Brown D., Chapman C., Hancock P.D., Leng G. (1984). Reversible fatigue of stimulus-secretion coupling in the rat neurohypophysis. *J Physiol* 248: 601–613

Bourque C.W., Ciura S., Trudel E., Stachniak T.J., Sharif-Naeini R. (2007). Neurophysiological characterization of mammalian osmosensitive neurons. *Prog Brain Res* 139: 85–94

Brown C.H., Bourque C.W. (2006). Mechanisms of rhythmogenesis: insights from hypothalamic vasopressin neurons. *Trends Neurosci* 29: 108–115

Brown C.H., Ghamouri-Langroudi M., Leng G., Bourque C.W. (1999). K-opioid receptor activation inhibits post-spike depolarising after-potentials in rat supraoptic nucleus neurones *in vitro*. *J Neuroendocrinol* 11: 825–828

Cazalis M., Dayanithi G., Nordmann J.J. (1985). The role of patterned burst and interburst interval on the excitation-coupling mechanism in the isolated rat neural lobe. *J Physiol* 369: 45–60

Chow R., Kingauf J., Neher E. (1994). Time course of Ca^{2+} concentration triggering exocytosis in neuroendocrine cells. *Proc Nat Acad Sci USA* 91: 12765–12769

Dutton A., Dyball R.E.J. (1979). Phasic firing enhances vasopressin release from rat neurohypophysis. *J Physiol* 290: 433–440

Dyball R. (1988). The importance of bursting in determining secretory response: how does a phasic firing pattern influence peptide release from neurohypophysial vasopressin terminals? G. Leng (ed), Pulsatility in Neuroendocrine Systems, Chapter 10. CRC Press

Gouzenes L., Desarmenien M.G., Hussy N., Richard P., Moos F.C. (1998). Vasopressin regularizes the phasic firing pattern of rat hypothalamic magnocellular neurons. *J Neurosci* 18: 1879–1885

Gionvannucci D., Stuenkel S. (1997). Regulation of secretory granule recruitment and exocytosis at rat neurohypophysial nerve endings. *J Physiol* 498: 735–751

Krsulovic J., Peruzzo B., Alvial G., Yulis C.R., Rodriguez E.M. (2005). The destination of the aged nonreleasable neurohypophyseal peptides stored in the neural lobe is associated with the remodelling of the neurosecretory axon. *Microsc Res Tech* 68: 347–359

Leng G., Bicknell R.J. (1984). Patterns of electrical activity and hormone release from neurosecretory cells. *Excerpta Medica International Congress Series* 655: 1020: 1023

Leng G., Bicknell R.J., Brown D., Bowden C., Chapman C., Russell J.A. (1994). Stimulus-induced depletion of proenkephalins, oxytocin and vasopressin and proenkephalin interaction with posterior pituitary hormone release *in vitro*. *Neuroendocrinology* 60: 559–566

Leng G., Brown C.H., Russell J.A. (1998). Physiological pathways regulating the activity of magnocellular neurosecretory cells. *Progr Neurobiol* 56: 1–31

Leng G., Brown D. (1997). The origins and significance of pulsatility in hormone secretion from the pituitary. *J Neuroendocrinol* 9: 493–513

Leng G. (2001). Responses of magnocellular neurons to osmotic stimulation involves co-activation of excitatory and inhibitory input: an experimental and theoretical analysis. *J Neurosci* 21: 6967–6977

Leng G., Ludwig M. (2008). Neurotransmitters and peptides: whispered secrets and public announcements. *J Physiol* 586: 5625–5623

Leng G., Mason W.T., Dyer R.G. (1982). The supraoptic nucleus as an osmoreceptor. *Neuroendocrinol* 34: 75–82

Ludwig M., Leng G. (1997). Autoinhibition of supraoptic nucleus vasopressin neurons *in vivo*: a combined retrodialysis/electrophysiological study in rats. *Eur J Neurosci* 9: 2532–2540

Morris J.F. (1976a). Hormone storage in individual neurosecretory granules of the pituitary gland: a quantitative ultrastructural approach to hormone storage in the neural lobe. *J Endocrinol* 68: 209–224

Morris J.F. (1976b). Distribution of neurosecretory granules among the anatomical compartments of the neurosecretory processes of the pituitary gland: a quantitative ultrastructural approach to hormone storage in the neural lobe. *J Endocrinol* 68: 225–234

Muschol M., Salzberg B. (2000). Dependence of transient and residual calcium dynamics on action potential patterning during neuropeptide secretion. *J Neurosci* 20: 6773–6780

Nordmann J.J. (1977). Ultrastructural morphometry of the rat neurohypophysis. *J Anat* 123: 213–2118

Nordmann J.J., Morris J.F. (1984). Method for quantitating the molecular content of a subcellular organelle: hormone and neurophysin content of newly formed and aged neurosecretory granules. *Proc Nat Acad Sci* 81: 180–184

Oliet S.H., Piet R. (2004). Anatomical remodelling of the supraoptic nucleus: changes in synaptic and extrasynaptic transmission. *J Neuroendocrinol* 16: 303–307

Sabatier N., Brown C.H., Ludwig M., Leng G. (2004a). Phasic spike patterning in rat supraoptic neurones *in vivo* and *in vitro*. *J Physiol* 558: 161–180

Sabatier N., Shibuya I., Dayanithi G. (2004b). Intracellular calcium increase and somatodendritic vasopressin release by vasopressin receptor agonists in the rat supraoptic nucleus: involvement of multiple intracellular transduction signals. *J Neuroendocrinol* 16: 221–236

Seward E., Chernevskaya N., Nowycky M. (1995). Exocytosis in peptidergic nerve terminals exhibits two calcium sensitive phases during pulsatile calcium entry. *J Neuro* 15: 3390–3399

Shaw F., Bicknell R.J., Dyball R.J. (1984). Facilitation of vasopressin release from the neurohypophsis by application of electical stimuli in bursts. *Neuroendocrinology* 39: 371–376

CHAPTER 12

CLINICAL ASPECTS OF VASOPRESSIN

Jacques Hanoune

Institut Cochin, 75014 Paris, France
Email: jacques.hanoune@inserm.fr

John Laycock

Division of Neuroscience and Mental Health
Faculty of Medicine, Imperial College London
Charing Cross Campus, London W6 8RF
Email: j.laycock@imperial.ac.uk

1. Introduction

The aim of this chapter is not to extensively describe all the clinical aspects of vasopressin's actions, nor the detailed diagnosis, prognosis and treatments of the various disorders. We will only broadly cover here the principal classical aspects of the pathologies linked to vasopressin action as well as a few very recent advances, since many of the known diseases are rather rare occurrences. Some additional clinical material will be found in other chapters when pertinent. Some relevant areas of potential clinical involvement of vasopressin and related agonists/antagonists are covered in other chapters of this book. Thus stress management and depressive disorders are briefly discussed in Chapter 9, and haemolytic disorders are briefly considered in Chapter 7. Readers will find a large number of clinical textbooks at their disposal if a more extensive documentation is required (Pinchera, 2001; Baylis, 2001), as well as a number of general reviews covering the usage of vasopressin receptor antagonists (Lemmens-Gruber and Kamyar, 2006; and others below).

2. Renal Disorders

a) *Central (hypothalamic) diabetes insipidus*

This rare disorder has a prevalence of about 1:25,000 and is characterized by the excretion of large volumes (up to 18 litres daily, i.e. the total glomerular filtrate delivered to the collecting ducts) of very dilute urine (less than 250 mOsmol.kg H_2O^{-1}). The vasopressin deficiency can be partial or complete. The absolute vasopressin deficiency is the most frequent case.

In most cases, diabetes insipidus is acquired and mainly secondary to lesions of the sellar region of the hypothalamus. Those lesions can be due to neurosurgery, various tumours or granulomatous diseases, encephalitis or meningitis etc., but often (one-third of all cases) the cause remains unknown (idiopathic diabetes insipidus).

Neurohypophysial familial diabetes insipidus is a rare autosomal dominant disease. The main clinical sign is the appearance of a delayed polyuria in early infancy and the vasopressin deficiency is never complete. Over the last few years, more than fifty different heterozygous mutations in the polypeptide precursor for vasopressin have been identified, essentially by the group of Bichet (see Fujiwara and Bichet, 2005). Those mutations result in the exchange or deletion of one or more aminoacids which alter the transport or the folding of the prohormone that accumulates in the endoplasmic reticulum and induces cellular degeneration. Why misfolding of the precursor protein leads to apoptotic cell death is unknown but it has been reproduced in animal models (Si-Hoe *et al.*, 2000; Russell *et al.*, 2003). It is interesting that misfolding is also the pathological mechanism for the mutations of the vasopressin receptor or the aquaporin 2 water channel.

Treatment includes the administration of natural vasopressin, or rather the specific V2 receptor agonist desmopressin, which has a longer duration of action and is devoid of side effects such as hypertension or angina. Desmopressin can be administered orally or intranasally, the latter with a 10-fold better bioavailability.

b) *Nephrogenic diabetes insipidus*

Nephrogenic diabetes insipidus (NDI) is usually acquired and is accompanied by a mild polyuria (3–4 litres per day). It is frequently observed in patients treated with the antibiotic dimethyl chlortetracycline (DMCT), on chronic lithium therapy for an affective disorder (about 50% of cases), or in patients suffering from hypokalemia or hypercalcemia. In all such cases, there is a reduction in the vasopressin-induced insertion of aquaporin 2 in the luminal membrane of the principal cell. Interestingly, the lithium-induced downregulation of aquaporin 2 receptors occurs independently of adenyl cyclase activity (Li *et al.*, 2006; Bichet, 2006) although lithium can affect many other signalling pathways in the kidney (Nielsen *et al.*, 2008). Treatment, which aims to reduce urinary output includes strict sodium reduction, and can be accompanied by the use of thiazide diuretics or prostaglandin inhibitors. Thiazide diuretics are believed to produce their paradoxical antidiuretic effect in diabetes insipidus because they induce an extracellular volume depletion consequent upon their action on the distal convoluted tubule, where they block sodium reabsorption. The volume depletion then induces various compensatory renal responses, including a decreased glomerular filtration rate, increased proximal sodium (and water) reabsorption and a decreased presentation of tubular fluid to the collecting duct. The antidiuresis is unlikely to decrease urine volume by more than 50%, and can be accompanied by potassium depletion. The latter problem is probably due to the increase in sodium reaching the collecting duct, where an enhanced sodium-potassium exchange occurs. Amiloride can be administered in conjunction with the thiazide to ameliorate this potassium-depleting effect.

Two different forms of congenital nephrogenic diabetes insipidus are known: X-linked and non-X-linked.

i) *X-linked nephrogenic diabetes insipidus*

The disease affects only males and is due to mutations in the vasopressin V2 receptor gene. Female carriers can sometimes show mild polyuria, which is probably due to an increased, unbalanced inactivation of the healthy chromosomal allele. Some mental retardation can be found in many adults probably caused by repeated episodes of unnoticed periods of dehydration in childhood, but this can be prevented by early diagnosis and treatment. All of these cases are due to mutations of the vasopressin V2 receptor gene. The mutations can be grouped according to the function and cellular location of the mutant protein after heterologous transfection (Morello and Bichet, 2001; Fujiwara and Bichet, 2005). Type 1 mutants reach the cell surface but display impaired vasopressin binding. Type 3 mutants are ineffectively transcribed and lead to unstable mRNA. Type 2 mutants, the most frequent, are trapped in the pre-Golgi apparatus due to impaired folding of the protein. Since the other functions of the renal cell are normal, this aggregation is not toxic to the cell (unlike that of vasopressin mutants). Extra-renal V2 vasopressin receptors are also affected by the mutations, with limited peripheral effects.

More than 180 mutations of the V2 vasopressin receptor are known in more than 280 families, including all kinds of types, such as missense, nonsense, frameshift or in-frame deletion or insertion, large deletion, splice-site, etc. In Quebec, the incidence of the disease is eight in one million male live births. Interestingly, a founder effect of two particular mutations, one in Ulster Scot immigrants (the 'Hopewell' mutation) and one in a large Utah family (the 'Cannon' pedigree) results in an elevated prevalence in Nova Scotia and in Utah, and it has spread across the North American continent (Fujiwara and Bichet, 2005; Bichet, 2008).

The misfolded protein problem can be potentially overcome by molecular chaperones, which convey the mutant protein to its final membrane site (Bernier *et al.*, 2004a, 2004b; Wüller *et al.*, 2004; Robert *et al.*, 2005; Hawtin, 2006). Cell culture studies by Morello *et al.* (2000) showed that while a cell-impermeant V2 receptor antagonist had no effect on rescuing mutant vasopressin receptors, nonpeptide V2 receptor antagonists acting intracellularly bound to, and stabilized, the defective receptor molecules and redirected them to the cell membrane. In a recent clinical study, the group of Bichet (Bernier *et al.*, 2006) administered the nonpeptide 1a receptor antagonist SR49059 for a limited period of time to patients with NDI, and observed a decrease in the urine volume and of water intake, with an increase of the urine osmolarity. Thus the use of nonpeptide chaperone vasopressin antagonists could provide an important method of treatment for such patients (Oueslati *et al.*, 2007; Robben and Deen, 2007).

ii) *Non-X-linked nephrogenic diabetes insipidus*
In a few families with NDI both men and women are affected. The administration of vasopressin V2 receptor agonists to these patients results in a normal increase in circulating coagulation factors and a normal vasodilatatory response, indicating the presence of a normal vasopressin V2 receptor. In these people, the cause is a mutation of the aquaporin 2 protein. To date, about 35 putative mutations have been identified in 40 families (Fujiwara & Bichet, 2005; Loonen *et al.*, 2008; Sahakitrungruang *et al.*, 2008). When the mutations are located throughout the gene, they result in misfolded proteins, retained in the endoplasmic reticulum and the disease is recessive. When the mutation is located on the carboxy terminus, the water channel is functional but misrouted to the basolateral surface of the principal cells instead of the apical plasma membrane (Kamsteeg *et al.*, 2003) and the mutation is dominant. Treatment is currently the same as for the other, non-genomic causes of NDI.

c) *Syndrome of inappropriate vasopressin secretion*
This condition, better known as the syndrome of inappropriate ADH (SIADH), is defined by hyponatraemia and natriuresis in the presence of euvolaemia and is classically used when no other cause for the hyponatraemia is found. The clinical symptoms are varied and mainly linked to encephalopathy and cerebral oedema.

The underlying cause is usually an unregulated or poorly regulated secretion of vasopressin. As reported by Schwartz *et al.* (1957) in a seminal paper, it was first found to be associated with the presence of a small-cell carcinoma of the lung. Because many other instances of such associations were reported later (see Bricaire *et al.*, 1965), it became the prototype for various paraneoplastic endocrine syndromes (see DeLellis and Xia, 2003, for a review) where the 'inappropriate' ectopic secretion of hormone originates from the tumour itself with a potentially autocrine stimulatory effect (Péqueux *et al.*, 2004). In fact, very often there is a true hypersecretion of vasopressin from the neurohypophysis. Whether the pulmonary decapeptide pneumadin (Batra *et al.*, 1990; Kosowicz *et al.*, 2003) which exerts an antidiuretic effect by increasing the secretion of vasopressin (Watson *et al.*, 1995) is involved in such cases is still an open question.

In addition to these well-defined cases, SIADH can be diagnosed in a large variety of clinical situations, such as pulmonary and central nervous system disorders, or as iatrogenic complications associated with many drugs. It occurs frequently in older people (Miller, 2006). The use of specific nonpeptide V2 vasopressin receptor antagonists (so-called aquaretic drugs) is currently under investigation (Bhardwaj, 2006; Miller, 2006).

Bearing in mind the control mechanisms involved in regulating vasopressin release, it is quite possible for a level of circulating vasopressin which is inappropriate for the existing plasma osmolality to exist; so-called 'physiological' SIADH. Thus, stressors (e.g. pain, etc.) and iso-osmolar hypotensive states, which involve pathways to the supraoptic and paraventricular vasopressinergic neurones which do not include osmoreceptor stimulation, would be examples of physiological raised circulating levels in the presence of normal plasma osmolality.

Finally, one should cite two instances of 'nephrogenic syndrome of inappropriate antidiuresis' in two infants whose clinical evaluation was consistant with SIADH but who had undetectable arginine vasopressin levels. The sequencing of their V2 vasopressin receptor genes revealed missense mutations, causing a constitutive activation of the receptor (Feldman *et al.*, 2005). This constitutes a new addition to the relatively long list of diseases caused by activating (gain of function) mutations of G protein-coupled receptors (Knoers, 2005).

3. Hyponatraemic Disorders

a) *Congestive heart failure and other oedematous, hyponatraemic states*

One common feature of congestive heart failure (CHF) is the excessive retention of water. In this condition, various hormones are present in raised circulating concentrations, including vasopressin and aldosterone. Other conditions such as cirrhosis of the liver are also associated with water retention and raised vasopressin concentrations in the blood. These disorders are hyponatraemic conditions in which vasopressin release is clearly not inhibited by the plasma hypoosmolality, as one might expect. Furthermore, in addition to the hyponatraemia, there is clear sodium retention which seems paradoxical. One hypothesis that has been advanced to account for these observations is that, in contrast with the total blood volume, there must be an 'effective blood volume' that is relevant to the release of hormones such as vasopressin and aldosterone, in addition to activation of the sympathetic nervous and ennin-angiotensin systems. Schrier has proposed that this effective blood volume, as distinct from the total blood volume, represents the blood in the arterial circulation which normally comprises approximately 15% of the total blood volume (see Schrier, 2006). Arterial underfilling, as would occur in heart failure (decreased cardiac output) would stimulate vasopressin release via the decreased tonic inhibition, following reduced arterial baroreceptor stimulation, i.e. non-osmotic vasopressin release. In other oedematous conditions (including pregnancy) Schrier explains the arterial underfilling as being the consequence of arterial vasodilatation, although it is unclear how this would be associated with the requisite decreased stimulation of the arterial baroreceptors. Whatever the precise mechanism for the non-osmotic release of vasopressin in these conditions, it is evident that unwarranted levels of the circulating hormone are present and that there is excessive stimulation of water reabsorption in the collecting ducts.

i) *V2 receptor antagonists*

While there are various treatments possible for hyponatraemic states such as CHF, there is currently much interest in the potential use of vasopressin receptor antagonists as a successful treatment for many of these disorders (see De Luca *et al.*, 2005; Palm *et al.*, 2001, 2006; Greenberg and Verbalis, 2006). As indicated in chapter 5 on pharmacological ligands for the vasopressin receptors, not only peptidergic but also nonpeptide antagonists (vaptans) are now available. One early study on the use of an orally active non-peptide V2 receptor antagonist in rats with experimentally induced heart failure showed beneficial effects such as an increased   ieresis without any effect on sodium excretion (Burrell *et al.*, 1998).   One measure of vasopressin's antidiuretic activity is the urinary excretion of the hormone-dependent aquaporin 2 (Kanno *et al.*, 1995). This measure has been used to determine how the nonpeptide vasopressin V2 antagonist VPA 985 (Lixivaptan) produces its observed diuretic effect in patients with CHF; Aquaporin 2 excretion decreases as urine output increases, in a dose dependent manner, indicating that antagonism of the V2 receptor is associated with a decreased transfer of the water channels to the apical membranes of the principal cells and their subsequent excretion (Martin *et al.*, 1999).

Another study on patients with various causes of hyponatraemia including cirrhosis/ascites, SIADH and CHF concluded that the antagonist now known as Lixivaptan is associated with an increased   ieresis and an increased serum sodium concentration without any serious adverse effects (Wong *et al.*, 2003). Another such V2 antagonist, tolvaptan, has been used in a few clinical trials to date. In one such randomised, double blind, placebo-controlled, Phase 2 trial tolvaptan was administered orally in one of three doses to hospitalised adult patients with CHF, who were already receiving a variety of standard treatments. While global assessment scales for the tolvaptan treatment groups did not show any significant improvement over the placebo group, there was a significant polyuria, a reduction in reported dyspnoea and post-hoc analysis indicated that mortality was reduced in patients with severe congestion in the tolvaptan groups compared with the placebo control (Gheorghiade *et al.*, 2004).

More recently the similar, larger multicentre EVEREST Clinical Status randomised, double blind, placebo-controlled trial on the use of a single dose of tolvaptan in patients hospitalised for heart failure also receiving standard treatments has been analysed and the results published. The overall finding of the short-term clinical effects of tolvaptan improves many of the signs and symptoms of heart failure without serious adverse effects, including acute dyspnoea and oedema by Day 7 or discharge (Ghorghiade *et al.*, 2007). A second part of the same study followed patients for up to nine months, and found that while some of the secondary end-points such as dyspnoea, body weight and oedema were still improved, there was no difference between this group and the placebo control group with respect to long-term mortality or heart-failure-related morbidity (Konstam *et al.*, 2007).

In contrast, another recent study by the same group on CHF patients with reduced systolic function following long-term treatment with tolvaptan showed a small but insignificant decrease in left ventricular volume, compared with the control group, but there was a significant beneficial combined effect on mortality and rehospitalisation for heart failure (Udelson *et al.*, 2007).

ii) *V1a receptor antagonists*
The use of V1 antagonists has also been studied in conscious dogs with experimental heart failure (Naitoh *et al.*, 1994). In general, the vasodilatory effect produced by these antagonists appeared to be beneficial. Interestingly, vasopressin appears to have a dose dependent stimulatory effect on myocyte contractile function, intracellular calcium concentration and IP3 production, and this seems to be V1a receptor-dependent (Chandrashakhar *et al.*, 2003). In the same study, cardiac cells from rats with experimental myocardial infarction showed reduced responsiveness to V1a receptor stimulation, as well as downregulated V1a receptor mRNA and density. The addition of a V1a receptor antagonist in the presence of vasopressin showed no beneficial effect on *in vivo* haemodynamics (heart rate, mean arterial blood pressure and left ventricular end diastolic pressure).

Interestingly, an earlier study on chronically nfracted rats had indicated that blockade of V1a receptors, but not V2 receptors, is associated with an improved left ventricular function as indicated by increased cardiac output (stroke volume), but no improvement in either the ventricular hypertrophy or capillary density (Van Kerckhoven *et al.*, 2002). A recent study using cultured neonatal mouse cardiomyocytes also indicates that vasopressin stimulates cardiac cell growth as shown by the enhanced atrial natriuretic peptide mRNA and protein expression, and that this is V1a-receptor mediated (Hiroyama *et al.*, 2007). In the same study, knockout mice for the V1a receptor had a diminished cardiac hypertrophy, again suggesting a vasopressin involvement. Thus at present there is no consensus on the overall effect of vasopressin on cardiac myocytes, and in particular on cardiac function, although it is generally agreed that any effects are related to V1a receptor mechanisms, and that V2 receptors are not involved.

iii) *Dual V1a/V2 receptor antagonists*
Naturally, it follows that there would be interest in knowing whether treatment using a combined V1a/V2 receptor antagonist has any benefit in hyponatraemic conditions such as CHF. One such non-peptide antagonist, conivaptan, has been shown to significantly increase urine volume and decrease urine osmolality, while also decreasing arterial blood pressure, right ventricular and lung weights in rats with experimental heart failure (Wada *et al.*, 2002). It also had beneficial effects in counteracting the acute haemodynamic changes induced by intravenous infusions of vasopressin in anaesthetized dogs (Yatsu *et al.*, 2002).

An early study in patients with advanced heart failure showed that a single intravenous dose of conivaptan significantly increased urine excretion during the 4 hours after administration and had beneficial effects on various cardiac parameters including right atrial pressure, but no effect on blood pressure (Udelson *et al.*, 2001). More detailed trials may be forthcoming.

A recent review on the clinical use of conivaptan for the treatment of euvolaemic hyponatraemic states based on three studies of heart failure concluded that the increased free-water excretion "offers a new option for the treatment of resistant hyponatraemia in the acute setting" (Walter, 2007).

Therefore, at present there seems to be a future for vasopressin antagonism in the treatment of a variety of disorders with the common underlying problem of hyponatraemia, specifically of the euvolaemic sort. For a recent consideration of the use of combined V1a/V2 receptor antagonists, see Goldsmith (2006).

The use of these various nonpeptide orally effective vasopressin receptor antagonists in liver cirrhosis also appears to be beneficial and therefore they may well play a therapeutic role in the future (see Fergusson *et al.*, 2003).

4. Essential Hypertension

As discussed elsewhere, vasopressin is one of the most potent naturally occurring vasoactive molecules that mammals produce, acting via its V1a receptors. It is also quite feasible that chronic water retention through excessive stimulation of the V2 receptors provides another mechanism by which vasopressin could induce a hypertensive state. However, it is not generally associated with essential hypertension in humans. On the other hand, there is plenty of evidence in animal models that this hormone is associated with clearly defined forms of hypertension such as deoxycorticosterone acetate (DOCA) salt hypertension, and one kidney one clip hypertension. Furthermore, in the young, spontaneously hypertensive rat V1a receptors are upregulated in renal resistance vessels, supporting the concept that vasopressin is linked to the developing raised arterial blood pressure in this genetic form of hypertension (Vagnes *et al.*, 2000).

In humans, the explanation has always been that vasopressin is not causally associated with hypertension because of the powerful compensatory mechanisms which exist to counteract its pressor activity, and that circulating levels of the hormone are not raised. In contrast to this point, it is interesting to note that as long ago as the 1980s, some small studies were showing that, while circulating vasopressin levels are not in the accepted pressor range, they are nevertheless significantly higher in moderately hypertensive males than in normotensive controls (Cowley et al., 1981). This increase in circulating vasopressin levels occurs despite the presumed increased inhibitory feedback of the raised arterial blood pressure, but presumably relates to the lower plasma sodium concentration and the raised sodium excretion measured in the hypertensive patients. Cowley and colleagues later showed that there might be a sex difference in the neuroendocrine predictors they examined, which included vasopressin and renin, which appeared to be good predictors in male and female hypertensives, respectively (Cowley et al., 1985).

More recently, the relationship between vasopressin and hypertension has been revisited. Again, significantly higher plasma vasopressin levels were found in middle-aged hypertensive patients in a study by Zhang et al. (1999); the values are lower than those measured by Cowley and his colleagues, maybe a reflection of the assay techniques used. There were significant correlations between the plasma vasopressin levels and systolic and diastolic blood pressures, the correlation being particularly strong in subjects with low renin levels. Another study has suggested that there are racial differences too, with African-American hypertensives having significantly higher plasma vasopressin levels than Caucasians (Bakris et al., 1997). Furthermore, in this study intravenous administration of a V1a receptor antagonist reduced the blood pressure of the African-Americans only.

Perhaps not surprisingly, there has been some interest in the potential use of the V1a antagonists. An early study by Kawan et al. (1997) concluded that the nonpeptide orally active V1 receptor antagonist OPC-21268 had little effect in reducing blood pressure in a small group of patients with mild essential hypertension. Thibonnier *et al.* (1999) showed that a single oral dose of nonpeptide SR49059 (relcovaptan) had no effect on resting arterial blood pressure in a small group of Stages I and II untreated essential hypertensive patients, although the peak increase in blood pressure following hypertonic saline infusion was significantly lower in the treatment group compared to the placebo effect. Relcovaptan was also associated with a small, but significantly greater, increase in plasma vasopressin (but not plasma renin or aldosterone) levels following the saline infusion compared with controls. Currently there are no known reported studies on the effect of V1a antagonists, short- or long-term, on arterial blood pressure in patients with higher stages of hypertension. However, there is little evidence to suggest that such treatments are likely to be particularly beneficial.

The other vasopressin mechanism that has to be considered for the development of hypertension is the one which links chronic V2 receptor stimulation with persistent enhanced water retention. One recent study suggestive of this mechanism in spontaneously hypertensive rats during the phase of developing raised arterial blood pressure showed that by Week 7 hypertension was already established and plasma vasopressin levels were raised (Buemi *et al.*, 2004). The urine volumes were reduced and urine osmolalities were raised, as was the excretion of aquaporin 2, indicating enhanced V2 receptor-mediated renal activity. Treatment of these hypertensive rats with a V2 receptor antagonist was associated with a significantly reduced arterial blood pressure and an improvement in renal function, as indicated by increased urine volume and a reduction in aquaporin 2 excretion. Further studies on the use of V2 receptor antagonists in hypertension, particularly in humans, are clearly required.

5. Haemolytic Disorders

Another involvement of vasopressin with the cardiovascular system is concerned with the effects this hormone has on aspects of platelet involvement in the vascular wound-healing process and blood clotting (see Chapter 7). Desmopressin has been used for the treatment of moderate/mild haemophilia A and von Willebrand disease since the late 1970s (Manucci *et al.*, 1977), as well as in a variety of other haemorrhagic disorders such as congenital platelet defects. While intravenous infusion is a common form of administration, the nasal spray is perfectly effective (Rose and Aledort, 1991). The use of this vasopressin analogue is particularly important because it is not a blood product and therefore its administration is not accompanied by concerns of blood-borne viral transmission. The main mechanism of action for desmopressin appears to be the production of von Willebrand Factor (vWF) and tissue plasminogen activator (tPA) from endothelial cells. However, since defective platelet aggregation appears to be corrected with desmopressin, along with an improved bleeding time (Cattaneo *et al.*, 1995), this may also be a relevant action of vasopressin via its V2 receptor.

There are a number of reviews on haemolytic disorders and their treatments, one recent one being by Franchini (2008) on the use of desmopressin.

a) *von Willebrand's disease*

Desmopressin is generally effective in type 1 of the disease (mild/moderate disorder due to partial vWF), but has a variable effect in patients with the various forms of type 2. For patients with types 2A and 2M of the disease, desmopressin should first be tested in the individual since some respond and others do not. The use of desmopressin in type 2B is still controversial because of the possible induction of thrombocytopaenia, as indicated in the Haemophilia Centre Doctors' Organisation current guideline document (Pasi *et al.*, 2004). Interestingly, in type 2N, desmopressin induces a large increase in plasma Factor VIII:C concentrations, but the half-life is greatly reduced because of the impaired binding to the stabilising vWF. Desmopressin treatment is not used in patients with type 3 because of the severity of the bleeding disorder (very low or absent vWF and Factor VIII:C).

b) *Mild haemophilia A*

Desmopressin is generally used in patients with mild to moderate forms of haemophilia although not all such patients respond. It is commonly used when these patients undergo dental extractions or other surgical procedures, or have acute bleeding. The therapeutic dose will be determined by Factor VIII levels and the type of bleeding episode.

c) *Other bleeding disorders*

Such disorders would include congenital platelet disorders, acquired forms of von Willebrand disease and haemophilia A, as well as patients with hepatic cirrhosis or chronic uraemia when appropriate (e.g. during surgery).

6. Conclusion

While the use of vasopressin, and particularly the V2 receptor agonist desmopressin, was initially focused on the treatment of cranial diabetes insipidus, it is clear that, with the advent of peptide and nonpeptide analogues, there is an increasing interest in the use of such compounds in the treatment of a number of clinical disorders. As our knowledge of the central physiological effects of vasopressin increases, it is interesting to speculate on whether therapeutic uses of these drugs will one day also be directed at modifying these actions on the brain.

Bibliography

Bakris G., Bursztyn M., Gavras I., Bresnahan M., Gavras H. (1997). Role of vasopressin in essential hypertension: racial differences. *J Hypertension* 15: 545–550

Batra V.K., Mathur M., Mir S.A., Kapoor R., Kumar M.A. (1990). Pneumadin: a new lung peptide which trigers antidiuresis. *Regul Pept* 30: 77–87

Baylis P.H (2001). Vasopressin, diabetes insipidus and syndrome of inappropriate antidiuresis. In De Groot L.J. and Jameson J.L. (eds), Endocrinology, pp 363–376, SW Saunders

Bhardwaj A. (2006). Neurological impact of vasopressin dysregulation and hyponatremia. *Ann Neurol* 59: 229–236

Bernier V., Lagacé M., Lonergan M., Arthus M.F., Bichet D.G., Bouvier M. (2004a). Functional rescue of the constitutively internalized V2 vasopressin receptor mutant R137H by the pharmacological chaperone action of SR49059. *Mol Endocrinol* 18: 2074–2084

Bernier V., Lagace M., Bichet D.G., Bouvier M. (2004b). Pharmacological chaperones: potential treatment for conformational diseases. *Trends Endocrinol Metab* 15: 222–228

Bernier V., Morello J.P., Zarruk A., Debrand N., Salahpour A., Lonergan M., Arthus M.F., Laperrière A., Brouard R., Bouvier M., Bichet D.G. (2006). Pharmacological chaperones as a potential treatment for X-linked nephrogenic diabetes insipidus. *J Am Soc Nephrol* 17: 232–243

Bichet D.G. (2006). Lithium, cyclic AMP signaling, A-kinase anchoring proteins and aquaporin 2. *J Am Soc Nephrol* 17: 920–922

Bichet D.G. (2008). Vasopressin receptor mutations in nephrogenic diabetes insipidus. *Semin Nephrol* 28: 245–251

Bricaire H., Joly J., Saltiel H., Peigné F., Hanoune J. (1965). Un cas de syndrome de Schwartz-Bartter au cours d'un carcinome bronchique. *Bull Mem Soc Hop Paris* 116: 1491–1506

Buemi M., Nostro L., Di Pasquale G., Cavallaro E., Sturiale A., Floccari F., Aloisi C., Ruello A., Calapai G., Corica F., Frisina N. (2004). Aquaporin-2 water channels in spontaneously hypertensive rats. *Am J Hypertension* 17: 1170–1178

Burrell L.M., Phillips P.A., Risvanis J., Chan R.K., Aldred K.L., Johnston C.I. (1998). Long-term effects of nonpeptide vasopressin V2 antagonist OPC-31260 in heart failure in the rat. *Am J Physiol* 275: H176–H182

Cattaneo M., Pareti F.I., Zighetti M., Lecchi A., Lombardi R., Manucci P.M. (1995). Platelet aggregation at high shear is impaired in patients with congenital defects of platelet secretion and is corrected by DDAVP: correlation with the bleeding time. *J Lab Clin Med* 125: 540–547

Chandrashekhar Y., Prahash A.J., Sen S., Gupta S., Roy S., Anand I.S. (2003). The role of arginine vasopressin and its receptors in the normal and failing rat heart. *J Mol Cell Cardiol* 35: 495–504

Cowley A.W., Cushman W.C., Quillen E.W., Skelton M.M., Langford H.G. (1981). Vasopressin elevation in essential hypertension and increased responsiveness to sodium intake. *Hypertension* 3: 193–200

Cowley A.W., Skelton M.M., Velasquez M.T. (1985). Sex differences in the endocrine predictors of essential hypertension. Vasopressin versus renin. *Hypertension* 7: 1151–1160

Delellis R.A., Xia L. (2003). Paraneoplastic endocrine syndromes: a review. *Endocr Pathol* 14: 303–317

De Luca L., Orlandi C., Udelson J.E., Fedele F., Gheorghiade J.E. (2005). Overview of vasopressin receptor antagonists in heart failure resulting in hospitalization. *Am J Cardiol* 96: 24L–33L

Feldman B.J., Rosenthal S.M., Vargas G.A., Fenwick R.G., Huang E.A., Matsuda-Abedini M., Lustig R.H., Mathias R.S., Portale A.A., Miller W.L., Gitelman S.E. (2005). Nephrogenic syndrome of inappropriate antidiuresis. *N Engl J Med* 352: 1884–1890

Ferguson J.W., Therapondos G., Newby D.E., Hayes P.C. (2003). Therapeutic role of vasopressin antagonism in patients with liver cirrhosis. *Clin Sci* 105: 1–8

Franchini M. (2007). The use of desmopressin as a hemostatic agent: a concise review. *Am J Hematol* 82: 731–735

Fujiwara T.M., Bichet D.G. (2005). Molecular biology of hereditary diabetes insipidus. *J Am Soc Nephrol* 16: 2836–2846

Ghearghiade M., Gattis W.A., O'Connor C.M., Adams K.F., Elkayam U., Barbagelata A., Ghali J.K., Benza R.L., McGrew F.A., Klapholz M., Ouyang J., Orlandi C. (2004). Effects of tolvaptan, a vasopressin antagonist, in patients hospitalized with worsening heart failure. *J Am Med Ass* 291: 1963–1971

Ghearghiade M., Konstam M.A., Burnett J.C., Grinfeld L., Maggione A.P., Swedberg K., Udelson J.E., Zannad F., Cook T., Ouyang J., Zimmer C., Orlandi C. (2007). Short-term clinical effects of tolvaptan, an oral vasopressin antagonist, in patients hospitalized for heart failure. *J Am Med Ass* 297: 1332–1343

Goldsmith S.R. (2006). Is there a cardiovascular rationale for the use of combined vasopressin V1a/V2 receptor antagonists? *Am J Med* 119: 593–596

Greenberg A., Verbalis J.G. (2006). Vasopressin receptor antagonists. *Kidney Int* 69: 2124–2130

Hawtin S.R. (2006). Pharmacological chaperone activity of SR49059 to functionally recover mis-folded mutations of the vasopressin V1a receptor. *J Biol Chem* 281: 14604–14614

Hiroyama M., Wang S., Aoyagi T., Oikawa R., Sanbe A., Takeo S., Tanoue A. (2007). Vasopressin promotes cardiomyocyte hypertrophy via the vasopressin V1a receptor in neonatal mice. *Eur J Pharmacol* 559: 89–97

Kamsteeg E.J., Bichet D.G., Konings I.B., Nivet H., Lonergan M., Arthus M.F., van Os C.H., Deen P.M. (2003). Reversed polarized delivery of an aquaporin-2 mutant causes dominant nephrogenic diabetes insipidus. *J Cell Biol* 163: 1099–1109

Kanno K., Sasaki S., Hirata Y., Ishikawa S., Fushimi K., Nakanishi S., Bichet D.G., Marumo F. (1995). Urinary excretion of aquaporin-2 in patients with diabetes insipidus. *New Engl. J Med* 332: 1540–1545

Kawano Y., Matsuoka H., Nishikimi T., Takishita S., Omae T. (1997). The role of vasopressin in essential hypertension. *Am J Hypertension* 10: 1240–1244

Knoers N.V.A.M. (2005). Hyperactive vasopressin receptors and disturbed water homeostasis. *New Engl J Med* 352: 1847–1849

Konstam M.A., Ghearghiade M., Burnett J.C., Grinfeld L., Maggione A.P., Swedberg K., Udelson J.E., Zannad F., Cook T., Ouyang J., Zimmer C., Orlandi C. (2007). Effects of oral tolvaptan in patients hospitalized for worsening heart failure. *J Am Med Ass* 297: 1319–1331

Kosowicz J., Miskowiak B., Konwerska A., Tortorella C., Nussdorfer G.G., Manlendowicz L.K. (2003). Tissue distribution of pneumadin immunoreactivity in the rat. *Peptides* 24: 215–220

Lemmens-Gruber R., Kamyar M. (2006). Drugs of the future: Review vasopressin antagonists. *Cell Mol Life Sci* 63: 1766–1779

Li Y., Shaw S., Kamsteeg E.J., Vandewalle A., Deen P.M.T. (2006). Development of lithium-induced nephrogenic diabetes insipidus is dissociated from adenylyl cyclase activity. *J Am Soc Nephrol* 17: 1063–1072

Loonen A.J., Knoers N.V., van Oc C.H., Deen P.M. (2008). Aquaporin-2 mutations in nephrogenic diabetes insipidus. *Semin Nephrol* 28: 252–265

Manucci P.M., Ruggeri Z.M., Pareti F.I., Capitanio A. (1977). 1-deamino-8-d-arginine vasopressin: a new pharmacological approach to the management of haemophilia and von Willebrand's disease. *Lancet* 8107: 869–872

Martin P.Y., Abraham W.T., Lieming X., Olson B.R., Oren R.M., Ohara M., Schrier R.W. (1999). Selective V2-receptor vasopressin antagonism decreases aquaporin-2 excretion in patients with chronic heart failure. *J Am Soc Nephrol* 10: 2165–2170

Miller M. (2006). Hyponatremia and arginine vasopressin dysregulation: mechanisms, clinical consequences and management. *J Am Geriatr Soc* 54: 345–353

Morello J.P., Salahpour A., Laperriere A., Bernier V., Arthus M.F., Lonergan M., Petaja-Repo U., Angers S., Morin D., Bichet D.G., Bouvier M. (2000). Pharmacological chaparones rescue cell-surface expression and function of misfolded V2 receptor mutants. *J Clin Invest* 105: 887–895

Morello J.P., Bichet D.G. (2001). Nephrogenic diabetes insipidus. *Ann Rev Physiol* 63: 607–630

Naitoh M., Susuki H., Murakami M., Matsumoto A., Arakawa K., Ishikara A., Nakamoto H., Oka K., Yamamura Y., Saruta T. (1994). Effects of oral AVP receptor antagonists OPC-21268 and OPC-31260 on congestive heart failure in conscious dogs. *Am J Physiol* 267: H2245–H2254

Nielsen J., Hoffert J.D., Knepper M.A., Agre P., Nielsen S., Fenton R.A. (2008). Proteomic analysis of lithium-nephrogenic diabetes insipidus: mechanisms for aquaporin-2 down-regulation and cellular proliferation. *Proc Nat Acad Sci USA* 105: 3634–3639

Oueslati M., Hermosilla R., Schonenberger E., Oorschot V., Beyermann M., Wiesner B., Schmidt A., Klumperman J., Rosenthal W., Schulein R. (2007). Rescue of a nephrogenic diabetes insipidus-causing vasopressin V2 receptor mutant by cell-penetrating peptides. *J Biol Chem* 282: 20676–20685

Palm C., Reimann D., Gross P. (2001). The role of V2 vasopressin antagonists in hyponatremia. *Cardiovasc Res* 51: 403–408

Palm C., Pistrosch F., Herbrig K., Gross P. (2006). Vasopressin antagonists as aquaretic agents for the treatment of hyponatremia. *Am J Med* 119: 587–592

Pasi K.J., Collins P.W., Keeling D.M., Brown S.A., Cumming A.M., Dolan G.C., Hay C.R.M., Hill F.G.H., Laffan M., Peake I.R. (2004). Management of von Willebrand disease: a guideline from the UK Haemophilia Centre Doctors' Organisation. *Haemophilia* 10: 218–231

Péqueux C., Keegan B.P., Hagelstein M.T., Geenen V., Legros J.J., North W.G. (2004). Oxytocin and vasopressin-induced growth of human small-cell lung cancer is mediated by the mitogen-activated protein kinase pathway. *Endocrine Related Cancer* 11: 871–885

Pinchera A. (2001). In: Endocrinology and Metabolism, McGraw-Hill, pp 102–115

Robben J.H., Deen P.M. (2007). Pharmacological chaperones in nephrogenic diabetes insipidus: possibilities for clinical applications. *Biodrugs* 21: 157–166

Robert J., Auzan C., Venura M.A., Clauser E. (2005). Mechanisms of cell-surface rerouting of an ER-retained mutant of the vasopressin V1b/V3 receptor by a pharmacological chaperone. *J Biol Chem* 280: 42198–42206

Rose E.H., Aledort L.M. (1991). Nasal spray desmopressin (DDAVP) for mild hemophilia A and von Willebrand disease. *Ann Intern Med* 114: 563–568

Russell T.A., Ito M., Yu R.N., Martinson F.A., Weiss J., Jameson J.L. (2003). A murine model of autosomal dominant neurohypophyseal diabetes insipidus reveals progressive loss of vasopressin-producing neurons. *J Clin Invest* 112: 1697–1706

Sahakitrungruang T., Wacharasindhu S., Sinthuwiwat T., Supornaitchai V., Suphapeetiporn K., Shotelesuk V. (2008). Identification of two novel aquaporin-2 mutations in a Thai girl with congenital nephrogenic diabetes insipidus. *Endocrine* 33:210–214

Schrier R.W. (2006). Water and sodium retention in edematous disorders: role of vasopressin and aldosterone. *Am J Med* 119: S47–S53

Schwartz W.B., Bennett W., Curelop S., Bartter F.C. (1957). A syndrome of renal sodium loss and hyponatremia probably resulting from inappropriate secretion of antidiuretic hormone. *Am J Med* 23: 529–542

Si-Hoe S.l., De Bree F.M., Nijenhuis M., Davis J.E., Howell L.M.C., Tinley H., Waller S.J., Zeng Q., Zalm R., Sonnemans M., Van Leeuwen F.W., Burbach J.P.H., Murphy D. (2000). Endoplasmic reticulum derangement in hypothalamic neurons of rats expressing a familial neurophypophyseal diabetes insipidus mutant vasopressin transgene. *FASEB J* 14: 1680–1684

Thibonnier M., Kilani A., Rahman M., DiBlasi T.P., Warner K., Smith M.C., Leenhardt A.F., Brouard R. (1999). Effects of the nonpeptide V1 receptor antagonist SR49059 in hypertensive patients. *Hypertension* 34: 1293–1300

Udelson J.E., Smith W.B., Hendrix G.H., Painchaud C.A., Ghazzi M., Thomas I., Ghali J.K., Selaru P., Chanoine F., Pressler M.L., Konstan M.A. (2001). Acute haemodynamic effects of conivaptan, a dual V1a and V2 vasopressin receptor antagonist, in patients with advanced heart failure. *Circ Res* 104: 2417–2423

Udelson J.E., McGrew F.A., Flores E., Ibrahim H., Katz S., Koshkarian G., O'Brian T., Kronenberg M.W., Zimmer C., Orlandi C., Konstam M.A. (2007). Multicenter, randomized, double-blind, placebo-controlled study on the effect of oral tolvaptan on left ventricular dilation and function in patients with heart failure and systolic dysfunction. *J Am Coll Cardiol* 49: 2151–2159

Vagnes O., Feng J.J., Iversen B.M., Arendshorst W.J. (2000). Upregulation of V1 receptors in renal resistance vessels of rats developing genetic hypertension. *Am J Physiol Renal Physiol* 278: F940–F948

Van Kerckhoven R., Lankhuizen I., van Veghel R., Saxena P.R., Schoemaker R.G. (2002). Chronic vasopressin V1a but not V2 receptor antagonism prevents heart failure in chronically infarcted rats. *Eur J Phramacol* 449: 135–141

Wada K-I., Tahara A., Arai Y., Aoki M., Tomura Y., Tsukada J., Yatsu T. (2002). Effect of the vasopressin receptor antagonist conivaptan in rats with heart failure following myocardial infarction. *Eur J Pharmacol* 450: 169–177

Walter K.A. (2007). Conivaptan: new treatment for hyponatremia. *Am J Health Syst Pharm* 64: 1385–1395

Watson J.D., Jennings D.B., Sarda I.R., Pang S.C., Lawson B., Wigle D.A., Flynn T.G. (1995). The antidiuretic effect of pneumadin requires a functional arginine vasopressin system. *Regul Pept* 576: 105–114

Wong F., Blei A.T., Blendis L.M., Thuluvath P.J. (2003). A vasopressin receptor antagonist (VPA-985) improves serum sodium concentration in patients with hyponatremia: a multicenter, randomized, placebo-controlled trial. *Hepatology* 37: 182–191

Wüller S., Wiesner B., Löffler A., Furkert J., Krause G., Hermosilla R., Schaefer M., Schülein R., Rosenthal W., Oksche A. (2004). Pharmacochaperones post-translationally enhance cell surface expression by increasing conformational stability of wild-type and mutant vasopressin V2 receptors. *J Biol Chem* 279: 47254–47263

Yatsu T., Kusayama T., Tomura Y., Arai Y., Aoki M., Tahara A., Wada K-I., Tskada J. (2002). Effect of conivaptan, a combined vasopressin V1a and V2 receptor antagonist, on vasopressin-induced cardiac and haemodynamic changes in anaesthetized dogs. *Pharmacol. Res* 46: 375–381

Zhang X., Hense H-W., Riegger G.A.J., Schunkert H. (1999). Association of arginine vasopressin and arterial blood pressure in a population-based sample. *J Hypertension* 17: 319–324

Index